NCHEC

National Commission for
Health Education Credentialing, Inc.

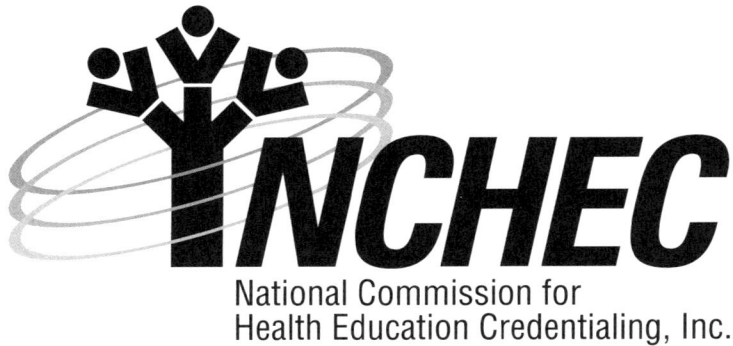

Credentialing Excellence in Health Education

The Health Education Specialist:
A Companion Guide for Professional Excellence

Seventh Edition

National Commission for
Health Education Credentialing, Inc.

The use of this companion guide is not a guarantee of successful completion of the Certified Health Education Specialist (CHES) or Master Certified Health Education Specialist (MCHES) examination. Please review the section, *How to Use this Book*, for a description of the purpose of this resource. Any expectation beyond the purpose stated in the Introduction is solely the responsibility of the user and not that of the *National Commission for Health Education Credentialing, Inc.*

Published by: National Commission for Health Education Credentialing, Inc.
1541 Alta Drive, Suite 303
Whitehall, PA 18052-5642
Local phone: (484) 223-0770
Phone: (888) NCHEC-4-U, (888) 624-3248
Fax: (800) 813-0727
www.nchec.org

ISBN 978-0-9652570-8-4

ACKNOWLEDGMENTS

In 1992, Sigred G. Deeds, DrPH, CHES, authored the original edition of *The Health Education Specialist: A Self-Study Guide for Professional Competence.* Her work was based on 25 years of experience in a variety of health education settings. In 1995, Dr. Deeds donated her book to the National Commission for Health Education Credentialing, Inc.

This edition marks the seventh revision to Dr. Deeds' original work. The sixth edition was revised by Chris Anne Rodgers Arthur, PhD, MPH, CHES; Donna Beal, MPH, CHES; Cam Escoffery, PhD, MPH, CHES; Patricia A. Frye, DrPH, MPA, CHES; Melissa Grim, PhD, CHES (author/editor); Leonard Jack, Jr, PhD, MSc, CHES (author/editor); Maurice "Bud" Martin, PhD, CHES; J. Dennis Kamholtz, PhD, CHES; Angela D. Mickalide, PhD, CHES; Christopher N. Thomas, MS, CHES; Rebecca Reeve, PhD, CHES; Tung-Sung Tseng, DrPH, MS, CHES; Katherine M. Wilson, PhD, MPH, CHES; and Kelly Wilson, PhD, CHES.

The difference in this companion guide is that it is based on the results of the Health Education Specialist Practice Analysis 2015. The resultant revised Areas of Responsibility, Competencies, and Sub-competencies identified in that project have been incorporated into this companion guide, and additional material on the new and revised Competencies has been included. The publication includes both entry- and advanced-level Competencies and Sub-competencies. In addition, the sample questions have been reviewed and revised, and questions have been added to reflect the new material.

The seventh edition of *Health Education Specialist: A Companion Guide for Professional Excellence* was compiled with efforts of health education specialists with expertise and experience in the Seven Areas of Responsibility identified in this companion guide. The authors refined and added to previous editions. Much gratitude to the co-editors, Melissa Grim, PhD, MCHES and Cam Escoffery, PhD, CHES for their tireless work to meet short deadlines in order to release this publication in a timely manner.

Sincere appreciation and recognition is extended to Carolyn Cox, PhD, MCHES and Kelly Wilson, PhD, MCHES for reviewing and assisting in polishing several drafts of practice examination questions.

Co-Editors:
Melissa Grim, PhD, MCHES
Cam Escoffrey PhD, MPH, CHES

Contributing Authors:

Chapter I: *Assess Needs, Resources, and Capacity for Health Education/Promotion*
C. Suzette McClellan, MPH, MCHES
Linda E. Forys, EdM, MCHES

Chapter II: *Plan Health Education/Promotion*
Angela Mickalide, PhD, MCHES

Chapter III: *Implement Health Education/Promotion*
Christopher N. Thomas, MS, MCHES
Martha Alexander, MPH, MCHES

Chapter IV: *Conduct Evaluation and Research Related to Health Education/Promotion*
Maurice "Bud" Martin, PhD, MCHES
Adam P. Knowlden, MBA, PhD, CHES

Chapter V: *Administer and Manage Health Education/Promotion*
Chris Arthur, PhD, MCHES
Patricia A. Frye, DrPH, MPA, MCHES
Leah Horn Roman, MPH, MCHES

Chapter VI: *Serve as a Health Education/Promotion Resource Person*
Cam Escoffery, PhD, MPH, CHES
Michelle Carvalho, MPH, CHES

Chapter VII: *Communicate, Promote, and Advocate for Health, Health Education/ Promotion, and the Profession*
Stacy Robison, MPH, MCHES
Amy Thompson, PhD, CHES

Study Companion-Practice Question Reviewers:
Carol Cox, PhD, MCHES
Kelly Wilson, PhD, MCHES

Study Companion Reviewers:
Cynthia Kusorgbor-Narh, MPH, CHES
Kerry Redican, MPH, PhD, CHES
Linda Lysoby, MS, MCHES, CAE
Melissa Opp, MPH, MCHES

Copy Editor:
Caitlin Rizzo

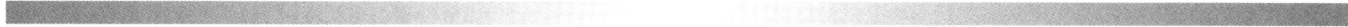

TABLE OF CONTENTS

INTRODUCTION

The purpose of this book is to guide health education specialists in advancing their knowledge and skills in the field of health education at both entry- and advanced-levels of practice. The title of the seventh edition, *Health Education Specialist: A Companion Guide for Professional Excellence,* incorporates the concept of "companion guide" to reflect the broad use of the publication. The companion guide may be used to help individuals prepare for the national examination for either the Certified Health Education Specialist (CHES) or Master Certified Health Education Specialist (MCHES) credentials. It can also be used as a professional development tool and as the basis for professional preparation programs. *The Health Education Specialist: A Companion Guide for Professional Excellence* can be used to help assess health education knowledge and direct continuing education studies. Employers can encourage their employees to use this book as a tool to determine whether additional professional development in specific areas is needed. Instructors in professional preparation programs may find the format and organization of this book to be a useful supplement to textbooks and classroom lectures. Students enrolled in health education professional preparation programs can utilize this guide as an excellent reference source. It should be understood that relying on this book as the only resource for studying for the CHES or MCHES exams is strongly discouraged.

The Health Education Specialist: A Companion Guide for Professional Excellence is organized to follow the Seven Areas of Responsibility, their related Competencies, and Sub-competencies at both entry- and advanced-levels as delineated in *A Competency-Based Framework for Health Education Specialists - 2015* (National Commission for Health Education Credentialing, Inc. [NCHEC] and Society for Public Health Education [SOPHE],

2015). That framework is based on the Health Education Specialist Practice Analysis 2015 (HESPA 2015) (NCHEC et al., 2015), an 18-month project to update, refine and validate the model of health education practice. The updated HESPA 2015 Model comprises 258 Sub-competencies organized into 36 Competencies within Seven major Areas of Responsibility. Of the Sub-competencies, 117 were validated as advanced-level only. The HESPA 2015 study expanded upon the two previous studies: the HEJA 2010 (Doyle) and Competency Update Project (CUP) (Gilmore, Olson, Taub, & Connell, 2005), which also utilized a model of three levels of practice (entry, advanced 1, and advanced 2) with each subsequent level building upon the previous level(s).

Extensive research involving health education specialists across the nation has verified the existence of entry- and advanced-levels of health education practice. NCHEC has been credentialing the advanced-level of certification since 2011. This proves to be an exciting time for the profession as we continue to understand the levels of practice of health education specialists.

Like earlier versions, the HESPA 2015 Model includes Responsibilities, Competencies, and Sub-competencies that are considered generic and independent of the setting in which the health education specialist works (NCHEC et al., 2015). The CHES examination addresses only those Competencies and Sub-competencies that were identified in the HESPA 2015 as entry-level. The MCHES examination addresses all of the Competencies and Sub-competencies: entry-, advanced 1-, and advanced 2-levels. Additional details regarding the role and history of credentialing can be found in Chapter VII of *The Health Education Specialist: A Companion Guide for Professional Excellence.*

HOW TO USE THIS BOOK

This book can be used to identify areas of practice that may require further study using nationally recognized scholarly references. Whether for purposes of exam preparation, part of academic preparation, or for professional development activities, study should not be limited to this one resource as it is a summary of many important topics that will require in-depth study through the use of additional resources. Texts, such as those listed in the reference section and on the NCHEC website, should be used to prepare for the certification examinations. Those preparing for the CHES or MCHES exam are reminded that these exams are national Competency-based tests that measure the possession, application, and interpretation of knowledge related to the Seven Areas of Responsibility. Further, the reader cannot consider the information included in this companion guide exhaustive. Additional optional readings that may also assist in study are listed on the NCHEC website: http://www.nchec.org. Textbooks from professional preparation programs in health promotion also are helpful resources to review.

Many CHES and MCHES who used previous NCHEC study companions reported that using the publication as a basic resource for a study group was very helpful. Using a discussion format to work through the practice questions was reported as a useful way to prepare not only for the exam but also for professional development activities.

As a starting point to assist in identifying gaps in one's formal preparation for health education practice a *Self-Assessment for Health Education Specialists: Perceived Competence* tool is included in the companion guide and follows the Introduction. After the self-assessment exercise, it may be helpful to review each chapter and note any other apparent weaknesses. Each chapter follows a logical organization: Area of Responsibility, followed by the role of a health education specialist relative to the Responsibility, examples of each role in the practice setting, key terms, and information germane to each of the corresponding Competencies and Sub-competencies. It is important to note that while key terms may appear in more than one chapter, users are advised that definitions within chapters may vary given the context in which it is being used.

Throughout the *Health Education Specialist: A Companion Guide for Professional Excellence*, there is a graphic differentiation between entry- and advanced-level Sub-competencies. Also, in some places, the editors felt that it was important to note that although the Sub-competency was advanced-level, content within the text was not beyond the scope of an entry-level health education specialist. After reviewing the material in each chapter, it may be beneficial to complete the practice questions. Practice questions for entry- and advanced-levels are located in Appendices C and D respectively.

The content of this publication reflects consensus about a common core of professional preparation leading to entry- and advanced-level practice as a health education specialist. This publication should be considered a supplemental tool, and not a primary source, for identifying areas of practice that may require further study using nationally recognized scholarly references. Study and preparation for the CHES and MCHES exams should not be limited to *Health Education Specialist: A Companion Guide for Professional Excellence*.

SELF-ASSESSMENT FOR HEALTH EDUCATION SPECIALISTS: PERCEIVED COMPETENCE

The Competency statement in this assessment describes the broadly defined skills that a qualified generic health education specialist is expected to be able to demonstrate at least at minimum levels. To assess individual skill level for each Competency statement, rate each Competency from 1 to 4, with 1 indicating not competent and 4 indicating very competent.

Area of Responsibility I:

ASSESS NEEDS, RESOURCES AND CAPACITY FOR HEALTH EDUCATION/PROMOTION

The health education specialist can:

		Not Competent		Very Competent	

COMPETENCY 1.1: Plan assessment process for health education/promotion

		Not Competent			Very Competent
1.1.1	Define the priority population to be assessed	1	2	3	4
1.1.2	Identify existing and necessary resources to conduct assessments	1	2	3	4
1.1.3	Engage priority populations, partners, and stakeholders to participate in the assessment process	1	2	3	4
1.1.4	❖ Apply theories and/or models to assessment process	1	2	3	4
1.1.5	Apply ethical principles to the assessment process	1	2	3	4

COMPETENCY 1.2: Access existing information and data related to health

1.2.1	Identify sources of secondary data related to health	1	2	3	4
1.2.2	❖ Establish collaborative relationships and agreements that facilitate access to data	1	2	3	4
1.2.3	Review related literature	1	2	3	4
1.2.4	Identify gaps in the secondary data	1	2	3	4
1.2.5	Extract data from existing databases	1	2	3	4
1.2.6	Determine the validity of existing data	1	2	3	4

COMPETENCY 1.3: Collect primary data to determine needs

1.3.1	Identify data collection instruments	1	2	3	4
1.3.2	Select data collection methods for use in assessment	1	2	3	4
1.3.3	Develop data collection procedures	1	2	3	4
1.3.4	Train personnel assisting with data collection	1	2	3	4
1.3.5	Implement quantitative and/or qualitative data collection	1	2	3	4

COMPETENCY 1.4: Analyze relationships among behavioral, environmental, and other factors that influence health

1.4.1	Identify and analyze factors that influence health behaviors	1	2	3	4
1.4.2	Identify and analyze factors that impact health	1	2	3	4
1.4.3	Identify the impact of emerging social, economic, and other trends on health	1	2	3	4

KEY: no symbol - entry level; ❖ advanced 1; ■ advanced 2

SELF-ASSESSMENT FOR HEALTH EDUCATION SPECIALISTS: PERCEIVED COMPETENCE

		Not Competent		Very Competent	

COMPETENCY 1.5: Examine factors that influence the process by which people learn

1.5.1	Identify and analyze factors that foster or hinder the learning process	1	2	3	4
1.5.2	Identify and analyze factors that foster or hinder knowledge acquisition	1	2	3	4
1.5.3	Identify and analyze factors that influence attitudes and beliefs	1	2	3	4
1.5.4	Identify and analyze factors that foster or hinder acquisition of skills	1	2	3	4

COMPETENCY 1.6: Examine factors that enhance or impede the process of health education/promotion

1.6.1	Determine the extent of available health education/promotion programs and interventions	1	2	3	4
1.6.2	Identify policies related to health education/promotion	1	2	3	4
1.6.3	Assess the effectiveness of existing health education/promotion programs and interventions	1	2	3	4
1.6.4	Assess social, environmental, political, and other factors that may impact health education/promotion	1	2	3	4
1.6.5	Analyze the capacity for providing necessary health education/promotion	1	2	3	4

COMPETENCY 1.7: Determine needs for health education/promotion based on assessment findings

1.7.1	❖ Synthesize assessment findings	1	2	3	4
1.7.2	Identify current needs, resources, and capacity	1	2	3	4
1.7.3	Prioritize health education/promotion needs	1	2	3	4
1.7.4	Develop recommendations for health education/promotion based on assessment findings	1	2	3	4
1.7.5	Report assessment findings	1	2	3	4

Area of Responsibility II:

PLAN HEALTH EDUCATION/PROMOTION

COMPETENCY 2.1: Involve priority populations, partners, and other stakeholders in the planning process

2.1.1	Identify priority populations, partners, and other stakeholders	1	2	3	4
2.1.2	Use strategies to convene priority populations, partners, and other stakeholders	1	2	3	4
2.1.3	Facilitate collaborative efforts among priority populations, partners, and other stakeholders	1	2	3	4
2.1.4	Elicit input about the plan	1	2	3	4
2.1.5	Obtain commitments to participate in health education/promotion	1	2	3	4

COMPETENCY 2.2: Develop goals and objectives

2.2.1	Identify desired outcomes using the needs assessment results	1	2	3	4
2.2.2	Develop vision statement	1	2	3	4
2.2.3	Develop mission statement	1	2	3	4
2.2.4	Develop goal statements	1	2	3	4
2.2.5	Develop specific, measurable, attainable, realistic, and time-sensitive objectives	1	2	3	4

SELF-ASSESSMENT FOR HEALTH EDUCATION SPECIALISTS: PERCEIVED COMPETENCE

		Not Competent		Very Competent	

COMPETENCY 2.3: Select or design strategies/interventions

2.3.1	❖ Select planning model(s) for health education/promotion	1	2	3	4
2.3.2	❖ Assess efficacy of various strategies/interventions to ensure consistency with objectives	1	2	3	4
2.3.3	❖ Apply principles of evidence-based practice in selecting and/or designing strategies/interventions	1	2	3	4
2.3.4	Apply principles of cultural competence in selecting and/or designing strategies/interventions	1	2	3	4
2.3.5	Address diversity within priority populations in selecting and/or designing strategies/interventions	1	2	3	4
2.3.6	Identify delivery methods and settings to facilitate learning	1	2	3	4
2.3.7	Tailor strategies/interventions for priority populations	1	2	3	4
2.3.8	Adapt existing strategies/interventions as needed	1	2	3	4
2.3.9	❖ Conduct pilot test of strategies/interventions	1	2	3	4
2.3.10	❖ Refine strategies/interventions based on pilot feedback	1	2	3	4
2.3.11	Apply ethical principles in selecting strategies and designing interventions	1	2	3	4
2.3.12	Comply with legal standards in selecting strategies and designing interventions	1	2	3	4

COMPETENCY 2.4: Develop a plan for the delivery of health education/promotion

2.4.1	Use theories and/or models to guide the delivery plan	1	2	3	4
2.4.2	Identify the resources involved in the delivery of health education/promotion	1	2	3	4
2.4.3	Organize health education/promotion into a logical sequence	1	2	3	4
2.4.4	Develop a timeline for the delivery of health education/promotion	1	2	3	4
2.4.5	Develop marketing plan to deliver health program	1	2	3	4
2.4.6	Select methods and/or channels for reaching priority populations	1	2	3	4
2.4.7	Analyze the opportunity for integrating health education/promotion into other programs	1	2	3	4
2.4.8	❖ Develop a process for integrating health education/promotion into other programs when needed	1	2	3	4
2.4.9	Assess the sustainability of the delivery plan	1	2	3	4
2.4.10	Design and conduct pilot study of health education/promotion plan	1	2	3	4

COMPETENCY 2.5: Address factors that influence implementation of health education/promotion

2.5.1	Identify and analyze factors that foster or hinder implementation	1	2	3	4
2.5.2	Develop plans and processes to overcome potential barriers to implementation	1	2	3	4

KEY: no symbol - entry level; ❖ advanced 1; ■ advanced 2

SELF-ASSESSMENT FOR HEALTH EDUCATION SPECIALISTS: PERCEIVED COMPETENCE

		Not Competent		Very Competent	

Area of Responsibility III:

IMPLEMENT HEALTH EDUCATION/PROMOTION

COMPETENCY 3.1: Coordinate logistics necessary to implement plan

3.1.1	Create an environment conducive to learning	1	2	3	4
3.1.2	Develop materials to implement plan	1	2	3	4
3.1.3	Secure resources to implement plan	1	2	3	4
3.1.4	Arrange for needed services to implement plan	1	2	3	4
3.1.5	Apply ethical principles to the implementation process	1	2	3	4
3.1.6	Comply with legal standards that apply to implementation	1	2	3	4

COMPETENCY 3.2: Train staff members and volunteers involved in implementation of health education/promotion

3.2.1	❖ Develop training objectives	1	2	3	4
3.2.2	Recruit individuals needed for implementation	1	2	3	4
3.2.3	❖ Identify training needs of individuals involved in implementation	1	2	3	4
3.2.4	❖ Develop training using best practices	1	2	3	4
3.2.5	❖ Implement training	1	2	3	4
3.2.6	❖ Provide support and technical assistance to those implementing the plan	1	2	3	4
3.2.7	❖ Evaluate training	1	2	3	4
3.2.8	❖ Use evaluation findings to plan/modify future training	1	2	3	4

COMPETENCY 3.3: Implement health education/promotion plan

3.3.1	Collect baseline data	1	2	3	4
3.3.2	❖ Apply theories and/or models of implementation	1	2	3	4
3.3.3	Assess readiness for implementation	1	2	3	4
3.3.4	Apply principles of diversity and cultural competence in implementing health education/promotion plan	1	2	3	4
3.3.5	Implement marketing plan	1	2	3	4
3.3.6	Deliver health education/promotion as designed	1	2	3	4
3.3.7	Use a variety of strategies to deliver plan	1	2	3	4

COMPETENCY 3.4: Monitor implementation of health education/promotion

3.4.1	Monitor progress in accordance with timeline	1	2	3	4
3.4.2	Assess progress in achieving objectives	1	2	3	4
3.4.3	Ensure plan is implemented consistently	1	2	3	4
3.4.4	Modify plan when needed	1	2	3	4
3.4.5	Monitor use of resources	1	2	3	4
3.4.6	Evaluate sustainability of implementation	1	2	3	4
3.4.7	Ensure compliance with legal standards	1	2	3	4
3.4.8	Monitor adherence to ethical principles in the implementation of health education/promotion	1	2	3	4

KEY: no symbol - entry level; ❖ advanced 1; ■ advanced 2

SELF-ASSESSMENT FOR HEALTH EDUCATION SPECIALISTS: PERCEIVED COMPETENCE

Area of Responsibility IV:

CONDUCT EVALUATION AND RESEARCH RELATED TO HEALTH EDUCATION/PROMOTION

COMPETENCY 4.1: Develop evaluation plan for health education/promotion

	Not Competent			Very Competent
4.1.1 ❖ Determine the purpose and goals of evaluation	1	2	3	4
4.1.2 ❖ Develop questions to be answered by the evaluation	1	2	3	4
4.1.3 ❖ Create a logic model to guide the evaluation process	1	2	3	4
4.1.4 ❖ Adapt/modify a logic model to guide the evaluation process	1	2	3	4
4.1.5 ❖ Assess needed and available resources to conduct evaluation	1	2	3	4
4.1.6 ❖ Determine the types of data (for example, qualitative, quantitative) to be collected	1	2	3	4
4.1.7 ❖ Select a model for evaluation	1	2	3	4
4.1.8 ❖ Develop data collection procedures for evaluation	1	2	3	4
4.1.9 ■ Develop data analysis plan for evaluation	1	2	3	4
4.1.10 ❖ Apply ethical principles to the evaluation process	1	2	3	4

COMPETENCY 4.2: Develop a research plan for health education/promotion

	Not Competent			Very Competent
4.2.1 ■ Create statement of purpose	1	2	3	4
4.2.2 ■ Assess feasibility of conducting research	1	2	3	4
4.2.3 ■ Conduct search for related literature	1	2	3	4
4.2.4 ■ Analyze and synthesize information found in the literature	1	2	3	4
4.2.5 ■ Develop research questions and/or hypotheses	1	2	3	4
4.2.6 ■ Assess the merits and limitations of qualitative and quantitative data collection	1	2	3	4
4.2.7 ■ Select research design to address the research questions	1	2	3	4
4.2.8 ■ Determine suitability of existing data collection instruments	1	2	3	4
4.2.9 ■ Identify research participants	1	2	3	4
4.2.10 ■ Develop sampling plan to select participants	1	2	3	4
4.2.11 ■ Develop data collection procedures for research	1	2	3	4
4.2.12 ■ Develop data analysis plan for research	1	2	3	4
4.2.13 ■ Develop a plan for non-respondent follow-up	1	2	3	4
4.2.14 ■ Apply ethical principles to the research process	1	2	3	4

■ COMPETENCY 4.3: Select, adapt and/or create instruments to collect data

	Not Competent			Very Competent
4.3.1 ■ Identify existing data collection instruments	1	2	3	4
4.3.2 ■ Adapt/modify existing data collection instruments	1	2	3	4
4.3.3 ■ Create new data collection instruments	1	2	3	4
4.3.4 Identify useable items from existing instruments	1	2	3	4
4.3.5 Adapt/modify existing items	1	2	3	4
4.3.6 ■ Create new items to be used in data collection	1	2	3	4
4.3.7 ■ Pilot test data collection instrument	1	2	3	4

KEY: no symbol - entry level;   ❖ advanced 1;   ■ advanced 2

		Not Competent		Very Competent	
4.3.8 ■ Establish validity of data collection instruments		1	2	3	4
4.3.9 ■ Ensure that data collection instruments generate reliable data		1	2	3	4
4.3.10 ■ Ensure fairness of data collection instruments (for example, reduce bias, use language appropriate to priority population)		1	2	3	4

COMPETENCY 4.4: Collect and manage data

4.4.1 ■ Train data collectors involved in evaluation and/or research		1	2	3	4
4.4.2 ■ Collect data based on the evaluation or research plan		1	2	3	4
4.4.3 Monitor and manage data collection		1	2	3	4
4.4.4 Use available technology to collect, monitor and manage data		1	2	3	4
4.4.5 Comply with laws and regulations when collecting, storing, and protecting participant data		1	2	3	4

COMPETENCY 4.5: Analyze data

4.5.1 ■ Prepare data for analysis		1	2	3	4
4.5.2 ❖ Analyze data using qualitative methods		1	2	3	4
4.5.3 ■ Analyze data using descriptive statistical methods		1	2	3	4
4.5.4 ■ Analyze data using inferential statistical methods		1	2	3	4
4.5.5 ■ Use technology to analyze data		1	2	3	4

COMPETENCY 4.6: Interpret results

4.6.1 ■ Synthesize the analyzed data		1	2	3	4
4.6.2 ■ Explain how the results address the questions and/or hypotheses		1	2	3	4
4.6.3 ■ Compare findings to results from other studies or evaluations		1	2	3	4
4.6.4 ■ Propose possible explanations of findings		1	2	3	4
4.6.5 ■ Identify limitations of findings		1	2	3	4
4.6.6 ■ Address delimitations as they relate to findings		1	2	3	4
4.6.7 ■ Draw conclusions based on findings		1	2	3	4
4.6.8 ■ Develop recommendations based on findings		1	2	3	4

COMPETENCY 4.7: Apply findings

4.7.1 Communicate findings to priority populations, partners, and stakeholders		1	2	3	4
4.7.2 Solicit feedback from priority populations, partners, and stakeholders		1	2	3	4
4.7.3 Evaluate feasibility of implementing recommendations		1	2	3	4
4.7.4 Incorporate findings into program improvement and refinement		1	2	3	4
4.7.5 ■ Disseminate findings using a variety of methods		1	2	3	4

KEY: no symbol - entry level; ❖ advanced 1; ■ advanced 2

SELF-ASSESSMENT FOR HEALTH EDUCATION SPECIALISTS: PERCEIVED COMPETENCE

Area of Responsibility V:

ADMINISTER AND MANAGE HEALTH EDUCATION/PROMOTION

COMPETENCY 5.1: Manage financial resources for health education/promotion programs

		Not Competent			Very Competent
5.1.1	❖ Develop financial plan	1	2	3	4
5.1.2	❖ Evaluate financial needs and resources	1	2	3	4
5.1.3	❖ Identify internal and/or external funding sources	1	2	3	4
5.1.4	❖ Prepare budget requests	1	2	3	4
5.1.5	❖ Develop program budgets	1	2	3	4
5.1.6	❖ Manage program budgets	1	2	3	4
5.1.7	❖ Conduct cost analysis for programs	1	2	3	4
5.1.8	❖ Prepare budget reports	1	2	3	4
5.1.9	❖ Monitor financial plan	1	2	3	4
5.1.10	❖ Create requests for funding proposals	1	2	3	4
5.1.11	❖ Write grant proposals	1	2	3	4
5.1.12	❖ Conduct reviews of funding proposals	1	2	3	4
5.1.13	❖ Apply ethical principles when managing financial resources	1	2	3	4

COMPETENCY 5.2: Manage technology resources

5.2.1	Assess technology needs to support health education/promotion	1	2	3	4
5.2.2	Use technology to collect, store and retrieve program management data	1	2	3	4
5.2.3	Apply ethical principles in managing technology resources	1	2	3	4
5.2.4	Evaluate emerging technologies for applicability to health education/promotion	1	2	3	4

COMPETENCY 5.3: Manage relationships with partners and other stakeholders

5.3.1	Assess capacity of partners and other stakeholders to meet program goals	1	2	3	4
5.3.2	❖ Facilitate discussions with partners and other stakeholders regarding program resource needs	1	2	3	4
5.3.3	Create agreements (for example, memoranda of understanding) with partners and other stakeholders	1	2	3	4
5.3.4	Monitor relationships with partners and other stakeholders	1	2	3	4
5.3.5	❖ Elicit feedback from partners and other stakeholders	1	2	3	4
5.3.6	Evaluate relationships with partners and other stakeholders	1	2	3	4

COMPETENCY 5.4: Gain acceptance and support for health education/promotion programs

5.4.1	Demonstrate how programs align with organizational structure, mission, and goals	1	2	3	4
5.4.2	Identify evidence to justify programs	1	2	3	4
5.4.3	Create a rationale to gain or maintain program support	1	2	3	4
5.4.4	Use various communication strategies to present rationale	1	2	3	4

KEY: no symbol - entry level;   ❖ advanced 1;   ■ advanced 2

		Not Competent		Very Competent	

COMPETENCY 5.5: Demonstrate leadership

5.5.1	❖ Facilitate efforts to achieve organizational mission	1	2	3	4
5.5.2	Analyze an organization's culture to determine the extent to which it supports health education/promotion	1	2	3	4
5.5.3	Develop strategies to reinforce or change organizational culture to support health education/promotion	1	2	3	4
5.5.4	❖ Facilitate needed changes to organizational culture	1	2	3	4
5.5.5	❖ Conduct strategic planning	1	2	3	4
5.5.6	❖ Implement strategic plan	1	2	3	4
5.5.7	❖ Monitor strategic plan	1	2	3	4
5.5.8	Conduct program quality assurance/process improvement	1	2	3	4
5.5.9	Comply with existing laws and regulations	1	2	3	4
5.5.10	Adhere to ethical principles of the profession	1	2	3	4

COMPETENCY 5.6: Manage human resources for health education/promotion programs

5.6.1	❖ Assess staffing needs	1	2	3	4
5.6.2	❖ Develop job descriptions	1	2	3	4
5.6.3	❖ Apply human resource policies consistent with laws and regulations	1	2	3	4
5.6.4	❖ Evaluate qualifications of staff members and volunteers needed for programs	1	2	3	4
5.6.5	Recruit staff members and volunteers for programs	1	2	3	4
5.6.6	❖ Determine staff member and volunteer professional development needs	1	2	3	4
5.6.7	❖ Develop strategies to enhance staff member and volunteer professional development	1	2	3	4
5.6.8	❖ Implement strategies to enhance the professional development of staff members and volunteers	1	2	3	4
5.6.9	❖ Develop and implement strategies to retain staff members and volunteers	1	2	3	4
5.6.10	❖ Employ conflict resolution techniques	1	2	3	4
5.6.11	❖ Facilitate team development	1	2	3	4
5.6.12	❖ Evaluate performance of staff members and volunteers	1	2	3	4
5.6.13	❖ Monitor performance and/or compliance of funding recipients	1	2	3	4
5.6.14	❖ Apply ethical principles when managing human resources	1	2	3	4

Area of Responsibility VI:

SERVE AS A HEALTH EDUCATION/PROMOTION RESOURCE PERSON

COMPETENCY 6.1: Obtain and disseminate health-related information

6.1.1	Assess needs for health-related information	1	2	3	4
6.1.2	Identify valid information resources	1	2	3	4
6.1.3	Evaluate resource materials for accuracy, relevance, and timeliness	1	2	3	4
6.1.4	Adapt information for consumer	1	2	3	4
6.1.5	Convey health-related information to consumer	1	2	3	4

SELF-ASSESSMENT FOR HEALTH EDUCATION SPECIALISTS: PERCEIVED COMPETENCE

			Not Competent			Very Competent

COMPETENCY 6.2: Train others to use health education/promotion skills

6.2.1	❖ Assess training needs of potential participants	1	2	3	4
6.2.2	❖ Develop a plan for conducting training	1	2	3	4
6.2.3	❖ Identify resources needed to conduct training	1	2	3	4
6.2.4	❖ Implement planned training	1	2	3	4
6.2.5	❖ Conduct formative and summative evaluations of training	1	2	3	4
6.2.6	❖ Use evaluative feedback to create future trainings	1	2	3	4

COMPETENCY 6.3: Provide advice and consultation on health education/promotion issues

6.3.1	❖ Assess and prioritize requests for advice/consultation	1	2	3	4
6.3.2	❖ Establish advisory/consultative relationships	1	2	3	4
6.3.3	❖ Provide expert assistance and guidance	1	2	3	4
6.3.4	❖ Evaluate the effectiveness of the expert assistance provided	1	2	3	4
6.3.5	❖ Apply ethical principles in consultative relationships	1	2	3	4

Area of Responsibility VII:

COMMUNICATE, PROMOTE, AND ADVOCATE FOR HEALTH EDUCATION/ PROMOTION, AND THE PROFESSION

COMPETENCY 7.1: Identify, develop, and deliver messages using a variety of communication strategies, methods, and techniques

7.1.1	Create messages using communication theories and/or models	1	2	3	4
7.1.2	Identify level of literacy of intended audience	1	2	3	4
7.1.3	Tailor messages for intended audience	1	2	3	4
7.1.4	❖ Pilot test messages and delivery methods	1	2	3	4
7.1.5	❖ Revise messages based on pilot feedback	1	2	3	4
7.1.6	Assess and select methods and technologies used to deliver messages	1	2	3	4
7.1.7	Deliver messages using media and communication strategies	1	2	3	4
7.1.8	Evaluate the impact of the delivered messages	1	2	3	4

COMPETENCY 7.2: Engage in advocacy for health and health education/promotion

7.2.1	Identify current and emerging issues requiring advocacy	1	2	3	4
7.2.2	Engage stakeholders in advocacy initiatives	1	2	3	4
7.2.3	Access resources (for example, financial, personnel, information, data) related to identified advocacy needs	1	2	3	4
7.2.4	Develop advocacy plans in compliance with local, state, and/or federal policies and procedures	1	2	3	4
7.2.5	Use strategies that advance advocacy goals	1	2	3	4

KEY: no symbol - entry level; ❖ advanced 1; ■ advanced 2

		Not Competent			Very Competent
7.2.6	Implement advocacy plans	1	2	3	4
7.2.7	Evaluate advocacy efforts	1	2	3	4
7.2.8	Comply with organizational policies related to participating in advocacy	1	2	3	4
7.2.9	Lead advocacy initiatives related to health	1	2	3	4

COMPETENCY 7.3: Influence policy and/or systems change to promote health and health education

7.3.1	Assess the impact of existing and proposed policies on health	1	2	3	4
7.3.2	Assess the impact of existing and proposed policies on health education	1	2	3	4
7.3.3	Assess the impact of existing systems on health	1	2	3	4
7.3.4	Project the impact of proposed systems changes on health education	1	2	3	4
7.3.5	Use evidence-based findings in policy analysis	1	2	3	4
7.3.6 ❖	Develop policies to promote health using evidence-based findings	1	2	3	4
7.3.7 ❖	Identify factors that influence decision-makers	1	2	3	4
7.3.8 ❖	Use policy advocacy techniques to influence decision-makers	1	2	3	4
7.3.9	Use media advocacy techniques to influence decision-makers	1	2	3	4
7.3.10	Engage in legislative advocacy	1	2	3	4

COMPETENCY 7.4: Promote the health education profession

7.4.1	Explain the major responsibilities of the health education specialist	1	2	3	4
7.4.2	Explain the role of professional organizations in advancing the profession	1	2	3	4
7.4.3	Explain the benefits of participating in professional organizations	1	2	3	4
7.4.4	Advocate for professional development of health education specialists	1	2	3	4
7.4.5	Advocate for the profession	1	2	3	4
7.4.6	Explain the history of the profession and its current and future implications for professional practice	1	2	3	4
7.4.7	Explain the role of credentialing (for example, individual, program) in the promotion of the profession	1	2	3	4
7.4.8	Develop and implement a professional development plan	1	2	3	4
7.4.9 ■	Serve as a mentor to others in the profession	1	2	3	4
7.4.10 ■	Develop materials that contribute to the professional literature	1	2	3	4
7.4.11 ■	Engage in service to advance the profession	1	2	3	4

KEY: no symbol - entry level; ❖ advanced 1; ■ advanced 2

This page was
intentionally left blank

Area of Responsibility I

Assess Needs, Resources, and Capacity for Health Education/Promotion

1.1: Plan Assessment Process for Health Education/Promotion

1.1.1   Define the priority population to be assessed
1.1.2   Identify existing and necessary resources to conduct assessments
1.1.3   Engage priority populations, partners, and stakeholders to participate in the assessment process
1.1.4 ❖ Apply theories and/or models to assessment process
1.1.5   Apply ethical principles to the assessment process

1.2: Access existing information and data related to health

1.2.1   Identify sources of secondary data related to health
1.2.2 ❖ Establish collaborative relationships and agreements that facilitate access to data
1.2.3   Review related literature
1.2.4   Identify gaps in the secondary data
1.2.5   Extract data from existing databases
1.2.6   Determine the validity of existing data

1.3: Collect primary data to determine needs

1.3.1   Identify data collection instruments
1.3.2   Select data collection methods for use in assessment
1.3.3   Develop data collection procedures
1.3.4   Train personnel assisting data collection
1.3.5   Implement quantitative and/or qualitative data collection

1.4: Analyze relationships among behavioral, environmental, and other factors that influence health

1.4.1   Identify and analyze factors that influence health behaviors
1.4.2   Identify and analyze factors that impact health
1.4.3   Identify the impact of emerging social, economic, and other trends on health

1.5: Examine factors that influence the process by which people learn

1.5.1   Identify and analyze factors that foster or hinder the learning process
1.5.2   Identify and analyze factors that foster or hinder knowledge acquisition
1.5.3   Identify and analyze factors that influence attitudes and beliefs
1.5.4   Identify and analyze factors that foster or hinder acquisition of skills

1.6: Examine factors that enhance or impede the process of health education/promotion

1.6.1   Determine the extent of available health education/promotion programs and interventions
1.6.2   Identify policies related to health education/promotion
1.6.3   Assess the effectiveness of existing health education/promotion programs and interventions
1.6.4   Assess social, environmental, political, and other factors that may impact health education/promotion
1.6.5   Analyze the capacity for providing necessary health education/promotion

KEY: no symbol - entry level; ❖ advanced 1; ■ advanced 2

1.7: Determine needs for health education/promotion based on assessment findings

1.7.1 ❖ Synthesize assessment findings
1.7.2   Identify current needs, resources, and capacity
1.7.3   Prioritize health education/promotion needs
1.7.4   Develop recommendations for health education/promotion based on assessment findings
1.7.5   Report assessment findings

The Role. The primary purpose of a needs, resources, and capacity assessment is to gather data and information to determine what interventions would be appropriate in a given setting. To successfully conduct a needs assessment, health education specialists must determine the purpose and scope of the assessment, collect appropriate data (i.e., primary and secondary), analyze the data, prioritize the needs, and identify the program focus. To assess the capacity of the priority population, health education specialists also must identify the available resources to address the needs and determine the extent of existing services and gaps in the provision of services.

Settings. The following text is presented to describe how assessment is used in different practice settings.

Community Setting. In a community setting, health education specialists rely on many sources of primary and secondary data to determine the needs of those in the priority population. Such data can come from health planning agencies, public health departments, census reports, data sets (e.g., Behavioral Risk Factor Surveillance Systems and Youth Risk Behavioral Surveillance Systems), and interviews with community leaders and members within the priority population. Data provide information about both real and perceived health needs. Depending on the types of needs identified, a well-planned health education program could be the way to address these needs. For example, if specific behaviors or health practices are

causally linked to the incidence of major health problems, then a health program can be planned to motivate and facilitate voluntary, desirable changes in those behaviors.

School (K-12) Setting. Local, state, and national data are used to determine the scope and sequence of curricula in a school setting, as well as to identify strengths and weaknesses that aid in developing a Whole School, Whole Community, Whole Child (WSCC) model program. National and state data may be considered and utilized, but local data are essential to good curriculum planning. Information about health knowledge, attitudes, skills, and practices can be gathered directly from students and used to improve health instruction, school policies, and school environment. Information gathered from parents, administrators, and school health personnel by a "School Health Team," consisting of representatives from each of the key areas of the WSCC model, may assist in identifying potential gaps in creating a healthy school community.

Health Care Setting. In a health care setting, complaints by health professionals about a growing number of emergency room visits might lead health education specialists to survey patients' medical records to determine whether the problem is general or limited to patients with particular kinds of emergencies or situational needs (e.g., patients without adequate health insurance or with limited access to primary care physicians). An assessment of the reasons for a given trend may help to determine what services or policies could improve the situation. Health

KEY: no symbol - entry level; ❖ advanced 1; ■ advanced 2

education specialists also may survey patients in a clinic to assess needs for, and interests in, educational programs offered in the clinical practice. When delivering health coaching in a clinic setting, health education specialists may assess patients' knowledge, perceptions, attitudes, and motivations regarding their current health status, as well as any potential changes the patients may be considering to improve or maintain their health. Health education specialists might accomplish this assessment by interviewing the patient and reviewing medical records of the patients.

Business/Industry Setting. In the workplace, health education specialists might work with medical professionals and/or health insurance carriers to analyze data that can be used to identify the health needs of workers. For example, this analysis might include data about health insurance claims, predictive modeling (future risk projections), disease prevalence, absenteeism and its causes, types of accidents and severity of injuries, and compensation claims. In addition, health education specialists in this setting may survey employees to discover their perceived needs and interests. Analysis of these data would indicate priority needs for health promotion programs.

College/University Setting. In the college or university setting, health education specialists are often involved in assessing student performance to meet state and national certification/licensure standards, as well as to meet program accreditation requirements. To revise curricula and meet accreditation standards, health education specialists track students' progress in meeting the standards, assess the learning environment, and analyze any links between the two.

College/University Health Services Setting. Health education specialists who practice in campus health services work closely with clinical practitioners in health, counseling, and fitness/wellness centers. Health education specialists assess the health needs of students, staff members, and faculty members through the use of focus groups, surveys, and interviews. In the assessment process, health education specialists develop avenues for obtaining information on knowledge, skills, perceptions, attitudes, beliefs, behaviors, learning preferences, and perceived needs in addition to health problems and practices. Once data are collected, health education specialists analyze them for factors that may impact the effectiveness of health education/promotion programs and interventions. The assessments form the basis of the priorities and recommendations for programs and interventions within the campus health services setting.

Key Terms

Capacity assessment is a measure of actual and potential individual, group, and community resources that can be inherent to and/or brought to bear for health maintenance and enhancement. The process of mapping community assets is included in the capacity assessment (Gilmore, 2012).

Needs assessment is the systematic identification of needs within a population and the determination of the degree to which those needs are being met (McKenzie, Neiger, & Thackeray, 2013).

Qualitative data is information that is difficult to measure, count, or express in numerical terms. For example, a participant's impression about the fairness of a program rule/requirement is qualitative data (United States Department of Health and Human Services [USDHHS], 2010).

Quantitative data is information that can be expressed in numerical terms, counted, or compared on a scale. Improvement in a child's reading level as measured by a reading test is one example (USDHHS, 2010).

Primary data are data gathered by health education specialists directly from or about the individual or population of interest. These data answer questions related to the specific needs assessment. Primary data are often collected by means of surveys, interviews, focus groups, and direct observation (McKenzie et al., 2013).

Secondary data are data that have already been collected by others that may or may not be directly gathered from the individual or population being assessed. Examples include existing research published in peer-reviewed journals and/or datasets, such as the United States Census, Vital Records, and Disease Registries (Gilmore, 2012).

Stakeholders are individuals or agencies that have a vested interest in the health education program (Bartholomew, Parcel, Kok, Gottlieb, & Fernandez, 2011).

Social determinants of health are conditions in which people are born, live, work, play, and age that affect their health risks, health, daily functioning, and quality of life (Centers for Disease Control and Prevention [CDC], 2013).

Competency 1.1: Plan Assessment Process for Health Education/Promotion

Needs assessment is the systematic identification of needs within a population and the determination of the degree to which those needs are being met (McKenzie et al., 2013). The program planner identifies and measures gaps between what is and what ought to be during needs assessment in order to provide direction in the development and support of an intervention. Some educators refer specifically to service needs and service demands or wants as a part of the needs assessment process (Windsor, Clark, Boyd, & Goodman, 2004). Service needs are those things health professionals believe a given population must have or be able to do in order to resolve a health problem. Service demands are those things people say they must have or be able to do in order to resolve their health problem. Both service needs and service demands are important.

KEY: no symbol - entry level; ❖ advanced 1; ■ advanced 2

In order to conduct a thorough needs assessment, health education specialists must carefully plan for the needs assessment process, including engaging the community, assessing resources, locating existing data, collecting data, and using research methods to guide data collection.

1.1.1 Define the priority population to be assessed

The foundation of any needs assessment process is to clearly identify the priority population to be assessed. Understanding the demographic qualities of the population such as age, sex, ethnicity, and income will impact the information gathered for the needs assessment. In addition to demographics, using a community perspective allows health education specialists to use specific criteria including geography (i.e., state, county, zip code), sector (i.e., school, worksite, faith-based), environmental conditions, culture and social aspects, size of population, and shared characteristics within the community to further and more comprehensively define the population for the needs assessment. It is also helpful to understand the health care context in terms of manpower, health care systems, and social service agencies.

1.1.2 Identify existing and necessary resources to conduct assessments

To save valuable time and to produce resources that will help in planning a program for the priority population, it is critical for health education specialists to conduct a needs assessment and collect health-related data from that population (Cottrell, Girvan, & McKenzie, 2014).

Many different approaches can be used to conduct a needs assessment. Often, the needs assessment may be limited by lack of time, personnel, and/or money. However, conducting a needs assessment is a critical step for health education programs.

McKenzie et al. (2013) identified the following six-step process for conducting a needs assessment:
1. Determine the scope of work and the purpose for the needs assessment
2. Gather the data
3. Analyze the data
4. Identify any factors linked to the health problem
5. Identify the focus for the program
6. Validate the need before continuing with the planning process

Developing an assessment plan will allow health education specialists to establish a roadmap that provides an overview of the process, resources needed, activities, and results that support the goals and objectives of the assessment. Resources for the conduct of an assessment may include human resources (e.g., staff, data collectors), supplies, incentives for participation, and travel costs. During the development of the assessment plan, health education specialists should research other needs assessments related to the targeted community that have been conducted in order to avoid duplication of efforts. Relevant assessments will add value to ensure a more comprehensive analysis of the community needs.

1.1.3 Engage priority populations, partners, and stakeholders to participate in the assessment process

Stakeholders and partners serve different purposes and make separate contributions. Partners are either individuals or organizations that bring knowledge, skills, or resources to the table and are willing to share risks, responsibilities, and rewards. Stakeholders are those who affect and are affected by change and those who have an interest in the results and/or what would be done with the results. Increasing the involvement of the priority population, partners, and stakeholders in the assessment process can not only result in an improved assessment but also increase the value of the results. Sometimes health education specialists or researchers might develop assessment plans using theories or their own experience; stake-holders can provide useful information or other ways of gathering information that might be relevant in that situation.

Identifying types of stakeholders allows health education specialists to develop relationships with stake-holders and help create an effective planning team to conduct a needs assessment, as well as to help with the development, implementation, and evaluation of programs.

❖ 1.1.4 Apply theories and/or models to assessment process

Given the complexity of health education and promotion practice, multi-level comprehensive interventions are needed to develop effective programs. Health education specialists need to consider many levels of influence including: behavioral, organizational, cultural, community, policy, and environmental. Theories and models can provide a framework for the needs assessment.

Theories are useful during the various stages of planning, implementing, and evaluating interventions. Program planners can use theories to shape answers to the questions of why, what, and how. In other words, health education specialists can use theories to guide the search for why people are not following public health and medical advice or not caring for themselves in healthy ways. Theories can help pinpoint what health education specialists need to know before developing and organizing an intervention program. Theories can provide insight into how to shape program strategies to reach people and organizations and make an impact on them. They also help to identify what should be monitored, measured, and compared in a program evaluation (Glanz, Rimer, & Viswanath, 2008b). Considering the role of theory based on how the constructs can be applied in practice can help health education specialists understand the behavior change at the community, interpersonal, or individual level.

The breadth and depth of information collected in needs assessments can vary depending on the needs assessment model used. Issel (2013) identifies five models for conducting a needs assessment: epidemiological model, public health model, social model, asset model, and rapid model.
- The *epidemiological* model focuses on epidemiological data (death rates, prevalence rates, birth rates, etc.).
- The *public health* model similarly attempts to quantify health problems and often uses epidemiological data. This model, however, can be more focused on a specific population and can be mindful of limitations of resources. Some planning models, such as PRECEDE-PROCEED, can be used as tools for this approach. See Sub-competency 2.3.1 for more information on planning models.
- The *social* model investigates social or political issues that influence health.

- The *asset* model focuses on the strengths of a community, organization, or population and looks to find ways to use existing assets to improve health.

- The *rapid* model is used when time and money are lacking for a needs assessment. This model offers some basic information, but is often lacking in detail.

These needs assessment models are not independent, and health education specialists might use several at once. Some program planning models include one or more steps involved in collecting data for needs assessment. Some models include:

- PRECEDE-PROCEED is specific in the order and types of information that should be collected (Green & Kreuter, 2005).

- Mobilizing for Action through Planning and Partnerships (MAPP) is a community driven strategic planning process for improving community health (NACCHO, 2013).

- Intervention Mapping Approach is a framework for health education intervention development. Intervention Mapping is composed of five steps: (1) creating a matrix of proximal program objectives, (2) selecting theory-based intervention methods and practical strategies, (3) designing and organizing a program, (4) specifying adoption and implementation plans, and (5) generating program evaluation plans (Bartholomew et al., 2011).

See Sub-competency 2.3.1 – Select planning model(s) for health education programs

Likewise, it is necessary to review behavior change models to understand the diverse influences on health and behaviors. See Sub-competency 2.5.1 for more information about factors that foster or hinder implementation.

Since health and health behaviors are influenced by many factors, it is important to collect data not only on what is happening but also why it is happening. Health education specialists should identify both a planning model and an implementation model in this stage as this will help to identify the types of data that need to be collected to fully understand the complex influences on health (Doyle, Ward, & Oomen-Early, 2010).

1.1.5 Apply ethical principles to the assessment process

It is important to consider ethical principles to guide the decision-making process of the assessment. While engaging the population, stakeholders, and partners, health education specialists may encounter conflicting priorities on the methodologies selected, data collected, and findings of the needs assessment. Issel (2013) provides an overview of six frequently applied ethical frameworks that can be applied to planning programs which includes needs assessment:

- Autonomy – personal right to self-determination and choice
- Criticality – the worst off benefit the most
- Egalitarian – all persons of equal value; minimize disparities
- Needs-based – equal opportunity to meet own needs, such as healthy life
- Resource sensitive – resources are scare
- Utilitarian – the greatest good for the greatest number; the end justifies the means

The application of ethical principles to the data collection needs to be carefully considered. The following discussion focuses on the ethics of data collection (Issel, 2013).

- Informed consent: This is the agreement to voluntarily and willingly participate in a study based on a full disclosure of what constitutes participation in the study, as well as identifies the risks and benefits involved in participation.
- Institutional Review Board (IRB): IRBs are composed of researchers and community members or stakeholders who review proposed research for compliance with federal regulations governing research involving human subjects.
- Health Insurance Portability and Accountability Act (HIPAA): The purpose of HIPAA is to protect personal health information. In order for health data to be used, individual permission must be granted, with some exceptions (CDC, 2003b).

Competency 1.2: Access Existing Information and Data Related to Health

A needs assessment is a critical part of program planning. A needs assessment allows health education specialists to determine what health problems exist in a particular setting or with a particular group of people. To obtain health-related data, multiple methods should be used. **Primary data** includes information health education specialists collect to answer unique questions about the specific purpose of the project. **Secondary data** have been collected previously for some other purpose and are available for use by others (McKenzie et al., 2013). However, not all collection methods and sources are appropriate in all practice settings.

1.2.1 Identify sources of secondary data related to health

Health education specialists locate and obtain valid and reliable data pertaining to a specific population. Most health education specialists identify needs of the priority population through a review of the current literature. Literature databases are available in libraries (specific computer databases) and through the Internet. Please refer to Sub-competency 6.1.2 for a description of databases for reviewing literature. Health education specialists need to be sure to gather data that refer to a population with characteristics similar to those of the priority population (McKenzie et al., 2013).

Health education specialists can use secondary data sources to gain important insight on community capacity, assets, and needs. Secondary data often involves gathering epidemiological data, such as health status, risk factors, incidence and/or prevalence rates, death rates, birth rates, and more.

Secondary Data Sources (McKenzie et al., 2013):
- Federal Government agencies
  - CDC
    - Morbidity/Mortality Weekly Report (MMWR)
    - Behavioral Risk Factor Surveillance System (BRFSS) data
    - Youth Risk Behavior Surveillance System (YRBSS) data
  - National Center for Health Statistics (NCHS)
    - Vital records

KEY: no symbol - entry level;   ❖ advanced 1;   ■ advanced 2

- United States Census Bureau
  - Population, employment, income, family size, education, housing, and other social indicators
  - The *Statistical Abstract of the United States* provides summary statistics of populations by metropolitan area, state, and the country as a whole, as well as information on health expenditures and health coverage (including Medicare and Medicaid), injuries, disability status, nutritional intakes, and food consumption
- USDHHS
  - Centers for Medicare and Medicaid Services (CMS)
  - Health Resources Service Administration (HRSA)
    - Social assistance programs
      - Social Security (SSA)
- State and local agencies
  - County, city, and state health departments or related agencies
    - Vital records, disease registries, police records, morbidity/mortality records, epidemiological studies, incident reports, safety surveys
    - Service, social, and religious organizations (e.g., Rotary Club, United Way)
- Nongovernment agencies and organizations
  - Health care system
    - Hospital discharge data, emergency room visit data, injury/hospitalization records
  - Voluntary health agencies or Disease-specific organizations, such as American Diabetes Association, American Heart Association, Arthritis Foundation, Susan B. Komen Breast Cancer Foundation
  - Professional health organizations (e.g., Society for Public Health Education, American Public Health Association)
  - Robert Wood Johnson Foundation-County Health Rankings
- Existing records
  - Health data that are collected as a by-product of services, such as clinical records, data from immunization programs, data from water pollution control programs, clinical indicators, data from physicians' offices, data on absenteeism, and data from insurance claims
- Literature
  - Peer-reviewed journals
  - Published scientific studies and reports

Health education specialists need to be able to assess and identify credible sources of data needed for the assessment. See Sub-competency 6.1.3 for more information about credible data sources and guidance on evaluating on-line data sources.

❖1.2.2 Establish collaborative relationships and agreements that facilitate access to data

There are a variety of ways to gather needs assessment data, including primary data from the community or priority population and secondary data from a literature review, federal, or local health agencies. Through collaborative relationships and agreements with stakeholders, agencies, or data resources, health education specialists have been able to facilitate access to data.

The collaborative relationship requires effort to identify common goals by which the organizations or groups could work together (Butterfoss, 2007). See Sub-competency 5.3.1 for more information about assessing capacity of partners and other stakeholders to meet program goals.

The level of that relationship could be identified as networking, cooperating, coordinating, or collaborating. Establishing an agreement with the organization or group outlining the intended outcome, audience, the purposes for which the data will be used, the ownership of data, confidentiality aspects, and conditions of the release of data can be an effective method to obtain or exchange needed data and practice data ethics. Data sharing agreement guides and templates are accessible online for health education specialists to integrate into their needs assessment process.

1.2.3 Review related literature

A **literature review** is a systematic method of locating, synthesizing and interpreting a collection of work by researchers and practitioners (Fink, 2013). An effective literature review is conducted in a systematic manner to uncover what is already known about a topic resulting in a summary and synthesis of the review. See Sub-competency 4.2.3 for more information about conducting searches for related literature.

Conducting a literature review during the needs assessment phase helps health education specialists understand the existing body of knowledge on the topic and populations, as well as identify information gaps to be included in the needs assessment. The topics for the literature review should be related to the key community assessment questions.

The basic components of the literature review process include:

1. Specify study aims. What questions do you want to answer?
2. Set inclusion criteria. What evidence will address the question?
3. Design the recruitment strategy. How will you find the evidence you want?
4. Screen potential partners. What evidence from the search process meets your criteria?
5. Decide on measures and design the data collection protocol. What characteristics will you code?
6. Select an appropriate metric to represent the strength of the findings. How will you represent findings from individual studies?
7. Collect the data. What are your coding procedures?
8. Analyze and display the data using appropriate methods.
9. Draw conclusions based on data and the limitations.

(Bartholomew et al., 2011)

1.2.4 Identify gaps in the secondary data

As data are analyzed, health education specialists might note there are little data that inform the key questions of the needs assessment that include certain health problems, health behaviors, attitudes, beliefs, or other theoretical constructs related to health behaviors. This observation might lead to further

KEY: no symbol - entry level;   ❖ advanced 1;   ■ advanced 2

data collection to gather the information or it might lead to the prioritization of health issues among a population based upon these gaps in data. Theories and models are useful for program planning, intervention, and evaluation. In this stage, health education specialists can apply explanatory theories and models to identify gaps in data, to help understand why a health problem exists, or to guide the search for modifiable factors (Glanz et al., 2008b).

1.2.5 Extract data from existing databases

Computerized reference databases are accessible at most universities and public libraries. Many reference databases are accessible to the public, such as the American FactFinder - United States Census Bureau, the BRFSS, the National Library of Medicine's PubMed, Google Scholar, and the Education Resources Information Center (ERIC).

1.2.6 Determine the validity of existing data

Valid and reliable data are necessary components in a thorough needs assessment. Health education specialists must be able to locate valid and reliable health and environmental data from a variety of sources if secondary data sources are to be used. If such instruments are used, then more meaningful comparisons of data can be made. These meaningful comparisons allow health education specialists to draw conclusions about needs for health programs.

Information is commonly obtained from the Internet, computerized reference databases, CD-ROMs, books, and peer-reviewed journals. The technology field is constantly producing new innovations, and the role of health education specialists is to make sound decisions about the appropriateness, credibility, and compatibility of the data. With knowledge from health behavior theories or models, health education specialists can make realistic decisions to meet the needs of the priority population.

There is an increasing demand for health information, and health education specialists may find a variety of sources. The roles of health education specialists include being a resource person and communicating information about the needs, concerns, and resources of the community. See Competency 6.1 – 6.3 for more information about serving as a health education/promotion resource person. Health education specialists must also have the skills to evaluate sources of information and must become a skeptical, critical consumer of health information.

Competency 1.3: Collect Primary Data to Determine Needs

Secondary data is important in defining the needs of the population. However, collecting primary data allows the health education specialist to obtain accurate data about problems, influences, and potential solutions to health issues specific to the community. Engaging community members in the needs assessment process helps to establish important relationships, which help to interpret the findings and support implementation of intervention (Doyle et al., 2010).

1.3.1 Identify data collection instruments

Primary data can be collected through a variety of sources and strategies at the individual, group, and community level. Health education specialists should become familiar with the various strategies to provide the framework to select the best method for data collection.

Primary Data Collection Strategies. A wide variety of strategies can be used to collect data. The strategies that can be used to collect primary data can be at the individual, group, or community level. The type of strategy used will depend upon the type of data needed for the needs assessment.

Individual:

Surveys are used to determine the knowledge, attitudes, beliefs, behaviors, skills, and health status of a priority population. Surveys should use well-constructed questionnaires that have been tested for validity and reliability, have a high response rate, and have been administered to a valid sample. According to Aday and Cornelius (2006), a "good" survey correlates with "good" planning.

Interviews are similar to surveys in that they can be conducted in a variety of ways. They can be completed by telephone, face-to-face, electronically, or in groups. Key informant interviews are conducted with individuals whom have knowledge of and the ability to report on the needs of a corporation, hospital, or organization. All methods require trained interviewers to ensure consistency and accuracy to conduct the interviews in an unbiased manner. Telephone interviews offer a relatively easy method of collecting data at moderate cost. They allow the interviewer to clarify questions, but do not have the advantage of visual cues the face-to-face method offers. Electronic (or Web-based) interviews are growing as a viable means of collecting data from a large number of individuals quickly and at low cost. However, the disadvantages—such as access to a limited population (only those with Internet access), lack of anonymity, and the fact that e-mails can easily be ignored—are difficult to overcome (McKenzie et al., 2013).

Self-assessment instruments can require people to answer questions about their health history, behavior, and screening results, such as blood pressure, cholesterol, height, and weight. These data are then compared against a database of individuals with similar characteristics, which provides a risk assessment for a number of diseases, as well as life expectancy. Individuals can detect disease or disease risk by performing other self-assessment techniques, including health assessments or health risk appraisals, breast self-examination, testicular self-examination, and self-monitoring for skin cancer (McKenzie et al., 2013).

Group:

Observations are used to gather data through direct surveillance of the population. Data collection is accomplished through watching and recording specific behaviors of the population being studied. At times, the observer becomes a part of the day-to-day activities. Examples of observations include watching factory workers for their use of safety equipment and/or precautions, observing the smoking behaviors of employees on a break, and checking food service workers' adherence to workplace health code regulations (McKenzie et al., 2013).

KEY: no symbol - entry level; ❖ advanced 1; ■ advanced 2

Community forums are public meetings. They bring together people in a particular population to discuss their perceptions of the community's health problems. It is important to remember the silent majority may not speak out, while more vocal individuals' views may wrongly be seen as the group's views (McKenzie et al., 2013).

Focus group techniques capitalize on communication among participants selected based on specific criteria. Individuals are invited to participate, and a skilled facilitator typically leads focus groups. In many instances, the facilitator encourages the participants to talk to one another, ask questions, give examples, and provide comments regarding a particular topic. Focus groups are designed so that participants share opinions and explain the reasons underlying those opinions. The number of participants for focus groups varies depending on the intended outcome; a focus group can be as small as two people or as large as the facilitator can manage. Analysis of results can be challenging. It may be difficult to infer consensus, and the results may not be generalizable (Neutens & Rubinson, 2010).

Nominal group process is a highly structured process in which a few representatives from the priority population are asked to respond to questions based on specific needs. This process uses small groups of five to seven people, with each member of the group having an equal voice in the discussion and voting. All participants share their opinions by privately ranking the ideas proposed and then sharing this ranking with the group in round-robin fashion. This is a time consuming process and may require a large meeting space, depending upon the number of people participating (Gilmore, 2012).

Delphi panel is a group process that generates consensus by using a series of mailed or e-mailed questionnaires. The process involves individuals from three groups: decision-makers, staff, and program participants. A questionnaire containing one or two broad questions is sent to the entire group. Their answers are then analyzed. Based on the analysis of the responses, a second questionnaire with more specific questions is developed. This questionnaire is sent to the same group of respondents, their responses are analyzed, and another questionnaire is developed. On average, questionnaires are analyzed and sent out three to five times (Gilmore, 2012).

Community:

Community capacity inventory and community asset maps are tools for identifying community resources and issues. Community capacity inventory typically involves developing a written list of the skills and talents of individual community members, associations, and other resources in the neighborhood as a whole. Simple survey, walking and windshield tours, interviews, community newspaper or directories, and other assessment methods can be used to gather information. Community members create community asset maps as they "map" local resources, abilities, and other building blocks for community growth and change. A community asset map is a visual representation of the physical assets of a community that may constitute important physical and social support structures for achieving community goals, such as libraries, playgrounds, schools, parks, and houses of worship (Minkler & Wallerstein, 2008).

PhotoVoice is a specific photographic technique to enable people to record and reflect personal and community strengths and concerns, as well as to promote critical dialogue and knowledge about personal and community issues through group discussion of photographs and to reach policy makers (Wang, 1997).

1.3.2 Select data collection methods for use in assessment

The method or strategy for collecting the primary data is based on the questions being asked, the data needed, the participants from whom the data will be collected, and the resources needed to collect data. Health education specialists should develop a comprehensive data collection and analysis plan. The data collection and analysis plan might apply multiple approaches based on program needs. For example, health education specialists should consider the feasibility of collecting data among different subpopulations in order to identify disparities. In addition, health education specialists should take into account potential bias results from data collection or analysis methods in the analysis plan. Please refer to Competency 4.2 for a description of research methods.

Data credibility can be improved by utilizing multiple methods for gathering data. Health education specialists can integrate primary and secondary data in order to obtain different, yet thorough perspectives on health needs and to compare data from the priority population with data from similar populations. The combination of data can help establish the rationale for program needs.

The selection of methods will include a consideration of the resources available, population characteristics and preferences, and timeframe to conduct assessment. Health education specialists' understanding of the advantages and disadvantages of the various data collection method assist in decision-making. Highlights of these considerations include:

Surveys (Neutens & Rubinson, 2010)
- Mail
  - Advantages: Eliminates interviewer bias, increases assurance of anonymity, allows respondents to complete at their convenience, increases accessibility to a wide geographic region, increases accuracy because respondent can consult records, encourages identical wording for all respondents, and promotes inter-rater reliability
  - Disadvantages: Lack of flexibility, likelihood of unanswered questions, low response rate, inability to record spontaneous reactions or nonverbal responses, lack of control over the order of responses, no guarantee of return by due date, inability to use complex questionnaire format, strong possibility of duplicate mailing, fear of loss of anonymity, and expense
- Telephone
  - Advantages: Cost savings compared with face-to-face survey, faster than mail survey or personal interview, accessibility to a wide geographic region, and increased monitoring and quality control

KEY: no symbol - entry level; ❖ advanced 1; ■ advanced 2

- Disadvantages: Respondents may see the call as a hoax or disruption, loss of visual component of reading the survey, interviewer has little control and respondent can hang up at any time, and low response rates due to unlisted numbers, caller ID, reduced use of land lines, "do not call" lists
- Face-to-Face
  - Advantages: Personalization of the survey to one participant, flexibility for further probing, higher response rates, control over question order, spontaneity, no possibility of help from others, and ability to use more complex questionnaires
  - Disadvantages: Expensive, time-consuming, increased change of interviewer bias, lack of anonymity, lack of standardization of questions, and difficulty in summarizing the findings
- Web or Internet
  - Advantages: Quick response, low cost to administer, automated data gathering process, administered to a large number of participants, and a forced-choice format
  - Disadvantages: Limited ability to monitor returned surveys, limited time frame within which respondent can access survey, forced-explicit choice responses, costly hardware and software, and the possibility that participants may not be anonymous

Interviews or focus group (University of Kansas, 2014a)
- Advantages: Help people learn more about group or community opinions and needs have more depth, nuance, and variety; nonverbal communications and group interactions can also be observed; and focus groups can therefore get closer to what people are really thinking and feeling
- Disadvantages: Responses may be harder to score on a scale

Observations (University of Kansas, 2014a)
- Advantages: actually looks at a place or event, can watch situations or interactions, and experience life of the community or a population
- Disadvantages: documenting observations may be harder to analyze

1.3.3 Develop data collection procedures

The evaluation or research design is the grand scheme that delineates when and from whom data are collected. Methods indicate the way in which data are collected as part of the evaluation and typically consist of strategies (Issel, 2013). When conducting needs assessments, health education specialists need to be mindful of sampling techniques, basic research designs used to collect and compare data, methods of collecting data, types of data needed to answer research questions, and the need for valid and reliable instruments to measure health status, behaviors, attitudes, beliefs, etc. A key part of assessment planning is the application of proper study design with appropriate methods and instruments. Please refer to Competency 4.2 for more information on research design and methods and Competency 4.3 for more information regarding instrumentation and data collection.

Table 1.1

Data Collection Phases

Phases	Components
Data Collection and Instrument Development	• Question development • Data collection method • Instrument protocol development • Instrument testing and revisions • Language requirements • Administration of data collection • Selection and preparation of data collectors
Data Analysis Plan	• Data system management • Data entry • Data verification • Quantitative analysis plan • Qualitative analysis plan • Data transfer
Findings or Results of Assessment	• Current results • Gaps • Existing strengths • Causal analysis
Written Reporting of Data	• Expected content or sections of report • Format of the report • Graphics and charts

Adequate planning and preparation are vital to successful data collection activities. Formulating and documenting procedures define standards and expectations that contribute to that success, and include: (a) data collection and instrument development, (b) data analysis plan, (c) findings or results of assessment, and (d) written reporting of data.

Sometimes health education specialists will be required to create a survey to collect data. The following provides steps in designing and completing a survey:

1. *Planning the survey.* This step includes determining (a) survey objectives, (b) monetary resources, (c) time resources, and (d) personnel resources.
2. *Designing the survey.* A survey should be designed to accomplish the objectives and should reflect data needs, data collection techniques, and resources.
3. *Collecting the data.* The method chosen should match the survey objectives and fit resource constraints.
4. *Planning data analysis.* An appropriate method of data analysis, consistent with the type of data being collected and the goals of the needs assessment, should be chosen.

KEY: no symbol - entry level;   ❖ advanced 1;   ■ advanced 2

5. *Drawing the sample.* From the survey objectives and design come (a) the population of interest, (b) the sample size and selection, and (c) appropriate interviewers if interviews are to be conducted.

6. *Constructing the questionnaire.* The questions formulated for a survey are of the utmost importance and require detailed attention. Use existing validated questions when possible. All questions should match the objectives.

7. *Pretesting the questionnaire.* The survey should be pretested with a sample comparable to the population of interest.

8. *Revising the questionnaire.* Revisions should be based on findings from the pretest. If there are extensive changes, a second pretest should be conducted.

9. *Administering the survey.* The method chosen (e.g., mail, e-mail, telephone) should fit the nature of the data to be gathered and the objectives of the survey.

10. *Preparing the data.* Data preparation includes coding the questions and responses for tabulation and designing contingent values (as necessary) to limit data entry errors.

11. *Verifying.* Data entered should be tested for accuracy and for errors in coding.

12. *Entering data.* The method of data entry will vary according to resources; the key is to use a software program that is user-friendly, advantageous for analysis, and that can be watched for errors.

13. *Tabulating.* A frequency count should be conducted to ascertain how many answers are in each of the categories for every question.

14. *Analyzing.* Analysis varies according to the purpose of the study, but it generally includes calculating percentages, averages, and relational indices, as well as performing tests of significance.

15. *Recording and reporting.* The report should reflect all of the previous steps outlined including the objectives, hypotheses, reliability of results, and recommendations for action. Reports often include an executive summary of the methods and major findings for the study.

(Neutens & Rubinson, 2010)

1.3.4 Train personnel assisting with data collection

Health education specialists train personnel and stakeholders regarding appropriate data collection methods in order to ensure the quality of data. Standardizing the procedure of data collection with frequent monitoring of the process will help ensure collection of data is accurate, complete, and conforms to program requirements.

1.3.5 Implement quantitative and/or qualitative data collection

Data collected for a needs assessment can be quantitative, qualitative, or both. Quantitative data are used to numerically describe what is occurring (Baumgartner & Hensley, 2012). Qualitative data are not numerical and are usually descriptions of what is occurring or why it is occurring (Baumgartner & Hensley, 2012). Both types of data are valuable to health education specialists throughout the program planning, implementation, and evaluation process.

To ensure quality, it will be important to find reliable, trustworthy, and skilled people to collect, enter, analyze, and manage the data. Other considerations for implementation are:

- Defining roles, responsibilities, and skills needed to collect, enter, and analyze qualitative data (focus groups, interviews, and community forums), which may differ from the needs related to quantitative data (surveys).
- Monitoring the data collection to ensure implementation of the process will assist in maintaining established timeframes and objectives. Identifying a committee or group would provide this oversight.
- Maintaining the integrity of the data you collect and ensure protocols address quality control measures not only on the collection but entry of data (See Competency 4.4 Collect and Manage Data).

Operational resources are essential to any data collection effort and must be considered during the planning stage. For example, use of incentives could add value to the response rates from populations/participants, access to software can help with qualitative analysis, and costs can cover use of facilities to conduct focus groups. Health educations specialists must also communicate with their partners and stakeholders to inform them of the implementation of the data collection process.

Competency 1.4: Analyze Relationships Among Behavioral, Environmental, and Other Factors that Influence Health

Planners need to identify and prioritize the behavioral, environmental, and social risk factors that are associated with health. These are called social determinants of health, or the conditions in which people are born, live, work, play, and age that affect their health risks, health, daily functioning, and quality of life (CDC, 2013). Modifying these factors or determinants is pertinent to improving the health status of individuals and communities (McKenzie et al., 2013). The types and number of risk factors are as varied as influences themselves.

1.4.1 Identify and analyze factors that influence health behaviors

Individual factors include educational, social, and cultural characteristics of the individual. Individual factors include a person's knowledge, attitudes, beliefs, and perceptions related to health. An individual's culture, religious or spiritual beliefs, and skill set must be considered when assessing influences on health behavior (McKenzie et al., 2013; Turnock, 2004).

Behavioral (lifestyle) factors are behaviors or actions of individuals, groups, or communities. Behavioral indicators may include compliance, consumption and utilization patterns, coping, preventive actions, and self-care (McKenzie et al., 2013).

Environmental factors are determinants outside the individual that can be modified to support behavior, health, and quality of life. Examples of environmental factors include economic factors, physical factors, and public services, as well as the accessibility, affordability, and equity of health services (McKenzie et al., 2013).

KEY: no symbol - entry level;   ❖ advanced 1;   ■ advanced 2

According to ecological models, behavior has multiple influences including factors at the intrapersonal, interpersonal, organizational, community, and public policy levels. Behavioral influences interact across these different levels (Sallis, Owen & Fisher, 2008). Once a health behavior has been determined and factors that influence the behavior have been identified, health education specialists need to gather more information to know how these factors influence the behavior. Health education specialists need to weigh the importance and changeability of the factors against available resources for the program. Using an ecological perspective can provide a multi-level and interactive approach as health education specialists explore the relationships between risk factors. Commonly there are five levels of influence for health behaviors:

- Individual: knowledge, attitudes, and beliefs that influence behavior
- Interpersonal: association with family, friends, and peers that define social identity, support, and role
- Institutional: rules, regulations, and policies which may constrain or promote recommended behaviors
- Community: social networks and norms
- Public policy: local, state, and federal policies and laws that regulate or support actions/ practices

Health education specialists can contribute to the impact of the program by understanding the relationships of the multidirectional flow of influence within and between levels and applying that understanding to the development of the intervention.

1.4.2 Identify and analyze factors that impact health

Health is impacted by a variety of different factors. The five major factors that contribute to determinant of the health of a population include:

- Genes and biology (e.g., sex and age)
- Health behaviors (e.g., healthy eating, physical activity, alcohol use, injection drug use, unprotected sex, and smoking)
- Social environment or social characteristics (e.g., discrimination, income, gender, and social support)
- Physical environment or total ecology (e.g., where a person lives, crowding conditions, and built environments)
- Health services or medical care (e.g., access to quality health care and having/not having insurance)

These various components are often interrelated, and their combined effect influences the likelihood of disease, functional capacity, health behavior, and well-being. Each determinant's level of influence on population health varies (Figure 1.2).

Figure 1.2. Estimates of how each of the five major determinants influence population health. From Centers for Disease Control and Prevention, 2014e, Social determinants of health. Reprinted with permission.

DETERMINANTS OF POPULATION HEALTH

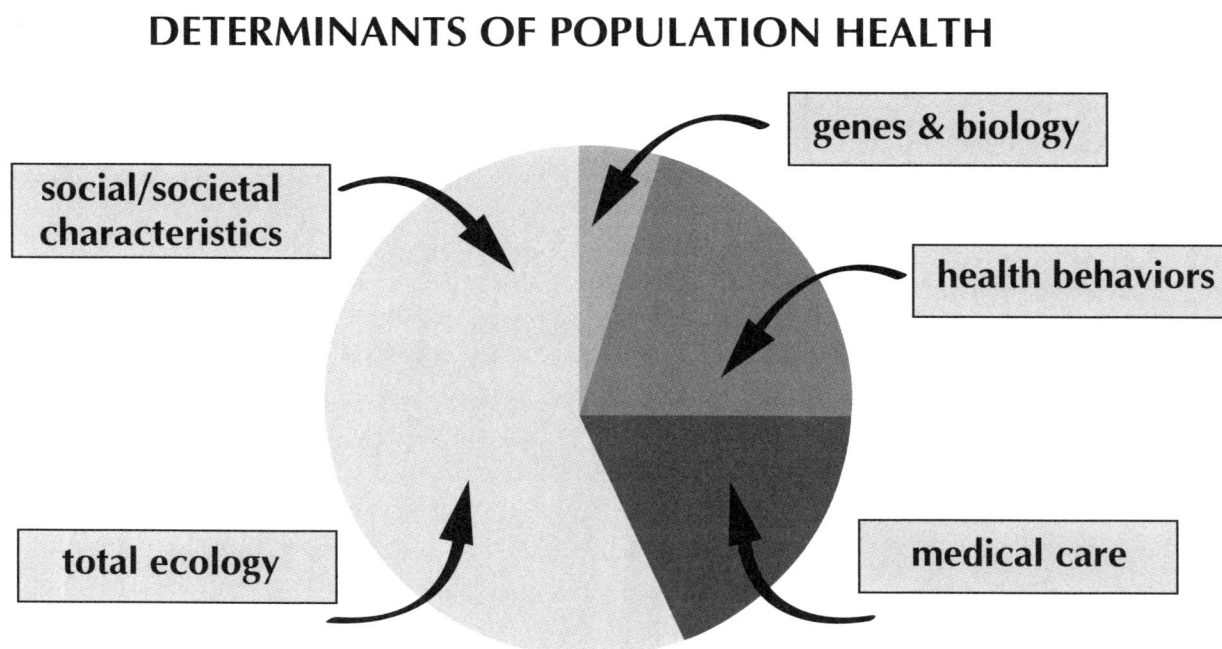

Once the factors that enhance or compromise health have been identified, there is a need to gather more information about how these factors impact health. Health education specialists can use data gathered from the needs assessment, data from the literature indicating risk factors and determinants of health, and data collected from surveys (i.e., YRBSS and BRFSS) to identify which factors are most important and changeable in order to determine the goals and objectives of the health promotion program.

1.4.3 Identify the impact of emerging social, economic, and other trends on health

There is a growing recognition that, while individual behavior plays a key role, opportunities to make healthy choices are shaped by the availability of choices. Social and economic conditions created by societal norms and policies in both health and nonhealth sectors determine these opportunities; such opportunities are not always distributed equitably across population groups (NACCHO, 2010). Strategies to improve population health need be developed and implemented where people live, learn, work, play, and worship.

The World Health Organization defines the social determinants of health as the conditions in which people are born, grow, live, work, and age (WHO, 2014b). These circumstances are shaped by the distribution of money, power, and resources at global, national, and local levels. Healthy People 2020 developed five key areas of social determinants of health:

- Economic Stability (e.g., poverty, employment, food security, housing stability)
- Education (e.g., high school graduation, enrollment in higher education, language and literacy, early childhood education and development)

KEY: no symbol - entry level; ❖ advanced 1; ■ advanced 2

- Social and Community Context (e.g., social cohesion, civic participation, perceptions of discrimination and equity, incarceration/institutionalization)
- Health and Health Care (i.e., access to health care and primary care, health literacy)
- Neighborhood and Built Environment (e.g., access to healthy foods, quality of housing, crime and violence, environmental conditions)

Healthy People 2020 (USDHHS, 2014) offers the following definitions of health disparities and health equity:

- Health disparities are "a particular type of health difference that is closely linked with social, economic, and/or environmental disadvantage."
- Health equity is the "attainment of the highest level of health for all people. Achieving health equity requires valuing everyone equally with focused and ongoing societal efforts to address avoidable inequalities, historical and contemporary injustices, and the elimination of health and health care disparities." Disparities are differences in health that are not only unnecessary and avoidable, but in addition are considered unfair and unjust.

It has been shown that tracking life expectancy by census track or zip code finds wide ranges of mortality between areas within a defined geographical area (USDHHS, 2014; Joint Center for Political and Economic Studies, 2012). Using this as an example, addressing these disparities by assessing the extent to which inequities exist among populations allows health education specialists to consider upstream factors in the social, physical, and built environments that are the root cause for differences in disease distribution and health outcomes among populations of different racial, ethnic, age related, and socioeconomic backgrounds.

Competency 1.5: Examine Factors that Influence the Process by Which People Learn

People learn in different ways. What works for one individual or group does not always work for everyone. People learn by making connections with previous knowledge and experiences. Therefore, health education specialists must acknowledge learning impacts and select methods for delivering health education, health promotion, and health messages that are tailored to specific individuals or groups.

1.5.1 Identify and analyze factors that foster or hinder the learning process

Health education specialists conduct needs and capacity assessments to better understand influences on the health and well-being of individuals and groups. As health education specialists understand the influences on health, they can help individuals and communities make informed decisions and take the appropriate steps to enhance health (Gilmore, 2012).

It is important to recognize factors that foster learning, such as attitudes, different learning styles, and readiness to adopt new strategies. When working with adults, health education specialists need to remember that adults and children learn in different ways (Knowles, Holton, & Swanson. 2005).

The following lists some key components of adult learning:
- Adults are motivated to learn when they have needs and interests that learning can satisfy
- Adults are oriented to learning that is life centered (i.e., based on life situations)
- Experience is the richest source of learning for adults
- Adults are self-directed learners
- Adult education considers individual differences as people age such as differences in time, place, and pace of learning

It is helpful to allow adult learners to be part of the decision-making process when planning learning experiences. In addition, health education specialists should explain why the participants are learning a topic, as well as the immediate value of the new knowledge and skills, and they approach teaching through problem solving techniques to engage the adult learner.

In order for learning to have the greatest chance of success, participant motivation and readiness must be assessed. Maslow's hierarchy of needs (Freitas & Leonard, 2011) and The Attention, Relevance, Confidence, Satisfaction (ARCS) Motivation Model (Gagne, Wager, Golas, & Keller, 2005) describe issues related to motivation.

In order for learners to be capable of learning, certain basic needs must first be met. Maslow's hierarchy of basic human needs holds that each level of needs must be met before the individual can move to the next levels. The levels of needs start at physiological needs and move up to self-actualization (Freitas & Leonard, 2011). The hierarchy of needs and its applications to training adults are presented in Table 1.2 below.

Table 1.2
Maslow's Hierarchy of Needs

Need	Application to Training
Physiological needs (food, water, warmth)	• Provide breaks and snacks/meals • Set a comfortable room temperature
Safety needs (security and safety)	• Offer safe training environment • Permit learners to ask questions throughout
Social belongingness (sense of belonging)	• Create a feeling of group dynamics and feeling of acceptance
Esteem (status, achievement)	• Recognize achievements. • Positively reinforce learning
Self-Actualization (personal fulfillment)	• Offer work or training that challenges learner • Offer skills to make progress on long term goals

KEY: no symbol - entry level; ❖ advanced 1; ■ advanced 2

The ARCS Motivation Model is a compilation of guidelines from many motivation theories. Causes of motivation may be either extrinsic (external to the learner) or intrinsic (internal to the learner). The intent of the ARCS Model is to provide learners with the necessary time and effort to acquire new knowledge and skills (Gagne, Wager, Golas, & Keller, 2005). The motivational categories of the ARCS Model are presented in Table 1.3 below (Gagne et al., 2005).

Table 1.3
Application of the Motivational Categories

Category	Application of the Motivational Category
Attention	• Capture the learners' interest • Maintain their attention
Relevance	• Know the learners' needs • Provide learners with opportunities to match activities to their motives for learning • Tie the instruction to learners' past experiences (e.g., analogies, prerequisite knowledge)
Confidence	• Build positive expectations of learning • Provide methods for learning to achieve success in mastery of knowledge and skill
Satisfaction	• Provide reinforcement to learners' successes • Encourage use of new knowledge and skills

The type of instruction also impacts the learning process. Gagne's Theory of Instruction presents a comprehensive view of instruction. He identifies categories of learning: (a) verbal information, (b) cognitive strategies, (c) intellectual skills, (d) motor skills, and (e) attitudes. He further proposes the nine events of instruction that provide conditions for learning. The nine events are presented below (Gagne et al., 2005). These hierarchies can help with developing the sequencing of instruction (See Table 1.4).

Table 1.4
Events of Instruction

Event of Instruction	Application to Training
1. Gain attention	Describe why training is important. Ask stimulating questions. Present a problem to be solved.
2. Inform learners of the objectives	Present the learning objectives.
3. Build on prior knowledge	Associate new content with prior knowledge.
4. Present the stimulus	Present the training content.
5. Provide guidance	Give illustrative examples, analogies, mnemonics, or basic steps in performance to help learner retain new knowledge or skill.
7. Provide feedback	Give immediate feedback on performance during the training.
8. Assess performance	Assess knowledge/skills gained.
9. Enhance retention and transfer	Provide supplemental materials (e.g., worksheets, problem sets, case scenarios, training manual) to reinforce learning. Discuss or ask how knowledge and skills can be applied on the job.

Bloom's Taxonomy relates to the classification of learning objectives developed for learners. He proposes that learning in the cognitive domain should apply the higher order processes instead of lower order objectives that are traditionally seen. Instruction should have higher ordered objectives that are mentally demanding. Table 1.5 presents the taxonomy, skills demonstrated, and examples of verbs for that level of objectives (Gronlund, 1995). Health education specialists can use these levels of skills when writing training objectives.

Table 1.5

Taxonomy and Skills Demonstrated

Event of Instruction	Skills Demonstrated	Verbs
Knowledge	Recall of information or major ideas Mastery of the subject matter	Define Describe Label List State Tell
Comprehension	Understand information	Explain Outline Restate Summarize
Application	Use information Solve problems using knowledge or skills	Apply Construct Demonstrate Illustrate Show Use
Analysis	Identification of components Recognition of patterns	Analyze Distinguish Compare Contrast Explain
Synthesis	Relate knowledge from several areas Predict and draw conclusions	Construct Create Devise Formulate Plan
Evaluation	Compare and discriminate between ideas Decide based on arguments	Choose Judge Justify Debate Assess

KEY: no symbol - entry level;   ❖ advanced 1;   ■ advanced 2

1.5.2 Identify and analyze factors that foster or hinder knowledge acquisition

After identification of factors that influence the learning process, health education specialists need to use the information gathered to make program-planning decisions. As health education specialists better understand the influences on learning, they can make informed decisions and develop appropriate learning experiences for programs. Knowing barriers to learning will help health education specialists develop methods for individuals and communities to overcome barriers and learn. These can include educational level, income, cultural factors, attitudes about the topics, etc. See Sub-competency 2.2.1 for more information on using assessment results to inform the planning process.

1.5.3 Identify and analyze factors that influence attitudes and beliefs

Attitudes and beliefs are shaped by physical, cultural, social, and community norms. Family values, religion, and the environment also shape attitudes and beliefs. Health education specialists must understand the dynamics of priority populations in order to build relationships, respect, and trust, as well as to identify ways to collaborate effectively on interventions. For health education and health promotion interventions to be successful, health education specialists must acknowledge diversity in backgrounds, experiences, and cultures to effectively engage priority populations and other stakeholders in interventions.

1.5.4 Identify and analyze factors that foster or hinder acquisition of skills

After identifying attitudes and beliefs that foster or hinder behavioral change, health education specialists can develop health promotion interventions that address these attitudes and beliefs both positive and negative. Health education specialists can then build trust with individuals and communities. Once trust has been established, health education specialists can assist the individuals and communities in developing their capacity and infrastructure for behavioral change and community action to take place. Health education specialists can provide the knowledge, technical assistance, and training for individuals and communities to make change happen.

Competency 1.6: Examine Factors that Enhance or Impede the Process of Health Education/Health Promotion

Factors that should be identified during the needs assessment include the following:
- Predisposing factors: individual knowledge and affective traits
- Enabling factors: factors that make possible a change in behavior
- Reinforcing factors: feedback and encouragement resulting from a changed behavior, perhaps from significant others

These factors may have a direct impact on health risk factors and how the health education program is planned and implemented (Green & Kreuter, 2005; McKenzie et al., 2013). Many of these factors can serve as either a facilitator or barrier. For example, knowledge that a behavior could lead to a health issue can facilitate change, but false information can be a barrier to change. These three factors (predisposing, enabling, and reinforcing) are important in combination. Knowledge regarding a health issue is an important facilitator, but the absence of knowledge, skills, or support in how to change can severely impact an individual's ability to change.

KEY: no symbol - entry level; ❖ advanced 1; ■ advanced 2

1.6.1 Determine the extent of available health education/health promotion programs and interventions

Health education specialists need to determine the health education programs, services, or policies that already exist for the priority population. Health education specialists need to use community-building processes, which focus on the identification, nurturing, and celebration of community assets.

A review of actual and potential availability of resources is essential for establishing realistic program/intervention starting points and determining how the programs/interventions can be sustained. The process of asset mapping or mapping community capacity can help the health education specialist identify available programs and interventions (Gilmore, 2012). See Sub-competency 6.2.5 for more evidence-based programs and resources.

1.6.2 Identify policies related to health education/promotion

Health policy and enforcement strategies come in a variety of formats, such as executive orders, laws, ordinances, position statements, regulations, and formal and/or informal rules. Policies related to health education/promotion occur at the national, state, local, and organizational levels. For example, tobacco use has been labeled the single most important, preventable cause of death and disease in the United States. One national health objective is to reduce public exposure to environmental tobacco smoke (ETS) or second hand smoke. There are objectives in the national plan that relate specifically to laws on smoke free air in restaurants. The CDC recommends smoking bans and restrictions in public places to reduce exposure to second hand smoke. The Task Force on Community Preventive Services, a nonfederal public health panel, which conducts in-depth systematic reviews on selected tobacco interventions, concluded that smoking bans and restrictions are the most effective measures to reduce exposure to second hand smoke. At the local level, advocates can educate citizens on the dangers and risks of second hand smoke exposure and empower them to support local campaigns to prohibit smoking in restaurants. Grassroots activities can also involve mobilizing citizens to advocate for smoke free ordinances at the city/county level (McKenzie et al, 2012).

Health education specialists can plan more effective interventions with a knowledge and understanding of policies related to health education/promotion. Policies are important to health promotion work. One of the core functions of public health is comprehensive public health policy development. The fifth essential public health service is to develop policies and plans that support individual and community health efforts (McKenzie et al, 2012).

1.6.3 Assess the effectiveness of existing health education/promotion programs and interventions

Health education specialists can collect recommendations throughout the development and evaluation of health promotion programs and interventions, so good ideas and insights are neither lost nor forgotten. When determining the effectiveness of programs and interventions, health education specialists can use recommendations from a variety of sources, such as scientific literature, program staff, program stakeholders, and program decision-makers. At the national level, health education specialists can use systematic reviews and meta-analysis of evidence-based practices. For example, the Guide to Community Preventive Services provides a summary of what is known about the effectiveness, economic efficiency, and feasibility of interventions to promote community health and prevent disease. It includes evidence-based recommendations for programs and policies to promote population-based health. The Community Guide includes evidence on topics, including alcohol, cancer, physical activity, obesity, and tobacco. The Community Guide (http://www.thecommunity guide.org/index.html) has been developed and continually updated by the nonfederal Task Force on Community Preventive Services, which is comprised of public health experts who are appointed by the director of the CDC (McKenzie et al, 2013).

Health education specialists can identify gaps or overlaps in existing programs by communicating with stakeholders in the community, looking at service use by clients, and observing levels and patterns of the provided services. At this stage, health education specialists should consider potential partnerships with other agencies or organizations that have similar goals. Working with existing partners and forming new partnerships can help agencies share resources as they work toward a common goal. See Sub-competencies 5.4.1, 5.4.7, and 5.5.3 for more information on health education specialists' role in developing partnerships.

1.6.4 Assess social, environmental, political, and other factors that may impact health education/promotion

In order to understand the "big picture" of how program processes fit together, health education specialists must understand the impact of social, environmental, and political factors (Issel, 2013). Building capacity to improve health involves the development of sustainable skills, resources, and organizational structures in the affected community. Building the capacity of the community is deeply rooted in the social, political, and economic environment and cannot be conducted without an understanding of the specific environment in which it will take place (National Institutes of Health [NIH], 2011).

Health education specialists must be aware of not only the biological risk factors affecting health but also the environmental, social, and behavioral contexts within which individuals and populations operate in order to identify factors that may hinder or promote the success of their interventions. Health education specialists need to understand that not all factors affecting an individual's health are under their control. People contribute to their health status, but it cannot be isolated from the environmental and social contexts in which it occurs (Gilmore, 2012). Factors affecting health status occur at multiple levels of social ecology. For example, the individual level for obesity prevention involves the selection of healthy food choices. The environmental level involves access to healthy food choices, such as the availability of fresh fruits and vegetables at farmers' markets and community gardens.

1.6.5 Analyze the capacity for providing necessary health education/promotion

Capacity, or asset-based, assessments can also be conducted to complement the needs assessment. These assessments focus on individual and group resources to analyze a community's strengths (Gilmore, 2012). Assets and resources are community contributions that may prevent the health problem from occurring or assist in its solution (Issel, 2013). Community empowerment through capacity building helps communities solve their own problems with their own resources (Doyle et al., 2010).

KEY: no symbol - entry level; ❖ advanced 1; ■ advanced 2

To implement an assets-based assessment to measure the community's capacity to solve its health problems, Beaulieu (2002) recommends the following steps:

1. Identify community resources (persons, groups, places), abilities, skills, networks, strengths, talents
2. Create or strengthen the relationships between community members and community organizations
3. Mobilize the community around its strengths/resources
4. Rally the community to develop a healthy vision of the future
5. Introduce any outside resources to fill gaps

Needs and capacity assessment results can guide health education specialists in the planning phases of program and intervention development. Key questions that can serve as a guide for the process include:

- What is the health problem and what are its consequences for the state or community?
- What is the size of the problem overall and in various segments of the population?
- What are the determinants of the health problem?
- Who are priority populations?
- What changes or trends are occurring?

(Gilmore, 2012)

Competency 1.7: Determine Needs for Health Education/Promotion Based on Assessment Findings

The final step in the needs assessment is validating the needs identified in the assessment. Health education specialists must confirm that the identified needs are the real needs of a population. The validation process involves "double checking" or making sure that an identified need is an actual need. Multiple methods can be used to determine the validity of assessment findings. Examples of methods include (a) rechecking the steps followed in the needs assessment to eliminate any bias, (b) conducting a focus group with some individuals from the priority population to determine their reaction to the identified need (if a focus group was not used to gather the data), and (c) getting a second opinion from other health professionals (McKenzie et al, 2013).

❖ 1.7.1 Synthesize assessment findings

The following steps can be used to infer the need for health education/promotion from obtained data:

- Analyze data, primary and secondary
- Compare data with local, state, national, or historical situation
- Consider the social, cultural, and political environment (relative needs)
- Set priorities by:
  - Assessing the size or scope of the problem
  - Determining the effectiveness of possible interventions
  - Determining appropriateness, economics, acceptability, resources, and legality of the possible intervention

(Doyle et al., 2010; McKenzie et al., 2013)

Summary tables can be used to present metadata or to triangulate data from multiple sources. Graphs, charts, and tables are pictorial resources that can be used to summarize key results from needs assessments.

1.7.2 Identify current needs, resources, and capacity

Health education specialists must involve community members in determining the goals of the assessment process. They must identify needs and build on community strengths. Knowing both the needs and assets of the community, health education specialists can work to identify the true concerns of the priority population and the capacity to work with them (McKenzie et al, 2013).

1.7.3 Prioritize health education/promotion needs

Health education specialists must confirm that health education needs match the program needs. For example, the health education needs must be determined appropriately for the right population. The needs assessment must be able to validate the community needs and to begin the process of assigning value to the various promotion efforts that need to be developed and implemented in the community (Healey & Zimmerman, 2010; University of Kansas, 2014a).

Health education specialists can prioritize health needs by using the following criteria.
- Assessing the size or scope of the problem
    - What percentage of the population directly affected?
    - How serious is the problem?
    - How urgent/critical is the nature of the problem?
    - How severe is the problem?
    - What is the morbidity/mortality severity, duration, and/or disability associated with the problem?
    - What medical costs are associated with the problem?
    - How many people are affected by the problem?
- Determining the effectiveness of possible interventions
    - How effective are health education interventions in addressing the problem? Are they meeting stated goals and objectives?
    - Are the potential interventions accessible to the affected population?
    - How were the needs for the potential programs determined? Are the needs of the population being met? If not, why?
- Determining appropriateness, economics, acceptability, resources, and legality of the possible intervention
    - What health education programs are presently available to the population(s) affected?
    - Are the programs being utilized? If not, why?
    - Given the population, is the intervention appropriate and in accordance with societal/group norms?
    - Are there sufficient resources for implementation?
    - Is the intervention legal?

(Healey & Zimmerman, 2010)

KEY: no symbol - entry level;   ❖ advanced 1;   ■ advanced 2

Health education specialists must identify emerging health education needs and address diverse health needs. A simple approach to prioritizing health education needs is to consider whether an intervention can actually make a change in the health problem and whether the health problem is important or worth addressing. Each health problem can be rated with regard to its degree of importance and changeability. Health problems classified as having both high changeability and high importance ought to be addressed first, as shown in Table 1.6 (Issel, 2013).

Table 1.6
Program Prioritization based on the importance and changeability of the health problem

	Highly Important	**Less Important**
High Changeability	High priority for intervention	Lower priority
Lesser Changeability	High priority with innovative program	No program

Note. Adapted from Green & Kreuter, 2005

1.7.4 Develop recommendations for health education/promotion based on assessment findings

Health education specialists can focus on positive aspects and areas that need improving based on the needs and/or capacity assessments. Health education specialists should frame recommendations so that the priority population can make decisions regarding what needs to or can be done and in what order of priority (Issel, 2013). For example, the Affordable Care Act (ACA) includes a mandate for nonprofit health care organizations to conduct a community health needs assessment. The purpose of the assessment is to identify gaps in services. The health care organization must then implement strategies to address the identified gaps in service (Issel, 2013).

1.7.5 Report assessment findings

After summarizing the findings of the assessment, health education specialists need to consider whom they will disseminate the findings to, such as the priority population, researchers, funding agencies, or other stakeholders. Health education specialists should use a variety of dissemination methods to present the information. Examples include:

- Preparing a user-friendly, easy to read report
- Writing a separate executive summary of the report
- Developing a press release, then holding a press conference in conjunction with the press release
- Creating a newsletter, newspaper article, or fact sheet
- Developing a power point presentation
- Making verbal presentations to community groups, the priority population, and stakeholders and using the power point, other demonstrations, or visual images to report the findings
- Constructing professionally designed graphics, charts, and displays for use in reporting sessions
- Making short videos or audiotapes for presenting the results
- Using social media to report information, such as Facebook, You Tube, or Instagram

(W.K. Kellogg Foundation, 2010)

This page was
intentionally left blank

CHAPTER II

Area of Responsibility II
Plan Health Education/Promotion

2.1: Involve priority populations, partners, and other stakeholders in the planning process
2.1.1   Identify priority populations, partners, and other stakeholders
2.1.2   Use strategies to convene priority populations, partners, and other stakeholders
2.1.3   Facilitate collaborative efforts among priority populations, partners, and other stakeholders
2.1.4   Elicit input about the plan
2.1.5   Obtain commitments to participate in health education/promotion

2.2: Develop goals and objectives
2.2.1   Identify desired outcomes using the needs assessment results
2.2.2   Develop vision statement
2.2.3   Develop mission statement
2.2.4   Develop goal statements
2.2.5   Develop specific, measurable, attainable, realistic, and time-sensitive objectives

2.3: Select or design strategies/interventions
2.3.1   ❖   Select planning model(s) for health education/promotion
2.3.2   ❖   Assess efficacy of various strategies/interventions to ensure consistency with objectives
2.3.3   ❖   Apply principles of evidence-based practice in selecting and/or designing strategies/interventions
2.3.4   Apply principles of cultural competence in selecting and/or designing strategies/interventions
2.3.5   Address diversity within priority populations in selecting and/or designing strategies/interventions
2.3.6   Identify delivery methods and settings to facilitate learning
2.3.7   Tailor strategies/interventions for priority populations
2.3.8   Adapt existing strategies/interventions as needed
2.3.9   ❖   Conduct pilot test of strategies/interventions
2.3.10   ❖   Refine strategies/interventions based on pilot feedback
2.3.11   Apply ethical principles in selecting strategies and designing interventions
2.3.12   Comply with legal standards in selecting strategies and designing interventions

2.4: Develop a plan for the delivery of health education/promotion
2.4.1   Use theories and/or models to guide the delivery plan
2.4.2   Identify the resources involved in the delivery of health education/promotion
2.4.3   Organize health education/promotion into a logical sequence
2.4.4   Develop a timeline for the delivery of health education/promotion
2.4.5   Develop marketing plan to deliver health program
2.4.6   Select methods and/or channels for reaching priority populations
2.4.7   Analyze the opportunity for integrating health education/promotion into other programs

KEY: no symbol - entry level;   ❖ advanced 1;   ■ advanced 2

2.4.8 ❖ Develop a process for integrating health education/promotion into other programs when needed

2.4.9   Assess the sustainability of the delivery plan

2.4.10   Design and conduct pilot study of health education/promotion plan

2.5: Address factors that influence implementation of health education/promotion

2.5.1   Identify and analyze factors that foster or hinder implementation

2.5.2   Develop plans and processes to overcome potential barriers to implementation

The Role. Program planning begins once the assessment of existing needs, resources, and capacity has been completed. The planning process involves individuals from the priority population, program partners, and other stakeholders. After the planning group is formed, the members of the group work to develop program missions, goals, and objectives, as well as create or adapt intervention strategies, locate the resources needed to implement and evaluate the program, develop a plan for delivery, and address the factors that influence the implementation of the intervention. This time is also when health education specialists begin the planning process for program evaluation.

Settings. The following text is presented to describe how planning is used in different practice settings.

Community Setting. In a community setting where a needs assessment has been used to identify a significant health problem, the role of health education specialists is to convene representatives of relevant groups for the purpose of planning a health education/promotion program to address these needs. In identifying committee members, health education specialists may seek input and promote involvement from those who will affect, and be affected by, the program. Another key responsibility of health education specialists is to lead efforts to

formulate goals and objectives and to develop evidence-based interventions that meet the needs of priority populations. Health education specialists identify and assess community resources and barriers affecting the implementation of the program to achieve a successful program or intervention in the community setting. The selection of program activities and interventions depends on the characteristics of the priority population: its constraints, concerns, budget, timeframe, and the fit between program schedules and other obligations of the participants.

School (K-12) Setting. Administrators, public policy, or law usually make or mandate the decision to provide health education in schools. School health education specialists organize an advisory committee consisting of teachers, administrators, members of the community, representatives from voluntary agencies, parents, youth group leaders, clergy, and students to select and develop health education curricula and materials. These decisions are based on research results and best practices. The advisory committee may consider available resources and barriers to implementation, such as time and space, and objectives based on the needs of school-aged children and adolescents. Ultimately, the curricula follow a logical scope and sequence, as well as focus on maintaining or improving health behaviors.

KEY: no symbol - entry level; ❖ advanced 1; ■ advanced 2

Health Care Setting. Health education specialists in the health care setting work with nurses, physicians, nutritionists, physical therapists, patients, and other health care professionals to plan patient and community education programs. This team develops education programs for patients and their families to assist with decision-making, promote compliance with medical directions, and enhance understanding of medical procedures and conditions. The role of health education specialists in this setting is to assist the team in establishing goals and objectives, identifying staff member roles in providing education, selecting teaching methods and strategies, evaluating results, documenting the education effort, designing promotion activities, and training interdisciplinary staff to conduct the program.

Business/Industry Setting. In the workplace, health education specialists analyze data from numerous sources, including insurance and safety records, workers' compensation claims, and self-reported employee questionnaires. These data provide the basis for a presentation to management outlining the benefits and costs of a health education program. After gaining management's support, health education specialists convene an employee committee with representatives from all levels of the organization to develop a strategic plan outlining program priorities, goals and objectives, schedules, publicity strategies, incentives, and fees, as well

as potential barriers and proposed solutions. Health education specialists lead the team in developing evidence-based interventions and strategies to meet the needs of employees.

College/University Setting. Health education specialists in a higher education setting analyze research results, current professional Competencies, accreditation standards, and certification requirements. Health education specialists use these results to design professional preparation programs that develop essential health education planning Competencies in candidates, regardless of their future practice setting.

College/University Health Services Setting. Using assessment results, health education specialists who practice in campus health services work closely with clinical practitioners in health, counseling, and fitness/wellness centers. This team works together to develop program goals and objectives, as well as to select and design strategies or interventions that address issues and improve health. Health education specialists develop partnerships with clinical practitioners, academicians, students, and others to integrate health education into other programs, including treatment regimens and campus wide activities. They also evaluate the efficacy of educational methods in achieving objectives.

Key Terms

Programs are defined as a set of planned activities over time designed to achieve specific objectives (Green & Kreuter, 2005).

Program planning is the process of identifying needs, establishing priorities, diagnosing causes of problems, assessing and allocating resources, and determining barriers to achieving objectives (Green & Kreuter, 2005).

A **vision statement** is a one-sentence or one-phrase statement that describes the long term desired change stemming from the efforts of an organization or program (Korlarr, 2012).

A **program mission statement** is a statement of the general focus or purpose of a program. A mission statement can be a one-sentence statement or a short narrative that broadly defines the program's purpose. Mission statements identify the scope or focus of the organization or program and are enduring over time (McKenzie et al. 2013).

Goals are general, long-term statements of desired program outcomes and provide the direction upon which all objectives are based (Rees & Goldsmith, 2009).

Objectives are statements that describe, in measurable terms, the changes in behavior, attitude, knowledge, skills, or health status that will occur in the intervention group as a result of the program. Objectives are small, specific steps that enable the goal to be met (McKenzie et al., 2013).

A **community-based organization** (CBO) is a public or private, nonprofit organization of demonstrated effectiveness that is representative of a community or significant segments of a community and provides educational or related services to individuals in the community (Sherow, Weinberg, Sloan, & Morin, 2002).

A **coalition** is a group of diverse organizations and constituencies working together toward a common goal (Butterfoss, 2013).

Cultural competence/competency refers to an ability to understand, communicate with, and effectively interact with people across cultures. Cultural competence comprises these components: a) awareness of one's own cultural worldview, b) attitude towards cultural differences, and c) knowledge of one's orientation affects different professional practices and relationships (Diaz-Cuellar & Evans, 2014).

Competency 2.1: Involve Priority Populations, Partners, and Other Stakeholders in the Planning Process

Often planners need to begin the planning process by gaining support from groups of key people to ensure that planning and implementation proceed smoothly and to ensure that they can acquire the necessary resource support. Groups of key people, or **stakeholders**, include those involved in the program operations, those served or affected by the program, and the primary users of the program (McKenzie et al., 2013). When seeking support from stakeholders, the planner should be able to explain to them why the program is necessary (McKenzie et al., 2013). Please refer to Sub-competency 1.1.3 for more information on the importance of selecting the right stakeholders in the program planning process.

KEY: no symbol - entry level;   ❖ advanced 1;   ■ advanced 2

2.1.1 Identify priority populations, partners, and other stakeholders

Needs assessment data is one avenue for identifying a priority population for a health education program (McKenzie et al., 2013). The priority population consists of the entire population if an intervention is being implemented for the total community. The audience for an intervention or program includes individuals who are part of the at-risk population. Participants are individuals who receive the intervention or participate in the program. The participants' roles are important, because they affect program evaluation (Issel, 2013).

Expressed, actual, perceived, and normative needs should all be addressed in the needs assessment, as community concerns may not always reflect empirical evidence (Doyle et al., 2010; Issel, 2013). Expressed needs can be observed through individuals' use of services, such as an exercise class taken by older adults at a senior center. Actual needs may be inferred through the discrepancy of services provided to one community group as compared to another, such as bicycling and walking lanes. Perceived needs refer to what individuals in a community state that they want, such as more healthy food choices in a school vending machine. Normative needs describe a discrepancy between an individual's or group's current status and that of others, such as smoke free environment in restaurants among different cities. Priority populations may also be identified as a result of a current health crisis, a public figure's "going public" regarding his health status, or requests of health officials and/or members of the community (McKenzie et al., 2013).

2.1.2 Use strategies to convene priority populations, partners, and other stakeholders

Well planned health education programs: (a) incorporate collected data about the health issues addressed and/or about other similar programs and (b) organize at the grassroots level to involve the populations that will be affected. A health education program will be most successful if the priority population feels it has been instrumental in program development. It is important to provide a sense of ownership and empowerment among those in the population of interest. In general, the community organization process includes community recognition of the issue, entrance of health education specialists into the community to help organize the citizens, community assessment, priority setting, selection and implementation of an intervention, and evaluation and reassessment of the action plan (McKenzie et al., 2013). Health education specialists can convene meetings through schools, workplaces, community, or health care settings; essentially these meetings should bring the program to the priority audience. Health education specialists should weigh the benefits and shortcomings of conference calls, webinars, face-to-face meetings, and strive to make participation seamless for priority populations, partners, and other stakeholders. Health education specialists should communicate about gatherings via oral messages, newsletters, and traditional and/or social media to ensure the broadest possible participation.

2.1.3 Facilitate collaborative efforts among priority populations, partners, and other stakeholders

Community groups and collaborative efforts are often referred to as **coalitions** (Butterfoss, 2007, 2013). Collaborative efforts provide the opportunity for program planners to bring together representatives from diverse organizations, segments, or constituencies within the community to work toward a common goal. Additionally, coalitions bring together a combination of resources and expertise (McKenzie et al., 2013).

No two coalitions or community efforts are formed or operate in the same way. Community efforts need to structure themselves to fit the goals and objectives of the program. Butterfoss (2009) identified the following as steps for an effective coalition:

1. Analyze the issue or problem on which the coalition will focus
2. Create awareness of the issue
3. Conduct initial coalition planning and recruitment
4. Develop resources and funding for the coalition
5. Create coalition infrastructure
6. Elect coalition leadership
7. Create an action plan

Ideally, the efforts and participation of a coalition will continue throughout the program and sustain community action. Health education specialists should develop a plan to encourage the coalition's participation in the entire programming process, from goal creation and resource allocation to project implementation and evaluation (Doyle et al., 2010).

Building a coalition or community wide effort can be a complex and sometimes challenging task. A simple partnership in which your organization pairs with just one community organization may be a quick and easy strategy to enhance health education efforts. To promote this type of collaborative effort, health education specialists need to research the partner organization's mission, establish clear goals, tasks, and communication methods, and continually monitor effectiveness (Doyle et al., 2010). The drawback of this approach is that resources are limited in comparison with a coalition approach.

2.1.4 Elicit input about the plan

The following people may be interested in being part of the **program-planning** process:

- Individuals who represent various groups within the priority population
- Representatives of other stakeholders not represented in the priority population
- Individuals who have key roles within the organization sponsoring the program

(McKenzie et al., 2013)

Obstacles to obtaining input from these individuals (lack of time, lack of awareness, lack of transportation or communication capabilities, lack of interest/apathy, inconvenient locations or times) need to be removed. To remove these obstacles, health education specialists should make personal contact with key representatives, provide incentives for participation, choose easily accessible meeting locations, and conduct training programs for them (Issel, 2013). In addition, they should use mixed methods for obtaining input, both global and specific, and vary modes of communication (email, face-to-face meetings, newsletters) to ensure widespread input about the plan.

2.1.5 Obtain commitments to participate in health education/promotion

It is essential for health education specialists to gain support from the community surrounding the priority population. Health education specialists need support from community leaders and groups, including:

KEY: no symbol - entry level; ❖ advanced 1; ■ advanced 2

- Local elected officials
- Clergy
- Influential members of the community
- Community-based organizations and civic associations
- Local departments of health or related agencies
- Social service organizations
- Print journalists and broadcast media representatives

Decision makers in the community are able to provide financial, organizational, and/or administrative support to the program planning process.

A comprehensive plan also includes identifying individuals in the community to be part of the planning committee. A planning committee may consist of the following:
- Representatives from all segments of the priority population
- Active community members
- Influential members of the community
- Representatives of the sponsoring agency
- School district faculty and staff
- Local government representatives
- Law enforcement
- Local health department representatives
- Business owners and managers
- Stakeholders
- Effective leaders

(McKenzie et al., 2013; Hodges & Videtto, 2011)

It is important to understand group dynamics and focus on team building to develop the support necessary for successful program planning (Johnson & Johnson, 2005). Planning groups, such as consortia and planning boards, help to increase community and stakeholder involvement in order to enhance the strategic plan. A group leader can be selected, appointed, or may emerge naturally; therefore, a standardized process for leadership selection should be stated at formation of the planning committee or team. The person in the leadership position may change as the task or stage changes (Issel, 2013). In addition, health education specialists should consider formalizing the relationship through shared agreements, memoranda of understanding (MOUs), and/or subcontracts to solidify participation commitments. Another strategy is for health education specialists to form a coalition or partnership among committed individuals and organizations.

Competency 2.2: Develop Goals and Objectives

All successful health education programs begin with the development of appropriate goals and objectives. **Goals** help to measure a program's processes and outcomes. Processes might include program components, activities, delivery, and time frame, while the outcomes could include short-term changes (e.g., knowledge, attitudes, skills, behaviors) or long-term changes (e.g., behavior adherence, health status). A shared understanding of the goals and objectives of health education programs among stakeholders, partners, and the priority audience is optimal.

2.2.1 Identify desired outcomes using the needs assessment results

Needs assessment data for the priority population and its health issue(s)/concern(s) should be carefully considered and used in planning a corresponding health education program. These data will not only justify the program to stakeholders (including potential funders) but they will also help "sell" the importance of the program to the priority population. The needs assessment research will help ensure the development of a program that avoids pitfalls experienced by other programs and prevents health education specialists from having to "reinvent the wheel" (McKenzie et al., 2013).

Data assists health education specialists in understanding the breadth and depth of the health issues in a community. Existing data such as archived, published literature or publicly accessible databases can be used in a secondary data analysis. Primary data that are collected by means of interviews, surveys, emails, letters, or forums provide information regarding community perceptions and attitudes about the health issues. Population-based data can be analyzed with computerized statistical tests and epidemiological techniques and used to develop a community profile. The profile provides a comprehendible statement of the results (Issel, 2013).

Data collection should not be conducted in a vacuum or without an end goal in mind. Needs assessment data can help health education specialists consider the level of intervention they want to address. **Primary prevention** is focused on protecting people from developing a disease or injury. Education about healthy diet is an example of primary prevention. **Secondary prevention** emphasizes early diagnosis of disease or potential injury (McKenzie et al., 2013). For example, secondary prevention might include recommending regular preventive exams or screening tests. Finally, **tertiary prevention** focuses on rehabilitation after the diagnosis of a disease or injury. The goals of tertiary prevention involve preventing further deterioration and maximizing quality of life through self-management or support groups (McKenzie et al., 2013). These levels of prevention can also help health education specialists consider interventions to address their desired outcome.

Without a defined goal for use, data collection wastes both financial and human resources. Prior to the data collection activity, researchers and practitioners must determine the outcomes to be achieved. These may include changing behavioral risks, modifying environmental characteristics, influencing public policies, and raising awareness among the media.

2.2.2 Develop vision statement

A **vision statement** is a one-sentence or one-phrase statement that describes the long-term desired change stemming from the efforts of an organization or program. Effective vision statements are clear, inspirational, memorable, and concise (Van Korlarr, 2012).

KEY: no symbol - entry level;   ❖ advanced 1;   ■ advanced 2

Sample Vision Statements
- Childhood Obesity Prevention Fund: To ensure that all children are physically fit and nutritionally fed in order to learn, play, and grow.
- I Love Literacy Foundation: To promote reading and financial literacy among all segments of the adult population.
- Safe Seniors Campaign: To prevent injuries among older adults in traffic, at home, and in the community.

2.2.3 Develop mission statement

In the program planning stages, it is important to develop and express a mission **statement** as well as goals and objectives to provide a direction for the program and a foundation for the program evaluation (McKenzie et al., 2013). Table 2.1 provides useful information for differentiating between a mission and a vision.

Table 2.1
Comparison of Mission and Vision Statements

Mission statement	Vision statement
Statement of the purpose of organization	Statement of the desired end state
Oriented to making decision, priorities, and actions of the organization	Oriented to group meeting the results of the organization
Questions answered: Why does your organization exist? What is the broadest way to describe the work of the organization?	Questions answered: What needs to be changed? What does success look like?

Note. Adapted from http://topnonprofits.com/vision-mission

A mission statement encompasses the distinctive purpose and unique "reason for being" of a program. A mission statement can be a one-sentence statement or a short narrative that broadly defines the purpose. Program mission statements identify the purpose or focus of the organization or program and are enduring over time (McKenzie et al. 2013).

Sample Mission Statements
- The mission of the South County Senior Services is to provide easy access to health information and health care resources to senior citizens in South County.
- The mission of Generations' employee wellness program is to improve the health status of our employees.
- The mission of Brookside elementary school's health program is to ensure that children are healthy, safe, and ready to learn.

2.2.4 Develop goal statements

Goals are general, long-term statements of desired program outcomes and provide the direction upon which all objectives are based (Rees & Goldsmith, 2009). Goals specify the priority population and often include action words such as increase, reduce, or eliminate (Chen, Sheu, & Chen, 2010).

Sample Goal

The goal of the program is to:

- Reduce the number of osteoporosis-related fractures among elderly men and women who live in the area served by the health department
- Increase the rate of mammography screening among women ages 50 and older
- Eliminate the number of new smokers among adolescents ages 18 and younger

2.2.5 Develop specific, measurable, attainable, realistic, and time-sensitive objectives

Program objectives are the specific actions that need to be undertaken in order to achieve the goal (Chen et al., 2010). Objectives are statements that describe in measurable terms, changes in health status, behavior, attitude, or knowledge that will occur in the intervention group as a result of the program. These are the small, specific factors that enable the goal to be met. Objectives are usually written to include: what will change (outcome), when or under what conditions the change will occur, how much change will occur, and who will change (McKenzie et al., 2013). SMART is the acronym for writing objectives: specific, measurable, attainable, realistic, and time-sensitive.

A program's objectives should be relevant to the program goal. There are many types of objectives, including program or outcome objectives, behavioral and environmental objectives, learning objectives, and administrative objectives. Table 2.2 outlines the different types of objectives.

Program or outcome objectives are related to the ultimate goal(s), but are specific, measurable statements of what the educator wants to accomplish at a given time. They represent the change in health status that is the desired result of the program or intervention. These are the ends rather than the means. Program or outcome objectives include items such as changes in health status, risk factors, morbidity, mortality, or quality of life (McKenzie et al., 2013).

Examples include:

- Within three years, osteoporosis-related fractures will decrease by 25 percent in the residents of South County
- By 2016, the rate of sports-related traumatic brain injury among soccer players in Goodwin, Pennsylvania will decrease by 10 percent

Behavioral objectives describe the behaviors or actions that the population will engage in to resolve the problem and lead to attainment of the program goal. They are statements of desired outcomes that indicate whom is to demonstrate how much of what action and by when (Green & Kreuter, 2005).

KEY: no symbol - entry level;   ❖ advanced 1;   ■ advanced 2

Examples include:
- Among those attending the program, weight-bearing activity will increase by 50 percent over the following six months
- Fast food consumption will be eliminated from the diet of all program participants after the second week of program implementation

Learning or **instructional objectives** are short-term, specific descriptions of awareness, knowledge, attitudes, and skills in relation to the content being taught (McKenzie et al., 2013). Health education specialists should formulate and state objectives with precision. Meaningful objectives should include implied or stated evaluation standards.

Examples include:
- The participants will be able to correctly identify three forms of weight-bearing activity after the first session
- After the completion of the program, the participants will be able to state the importance of calorie control for weight loss

Behavioral and learning objectives may also be referred to as impact objectives: short-term/intermediate, measurable, and realistic guidelines to help accomplish the health goal (Doyle et al., 2010).

Administrative or **process objectives** detail the tasks or activities completed by program facilitators for the program to succeed. They are the daily tasks and work plans that lead to the accomplishment of all other planned objectives. Administrative objectives are also referred to as process objectives (McKenzie et al., 2013).

Examples include:
- Before the start of the program, the planning committee members will place physical-activity resources in each of the communities served by the health department
- Prior to the start of the program, planners will contact ten OB/GYN physicians to gather support for the program

Environmental objectives refer to environmental or nonbehavioral influences on a health problem. These factors include social, physical, psychological, policy, and service environments (McKenzie et al., 2013).

Examples include:
- By 2025, the number of high air pollution alert days in the city will decrease by 10 percent
- By 2020, the number of bicycle lanes on streets in River City will increase by 35 percent

The following is a guide to determine the appropriateness of objectives. Objectives should:
- Be clear statements
- Include just one indicator
- State reasonable time frames
- Be stated in terms of performance, not effort
- Be realistic and within the control of those responsible
- Be relevant, logical, feasible, observable, and measurable

Writing measurable objectives. To ensure that objectives are measurable, health education specialists must add criteria for measurement. This can be accomplished by using verbs that show action, including verbs that describe the expected behavior or performance. These action verbs make objectives more precise, less likely to be misinterpreted, and easier to evaluate. Examples of these verbs can be drawn from nearly every letter in the alphabet: analyze, build, contrast, demonstrate, enumerate, find, generate, hypothesize, infer, list, measure, name, observe, predict, query, recognize, state, test, unite, visit, and weigh (McKenzie et al., 2013).

Table 2.2
Types of Objectives

Objective	Result	Evaluation
Program objective	Changes in health status, morbidity, mortality, quality of life	What is the outcome? Is there a change in health status and is it attributed to the program?
Environmental objective	Changes in environment	How has the environment changed to improve behavior and health?
Behavioral objective	Changes in behavior or actions of the priority population	What is the impact? Is there adoption of a new healthier behavior and can it be attributed to the program?
Learning objective	Changes in awareness, knowledge, attitude, skills, etc.	Is there the requisite change in knowledge, attitudes, habits, and skills needed for behavior change?
Administrative objective	Adherence to time line tasks, completion of activities, efficient use of resources	Is the program working? Are people attending? Are the methods appropriate?

Note. Adapted from McKenzie et al., 2013

Competency 2.3: Select or Design Strategies/Interventions

Designing effective health education programs requires careful planning regarding the content, process, and amount of time needed to deliver an intervention. Health education specialists need to consider their priority population's needs and interests, as well as evidence-based strategies when planning a program.

2.3.1 Select planning model(s) for health education/promotion

There is no shortage of planning models for health education specialists to use in designing health education and promotion programs. Advanced-level health education specialists are typically responsible for selecting planning models to be used in health education interventions and programs. Entry-level health education specialists should have knowledge of planning models that are commonly used in health education. Although health education specialists address goals and objectives in program planning, other components should not be ignored. Important components of program planning include:

- Understanding and engaging the priority population
- Conducting a needs assessment
- Developing goals and objectives
- Creating an intervention
- Implementing the intervention
- Conducting program evaluation

(McKenzie et al., 2013)

Program planning includes designing an appropriate intervention. Health education specialists need to select the level of prevention (i.e., primary, secondary, or tertiary) and the level of influence (i.e., intrapersonal, interpersonal, institutional, organizational, community, or policy) on which the program will focus. Programs should be based on sound and appropriate learning and educational theories and tailored to meet the needs of the participants (McKenzie et al., 2013).

Individuals often confuse theories with planning models. Planning models help lay out the program planning steps to ensure that health education specialists have anticipated potential problems in a program and developed solutions accordingly. The planning models in this chapter are ones that have been commonly used by health education specialists when planning programs for individuals and communities (Cottrell et al., 2009). Health education specialists use models early in the planning process to help create an "ideal" or "real world" strategy for future implementation of their program (Goodson, 2010).

Other items to consider in intervention design include:

- Available resources
- Previously used effective strategies
- Single or multiple strategies

(McKenzie et al., 2013)

Three proven theories and/or models are described below. Please refer to Sub-competency 3.3.2 for a description of behavior change theories.

The **PRECEDE-PROCEED Model.** The PRECEDE-PROCEED model (Green & Kreuter, 2005) is currently the most often used formal planning model in health education. This model, developed as PRECEDE in the 1970s, was expanded in the 1980s to incorporate PROCEED. The model has eight phases:

PRECEDE

Phase 1:   *Social assessment* – define the quality of life of the priority population.

Phase 2:   *Epidemiological assessment* – identify the health problems of the priority population and determine and prioritize behavioral (individual) and environmental (external) risk factors associated with the health problem.

Phase 3:   *Educational and ecological assessment* – determine predisposing (individual knowledge and affective traits), enabling (those that make possible a change in behavior, such as skills), and reinforcing (feedback and encouragement for a changed behavior, perhaps from significant or important others) factors.

PROCEED

Phase 4:   *Administrative and policy assessment* – determine the resources (funding, staff, other) available for the program.

Phase 5:   *Implementation* – select strategies and activities; begin program.

Phase 6:   *Process evaluation* – document program feasibility.

Phase 7:   *Impact evaluation* – assess the immediate effect of an intervention.

Phase 8:   *Outcome evaluation* – determines whether long-term program goals were met.

(Green & Kreuter, 2005)

Multilevel Approach to Community Health (MATCH). MATCH, a multi-level community-planning model, consists of five phases with several steps within each stage (Simons-Morton, Simons-Morton, Parcel, & Bunker, 1988). The phases include:
1. Goals selection
2. Intervention planning
3. Program development
4. Implementation preparation
5. Evaluation

The model recognizes that intervention planning should be aimed at multiple objectives and a variety of individuals. MATCH can be used in a variety of settings (Simons-Morton, Greene, & Gottlieb, 1995).

CDCynergy. The CDCynergy community-level model, often used for social marketing, has six phases of program planning:
1. Define and describe the problem
2. Analyze the problem
3. Identify and profile the audience

KEY: no symbol - entry level;   ❖ advanced 1;   ■ advanced 2

4. Develop communication strategies
5. Develop evaluation plan
6. Launch the plan and obtain feedback

These interrelated phases help health education specialists to understand the priority population as well as the communication strategies that will best help individuals in the priority population to change their behaviors (CDC, 2003; 2007).

2.3.2 Assess efficacy of various strategies/interventions to ensure consistency with objectives

It is essential to ensure that interventions or strategies that have been selected yield the desired outcomes or meet the desired objectives, whether these objectives are individual or behavioral change, environmental modifications, or policy shifts. For example, educating youth on healthy food choices in order to stop the prevailing trend of obesity among children will be useless if their school, home, and community environments do not make healthier options such as fruits, vegetables, and grains available to them. Alternately, the enactment and enforcement of policies within the school (e.g., removal of soda and candy machines) or social environment (e.g., tax on sugary snacks and funding for recreational areas) will facilitate the desired outcome of obesity prevention or mitigation. Promoting the use of smoke alarms in homes to protect families during a fire will not be successful unless the families know proper guidelines for installation, placement, and regular maintenance. Other criteria to consider in assessing the efficacy of strategies/interventions are fit with the organization, feasibility of implementation and costs, and acceptability to the priority population.

2.3.3 Apply principles of evidence-based practice in selecting and/or designing strategies/ interventions

Once goals have been set and objectives determined, health education specialists should select the most effective evidence-based strategies to meet the goals and objectives. The most appropriate interventions should be based on theory, available resources, and reasonable fit. A variety of strategies can be used to meet the objectives of a program. These include educational, health engineering, community mobilization, health communication, health policy and enforcement, and health-related community service strategies. A more detailed discussion of each type of strategy is found in Table 2.3 on the next page.

Table 2.3
Types of Strategies

Educational strategies are activities usually associated with classroom-based courses, workshops, distance learning courses, or seminars. Some examples of educational strategies are: audiovisual materials; printed materials; e-learning courses; social networking such as Twitter, Facebook, and MySpace; classroom techniques; brainstorming; case studies; lectures; panel discussions; role playing; simulations; outside classroom techniques; health fairs; and field trips (Gilbert, Sawyer, & McNeill, 2011).

Health engineering strategies change the social or physical environment in which people live or work. They usually affect a large number of people and may change behavior by influencing awareness, attitudes, and knowledge or through guided choice. An example of a health engineering strategy includes modification of offerings (inclusion of only healthy foods or beverages) in vending machines (Butterfoss, 2007).

Community mobilization strategies directly involve participants in the change process. These strategies include initiatives such as coalition building and lobbying. Other examples of community mobilization strategies are community organization, community building, and community advocacy (McKenzie et al., 2013).

Health communication strategies use all types of communication channels (for example, print media, radio, television, billboards, newsletters, flyers, direct mail, e-mail, and self-help materials) to change behavior. These activities can impact knowledge, awareness, or attitudes. Communication may also provide cues for action and provide reinforcement of behaviors (McKenzie et al., 2013).

Health policy and enforcement strategies mandate actions through laws, regulations, policies, or rules. Such actions are justified on the basis of "the common good;" that is, they are actions implemented to protect the public's health (McKenzie et al., 2013).

Health related community service strategies include services, tests, or treatments to improve the health of the priority population (McKenzie et al., 2013). Examples include activities that enable individuals to evaluate their personal level of health through the use of health-risk appraisals, screenings (such as blood pressure screenings), and self-examination (such as breast self-examination).

2.3.4 Apply principles of cultural competence in selecting and/or designing strategies/ interventions

Regardless of the type of strategy used, the method must "fit" or meet the needs of the priority population in order for a program to be effective. The characteristics of the priority population will dictate how the intervention is received. Cultural competence is the "ability of a person to understand and respect values, attitudes, and beliefs that vary across cultures, and to consider and address appropriately to these differences in planning, implementing, and evaluating health education and promotion programs and interventions" (Joint Committee on Health Education Terminology, 2012). It is important for health education specialists to identify how the characteristics of a chosen strategy fit the population's culture and are relevant to the priority population (McKenzie et al., 2013).

Education and training on cultural competency may be obtained through federal agencies (e.g., Office of Minority Health, Health Resources and Services Administration), academic institutions (e.g., Georgetown University's National Center for Cultural Competence), articles published in peer-reviewed journals (e.g., European Journal of Cross-Cultural Competence and Management), and at conferences (e.g., Society for Public Health Education), among other sources. Other strategies to enhance organizations' cultural competency include assessing needs for bilingual staff, adopting/adapting/creating materials for specific populations, considering the priority populations' learning and programmatic preferences, providing translators, if necessary, through use of in-person resources or language lines, and evaluating the use of health workers and advisors from the communities served.

2.3.5 Address diversity within priority populations in selecting and/or designing strategies/interventions

The ability to match a particular program to the needs of the priority population is an essential skill for health education specialists. Disparities or inequities may be identified by gender, income, education, disability, geographic location, sexual orientation, and race/ethnicity (Mas, Allensworth & Jones, 2010).

According to the Prevention Institute (2014), the root causes of racial and ethnic disparities or inequities fall into four discrete yet often overlapping categories:

- Societal factors
    - Poverty
    - Racism
    - Economics
    - Health illiteracy
    - Limited education
    - Educational inequality

- Environmental factors
    - Poor and unsafe physical and social environments
    - Viral and microbial agents
    - Exposure to toxins
    - Inadequate access to nutritious food
    - Limited options for exercise
    - Community norms which do not support prevention

- Individual and behavioral factors
    - Sedentary lifestyles
    - Poor eating habits

- Lack of seat belt use
- Smoking
- Other high-risk behaviors

- Medical care factors
  - Limited access to health care
  - Lack of quality health care
  - Gaps in cultural competence among providers

(Adapted from Mas, Allensworth & Jones, 2010)

Health education specialists need to involve the priority population in all aspects of program planning and delivery to ensure that the program addresses their identified health care needs, cultural preferences, and best modes of implementation. Health education specialists should also recruit and mentor diverse program staff to enhance the likelihood of success in reducing morbidity and mortality in any given community.

2.3.6 Identify delivery methods and settings to facilitate learning

Once goals and objectives are established, health education specialists must consider a range of options and then select the most appropriate methods and environments to deliver the program in a way that ensures success. These decisions must be based on the theory or model underpinning the program. For example, if health education specialists choose a social cognitive theory, then the health promotion program should emphasize self-efficacy, modeling, and reinforcements (Hodges & Videto, 2011). Program delivery methods might include activities related to communication, education, behavior modification, environmental change, regulation, and community advocacy (Hodges & Videto, 2011). Health education specialists should next decide which setting or combination of settings are most appropriate for the intervention from individual, community, worksite, school, and house of worship settings in order to most effectively yield desired outcomes.

2.3.7 Tailor strategies/interventions for priority populations

Health promotion programs should be customized to meet the needs of the members of priority population in terms of their age, gender, race, ethnicity, culture, literacy level, income, learning styles, knowledge, attitudes, and beliefs, among other characteristics. Interventions tailored to the population's unique features are more likely to be accepted and possess greater potential for behavioral change and positive health outcomes. Gardner's theory of multiple intelligences purports that instruction should dovetail with the learning styles of the individuals served (Gardner, 2011). For example, a person with interpersonal intelligence might benefit from group exercise or social media strategies, while another person with logical-mathematical intelligence might respond more readily to epidemiological data to influence behavioral change (Hodges & Videto, 2011). Please see Chapter VII (Sub-competencies 7.1.2 and 7.1.3) for more information on cultural competency as well as health literacy.

KEY: no symbol - entry level; ❖ advanced 1; ■ advanced 2

2.3.8 Adapt existing strategies/interventions as needed

Few programs are planned perfectly from their inception; most need multiple modifications to enhance their effectiveness and efficiency. For example, a carbon monoxide prevention program may be initially designed for elementary school children and delivered through the classroom. As a part of the intervention, coloring books, a DVD, activity sheets, and stickers may raise awareness among the children of the dangers of this odorless, colorless, and tasteless gas. Yet, after initial implementation, program planners may determine that parents and caregivers need to be involved as well because they are in the best position to purchase, install, and maintain carbon monoxide (CO) alarms. Only by modifying the prevention program can health education specialists enhance the health of the entire family. When adapting an existing strategy or intervention, health education specialists should review the materials or processes to see which changes, such as content (e.g., statistics, images), delivery, or logistics, may better fit with their population of interest. Health education specialists should refer to implementation guides or protocol to see if the intervention developer has provided guidance on how to make adaptations.

Health education specialists should examine how changes to existing strategies and interventions may impact the program's timeline, budget, and relationships with the funders and stakeholders before making any final decisions.

❖ 2.3.9 Conduct pilot test of strategies/interventions

Pilot testing is a type of formative evaluation that is conducted before the program is rolled out on a large scale. It sheds valuable light on whether materials, strategies, and interventions are feasible, appropriate, and acceptable to the priority audience. Although pilot testing has the advantage of testing a program before it is launched, only a few respondents may be involved and the results may not be entirely generalizable (McKenzie et al., 2013). To minimize the drawbacks, participants should be drawn from and be similar to the priority population served by the health promotion program (Harris, 2010). Pilot testing may be conducted face-to-face in focus groups, through one-on-one interviews, with paper-and pencil instruments, and via computerized surveys.

❖ 2.3.10 Refine strategies/interventions based on pilot feedback

Once the pilot testing is completed, health education specialists should make any necessary modifications to materials, strategies, and interventions. Health education specialists should view any barriers or deficiencies identified in the pilot test results as positive rather than negative because feedback allows planners to refine the program before it is launched. Necessary modifications emerging from the pilot test results should be shared with stakeholders, sponsors, and the priority population. Such transparency will reinforce health education specialists' aim to steward funding wisely and optimally improve the health status of the audience of interest.

2.3.11 Apply ethical principles in selecting strategies and designing interventions

Health education specialists are expected to abide by a Code of Ethics for the Health Education Profession (Coalition of National Health Education Organizations [CNHEO], 2011). The Code of Ethics helps to ensure that the integrity and ethos of the profession are upheld as difficult ethical challenges emerge. Health education specialists must use their knowledge and experience to fulfill their responsibilities to the public, profession, and employers in the delivery of health education, in research and evaluation, and in professional preparation. For example Article IV, Responsibility in the Delivery of Health Education, holds that health education specialists should be sensitive to cultural diversity and be informed of the latest science of theory and practice (CNHEO, 2011). Please see Appendix A for the Code of Ethics.

2.3.12 Comply with legal standards in selecting strategies and designing interventions

All health professionals wrestle with legal standards, and health education specialists are no exception. Liability insurance to cover the cost of any physical or psychological risks to program participants is highly recommended. Some steps to reduce the risk of legal liability include the following:

- Ensure that all informed consent procedures are implemented
- Maintain the privacy of participants' personal health information (i.e., HIPPA)
- Choose currently certified instructors to teach classes
- Provide written guidelines for emergency medical procedures for participants
- Ask program participants to be cleared by health professionals before modifying their diet or engaging in strenuous exercise
- Make sure classrooms and other facilities comply with building codes and are regularly maintained

(Partially adapted from McKenzie et al., 2013)

Competency 2.4: Develop a Plan for the Delivery of Health Education/Promotion

To maximize successful outcomes, it is essential that health education specialists do some initial planning to help ensure the smooth delivery of the program. In this process, health education specialists need to include theories and/or models to guide implementation, identify needed resources, use logical sequence tools to organize the program delivery, create and adhere to a timeline, develop a sound marketing plan, select the right methods to reach the priority population(s), consider integration with other programs, evaluate the sustainability of the plan, and pilot test the program.

2.4.1 Use theories and/or models to guide the delivery plan

In the absence of a theoretical perspective underpinning health interventions, researchers and practitioners will be hampered in their efforts to understand what worked, what did not, and the possible reasons for success and failure. Without a theoretical framework, health education specialists will not be able to modify a program's design or delivery in order to better achieve desirable outcomes in the priority population. Please refer to Sub-competency 2.3.1 above for planning theories and models (PRECEDE-PROCEED, MATCH, and CDCynergy) and Chapter VII (Sub-competency 7.1.1) for communication and social marketing theories.

2.4.2 Identify the resources involved in the delivery of health education/promotion

Both researchers and practitioners need to give careful attention to the resources necessary to achieve the desired objectives. These resources may include individuals whom have varying skills in finance

KEY: no symbol - entry level; ❖ advanced 1; ■ advanced 2

and budgeting, statistics, social and behavioral theory, communications, or administration. Human resources could include an organization's staff, partners, or community volunteers. In addition, tangible resources will require thoughtful planning. These resources can include computers, paper, writing implements, office space, and transportation, among others.

2.4.3 Organize health education/promotion into a logical sequence

Health education specialists are responsible for deciding what and how much information will be discussed regarding specific health content during a health education program. This is determined by considering:

- Needs assessment data
- Culture of the priority population
- Literacy level of the priority population
- Priority population's previous experience regarding the health issue
- Budget constraints
- Time restrictions of program participants
- Availability of space to conduct programs

Regardless of the health education setting, health education specialists should plan instruction for optimal educational effectiveness. The plan for action should sequence the units or modules (including objectives, health topic content, and teaching strategies) for the specific health education course or workshop being facilitated. The plan of instruction should focus on continuity, sequence, and integration (Fodor, Dalis, & Giarratano, 2010). The instruction plan should provide the scope and sequence, or "bigger picture," for what the program will look like. In addition to the following information, please refer to Competency 1.5 for more information on factors that influence learning.

Learning Principles. People who do not want to learn can be difficult to teach. To facilitate the learning process, health education specialists should focus on increasing participants' motivation to learn. Health education specialists may use the following ten principles to help (Minelli & Breckon, 2009).

- *Use several senses.* People retain:
  - 10 percent of what is read
  - 20 percent of what is heard
  - 30 percent of what they see
  - 50 percent of what they hear and see
  - 70 percent of what they say
  - 90 percent of what they do and say
- *Actively involve participants.* Use methods that enable them to be active, rather than passive participants. For example, use discussion rather than lecture.
- *Provide an appropriate learning environment.* Keep extraneous interference and distractions to a minimum and ensure comfortable accommodations.
- *Assess learner readiness.* People learn only when they are physically and emotionally ready.

- *Establish the relevance of the information.* People tend to learn what they perceive is important to them. Knowing what is important to participants can help you make the information meet their needs.
- *Use repetition.* Learning is enhanced if information is repeated several times in a variety of ways.
- *Strive for a pleasant learning experience.* Encouragement through frequent, positive feedback and recognizable progress contributes to a positive experience.
- *Start with the known and move toward the unknown.* Present information that builds from the simple to the complex in an organized manner.
- *Generalize the information.* Learning is more likely to occur if the information is applied to more than one setting or situation.
- *Appropriately pace delivery of the information.* Adjust the rate at which information is covered to meet the needs of the participants.

Health education specialists must be mindful that environments conducive to learning have both psychological and physical characteristics. Psychologically, students must feel comfortable with the pace of teaching, mix of didactic and experiential instruction, and methods of examination. Other factors that affect the learning environment include meaningfulness, openness of the community, learning aids, and consistency. Physically, the learning environment must be clean, safe, lighted, and equipped with furniture in good repair and adequate audiovisual equipment, as well as heated or cooled to the right temperature. Clients or participants of a health education program may associate comfort with the learned information. Health education specialists should strive to ensure that their students are instructed in an environment conducive to learning and should make learning satisfying.

Health education programs must be carefully planned, implemented, and evaluated. The templates in basic logic models can allow evaluators to move freely back and forth among the elements of a flowchart to determine reasons for success and failure of a program (Healy & Zimmerman, 2010). Through examination of the logical sequence of inputs, activities, outputs, outcomes, and impact, health education specialists are armed with the necessary information to make recommended changes to improve programmatic effectiveness and efficiency. Programmatic effectiveness (success in achieving outcomes) and efficiency (success in using resources, both human and financial) can be easily measured through logic models.

According to Harris (2010), a logic model can be used in many ways, including:
- To map a program during the planning and evaluation phases
- To process for understanding the program's components and their relationship to outcomes
- To serve as a graphic to enhance stakeholders' understanding and engagement
- To be a tool to help develop and monitor programmatic benchmarks

Please refer to Competency 4.1 for more information about logic models.

KEY: no symbol - entry level;   ❖ advanced 1;   ■ advanced 2

2.4.4 Develop a timeline for the delivery of health education/promotion

Every project or program conducted by health education specialists requires an orderly sequence of milestones and deliverables, such as a **Gantt chart** or **Program Evaluation and Review Technique (PERT) chart.** It is essential that these sequences be determined in advance, so that all parties involved can anticipate what to expect and when. This is particularly important for funded projects in which payment is "triggered" by the delivery of products and services such as interim progress and final reports. By scheduling tasks and responsible parties a priori, adjustments can be made to achieve desired outcomes. In creating this timeline, health education specialists need to consider the length of time and resources necessary to deliver an effective intervention. Health education specialists will have to make difficult decisions regarding the possible content that can be covered in the timeframe, as well as the logical sequence of it, so that the learning modules can be developed.

2.4.5 Develop marketing plan to deliver health program

Information and resources that are used in any health education program should be developmentally and culturally appropriate for the priority population. During the planning process, health education specialists will need to assess whether appropriate health promotion and education materials are available, how to attain them, and how to market them. If they are not available, materials will need to be developed to meet program objectives. Information and resources should be researched early in program planning to ensure that there is time to develop adequate materials if needed (Plomer & Bensley, 2009). Health education specialists should consider reaching out to their priority population or wider community for pro bono marketing and public relations expertise.

Healey & Zimmerman (2010) describe the key components in the marketing process, which helps to ensure successful program planning, implementation, and evaluation (Table 2.4).

Table 2.4
Stages of the Marketing Process

I. Planning
- Step 1: Analyze the situation:
    - ✓ Identify problems and populations affected.
    - ✓ Analyze current and possible replacement behaviors.
    - ✓ Outline all components for a solution (education, law, marketing).
    - ✓ Assess the environment in which change will occur.
- Step 2: Select approaches and determine the role of marketing.
- Step 3: Set goals and objectives:
    - ✓ Specify behaviors, conditions, or policies to be changed.
- Step 4: Segment and select priority audiences:
    - ✓ Determine the priority populations for each desired change, and within each population, the audience segment(s) on which you will focus.

✓ Identify current and competitive behaviors and how they satisfy needs, desires, and values.

✓ Identify barriers to the public health behavior.

- Step 5: Design public health offering(s)

✓ Product: Identify and develop a bundle of benefits that you can deliver that differentiates the desired behavior from competitors. Develop any necessary supporting goods and services.

✓ Price: Determine how to make costs manageable for audience members.

✓ Place: Determine how you will access channels that deliver the product so that it is easily available to audience members at prices (financial, time, psyche, social, etc.) that they are willing and able to pay.

✓ Promotion: Develop a communication strategy to position the public health offering as something consistent with the audience's core values that delivers a key benefit.

- Step 6: Plan evaluation.

II. Development
- Develop budgets and distribution and promotion plans.
- Develop prototype products, services and/or communication materials.
- Pretest with priority audience members.
- Refine as necessary.
- Build in process evaluation measures.

III. Implementation
- Produce offerings and materials.
- Coordinate with partners.
- Implement intervention.
- Use process evaluation to monitor implementation.
- Refine offerings, promotions, and distribution channels as needed.

IV. Assessment
- Conduct outcome evaluation.
- Refine intervention as needed.

Note. Adapted from Healey & Zimmerman, 2010

2.4.6 Select methods and/or channels for reaching priority populations

In order to reach a program's priority populations, health education specialists need to carefully select the best routes of message delivery. The audience of interest must be both receptive to the message and able to act upon the advice provided. There are several methods and channels available to health education specialists including:

KEY: no symbol - entry level;   ❖ advanced 1;   ■ advanced 2

- Interpersonal (e.g., health care professionals, family, friends)
- Group (e.g., neighborhood associations, work sites, houses of worship, social clubs)
- Community (e.g., meetings, conferences, events)
- Mass media campaigns (e.g., radio, television, newspapers, magazines)
- Interactive media (e.g., webinars, blogs, e-mail, text messages, social networking sites such as Facebook, Pinterest, and Twitter)

(Ammary-Risch et al., 2010)

Health education specialists can help to improve reach, potentially change behavior, and steward limited budgets and human resources by pilot testing the channels of message delivery as well as soliciting advice from the priority population(s).

2.4.7 Analyze the opportunity for integrating health education/promotion into other programs

Whenever there is an opportunity to present health education as a prevention option within a health program, health education specialists should be prepared to do so. This opportunity may develop an avenue to market health education. In addition, this opportunity allows for the coordination of community resources to be used within the health education component of an existing program. For example, a pedestrian safety initiative could simultaneously aim to instill cautious pedestrian behavior and promote driver awareness of the risks of speeding, texting, and drinking, as well as reduce obesity by promoting walking.

❖ 2.4.8 Develop a process for integrating health education/promotion into other programs when needed

The most effective health education programs are planned with the aid of a planning model and incorporate theory in creating the intervention. These steps, however, will not be enough to ensure the program is meeting the priority population's needs. Several extensive, well-researched documents have been published to keep health education programs moving in a direction to positively affect individual and community behavior change. Healthy People 2020 (USDHHS, 2014) includes national and state standards, benchmarks for school health education, and important data to inform agency/organization mission statements. It can be consulted when planning for program development. After researching standards, benchmarks, and mission statements, health education specialists can contact agencies already working with the priority population to see if they can integrate health education efforts into ongoing programs.

2.4.9 Assess the sustainability of the delivery plan

Long-term sustainability of a program is often beset with many challenges. These challenges can include staff turnover, the emergence of more pressing health concerns in the community, a lack of sustained interest among members of the priority population, political upheavals, and an erosion of funding streams (Chen, Sheu, & Chen, 2010). To minimize budgetary shortfalls, health education specialists should maintain strong relationships with funders by keeping them informed of program achievements, keeping excellent financial records, and requesting opportunities to leverage their investment through introductions to other potential donors (Fertman, Spiller, & Mickalide, 2010). In order to sustain effective programs, Sleet and Cole (2010) recommend that program staff, stakeholders, and the priority audience ask themselves the following questions:

- Does the health promotion program have a clear and honest understanding of its current reality?
- Is the understanding of the current reality shared throughout the health promotion program and used to sustain and improve the program?
- Is that knowledge translated into effective action toward a desired future?

Schell and colleagues (2013) undertook a thorough literature review, sought advice from subject matter experts, and engaged in concept mapping to determine the essential factors for program sustainability. The authors identified nine core domains: political support, funding stability, partnerships, organizational capacity, program evaluation, program adaptation, communications, public health impacts, and strategic planning. This sustainability framework may benefit health education specialists as they develop and implement health education and promotion programs.

2.4.10 Design and conduct pilot study of health education/promotion plan

Using formative evaluation techniques to pilot test strategies and interventions is essential to program planning. Pilot testing can help ensure that messages and images are clear and consistent, culturally relevant, and motivational. Focus groups, self-reported knowledge, attitudes, and behavior surveys can help reveal what the priority audience understands and what barriers and facilities to behavioral change exist. Data and information gathered from a pilot test can help refine a program to increase likelihood of success.

Competency 2.5: Address Factors that Influence Implementation of Health Education/Promotion

All of the strategies that make up an intervention require resources for implementation. There are a number of additional logistical activities that must also be carried out such as participant recruitment, intervention development and pilot testing, or partnership development. Health education specialists must be able to assess what is needed for program creation and delivery prior to implementation.

2.5.1 Identify and analyze factors that foster or hinder implementation

There are many potential barriers to the implementation of health education programs, which should be anticipated early in the planning process. Barriers might include lack of community support, agency administration support, or funding. Other barriers might be overextended health education specialists with limited time for program planning, a lack of coordination of resources within the community, or territorial issues among local agencies. A skillful planner is familiar with, or becomes familiar with, the community and its potential issues. A successful planner will foresee and overcome challenges that may lie ahead. A positive attitude, sense of humor, and willingness to accept the community process will aid in the successful implementation of health education programs (Roe, Roe, & Strona, 2009).

KEY: no symbol - entry level;   ❖ advanced 1;   ■ advanced 2

Although a program may be fully funded and perfectly designed, there may be factors that affect implementation, both negatively and positively. For example, a priority audience may be reluctant to participate in a program, such as families who refuse to allow fire fighters to enter their home to conduct a home safety check or install free smoke alarms. These families may fear scrutiny of their living situation by authority figures. In addition, there may not be enough time for health education specialists to carry out a program in its entirety due to schedule, changes of personnel, or budget cuts in an eroding tax base in a declining economy. In other instances, the audience may be highly receptive to the program, such as parents who voluntarily attend a car seat checkup event shortly after the birth of their child. Health education specialists need to seize this "teachable moment" to recognize and take advantage of the educational opportunity, in this case to ensure that parents appropriately restrain their infant.

2.5.2 Develop plans and processes to overcome potential barriers to implementation

Careful planning can provide enormous benefits in ensuring that program design and implementation are sound. Often, however, real world experience indicates that the program needs to be further refined to truly be effective. In a pilot study, health education specialists might find that content could not be delivered in the specified time period, the audience could not understand certain concepts, or the method of instruction was not the most preferred method for participants. Health education specialists should take information from the pilot study and modify content or delivery method for full implementation of the program. In this way, program planners can be more effective in stewarding resources, helping the priority population change its unhealthy behaviors, and ultimately reduce morbidity and mortality. Health education specialists should consider involving new stakeholders in the implementation as needed, seek opportunities to leverage existing resources, and ask the priority audience for advice on overcoming barriers.

A Gantt chart, PERT chart, or other timeline can help all parties involved keep track of program implementation milestones and deliverables (McKenzie et al., 2013). Throughout the program, maintaining regular communication with the team through e-mails, phone calls, and mail keeps everyone updated and helps to troubleshoot obstacles to program delivery. In addition, health education specialists should schedule regular, face-to-face meetings with stakeholders to solve emerging challenges and, most importantly, celebrate successes.

This page was
intentionally left blank

CHAPTER III

Area of Responsibility III
Implement Health Education/Promotion

3.1 Coordinate logistics necessary to implement plan

3.1.1   Create an environment conducive to learning
3.1.2   Develop materials to implement plan
3.1.3   Secure resources to implement plan
3.1.4   Arrange for needed services to implement plan
3.1.5   Apply ethical principles to the implementation process
3.1.6   Comply with legal standards that apply to implementation

3.2 Train staff members and volunteers involved in implementation of health education/promotion

3.2.1   ❖ Develop training objectives
3.2.2   Recruit individuals needed for implementation
3.2.3   ❖ Identify training needs of individuals involved in implementation
3.2.4   ❖ Develop training using best practices
3.2.5   ❖ Implement training
3.2.6   ❖ Provide support and technical assistance to those implementing the plan
3.2.7   ❖ Evaluate training
3.2.8   ❖ Use evaluation findings

3.3 Implement health education/promotion plan

3.3.1   Collect baseline data
3.3.2   ❖ Apply theories and/or models of implementation
3.3.3   Assess readiness for implementation
3.3.4   Apply principles of diversity and cultural competence in implementing health education/
         promotion plan
3.3.5   Implement marketing plan
3.3.6   Deliver health education/promotion as designed
3.3.7   Use a variety of strategies to deliver plan

3.4 Monitor implementation of health education/promotion

3.4.1   Monitor progress in accordance with timeline
3.4.2   Assess progress in achieving objectives
3.4.3   Ensure plan is implemented consistently
3.4.4   Modify plan when needed
3.4.5   Monitor use of resources
3.4.6   Evaluate sustainability of implementation
3.4.7   Ensure compliance with legal standards
3.4.8   Monitor adherence to ethical principles in the implementation of health education/promotion

---

KEY: no symbol - entry level;   ❖ advanced 1;   ■ advanced 2

The Role. Health education specialists, regardless of the setting in which they work, implement planned programs to assist those in priority populations with maintaining or improving their health. To do so, health education specialists must coordinate the logistics to implement the plan, train volunteers and staff members involved in the implementation, deliver the program, monitor the progress of the program, and evaluate the sustainability of the program. Each of these steps must be completed while ensuring compliance with legal standards and while adhering to the ethical principles of the profession).

Settings. The following text is presented to describe how implementation is used in different practice settings.

Community Setting. Once a health education program has been created for a priority population, health education specialists must work to identify and obtain the resources to implement the program. Personnel are a primary resource in implementing any such program. Health education specialists will need to train staff members and volunteers or obtain assistance from a community coalition to implement the program. After launching the program, health education specialists continue to monitor progress and consider various strategies for sustaining the program over time.

School (K-12) Setting. In a school setting, health education specialists work to increase students' knowledge and to promote positive attitudes and behaviors regarding health. The school administration typically provides a curriculum to school-based health education specialists. From the curriculum, health education specialists infer objectives appropriate to students' learning potential and abilities, as well as decide on appropriate teaching techniques.

Health education specialists' awareness of the students' learning needs, health behaviors, and related factors inform lesson plans. Health education specialists assess and monitor student learning to facilitate revisions in curricula and instructional methods, and also work with administrative staff members, faculty members, parent groups, and community groups to encourage school policies that support healthy behaviors.

Health Care Setting. Health education specialists employed in health care often serve as liaisons between patients and providers to enhance patient education. In addition, they can serve as outreach coordinators and provide patient education programs in the health care facility. Thus, health education specialists in this setting might conduct a program to support patients' weight-loss efforts. They may offer classes, supported by presentations from the health care providers, and make use of educational materials consistent with the patients' needs. Health education specialists arrange opportunities to apply information learned through cooking classes or a grocery store tour to improve ability to read food labels. They may monitor participant outcomes and providers' reactions and the process of delivering such activities to make changes to the program and objectives as warranted.

Business/Industry Setting. In the workplace, health education specialists work with employers to offer educational programs that respond to employees' health and lifestyle needs in a manner conducive to employee participation. Health education specialists must understand the needs and interests of employees, the workplace culture, and the ways of doing business that might affect healthy behaviors. Health education specialists may offer healthful

KEY: no symbol - entry level; ❖ advanced 1; ■ advanced 2

food choices in the company cafeteria, exercise classes, stress reduction counseling, and smoking cessation therapy, all supplemented by educational materials.

College/University Setting. Once a professional preparation program is created, health education specialists working in a higher education setting use their knowledge and skills to implement academic programs and prepare future health education specialists. Specifically, they use a variety of teaching methods, including lectures, discussions, simulations, practical experiences, and focused assignments. These methods and curricula help their students develop the essential health education implementation Competencies regardless of their future practice setting.

College/University Health Services Setting. In this setting, health education specialists work with others on campus to implement programs that address established needs utilizing best practices, appropriate theories, and a variety of strategies. Health education specialists may coordinate special events, develop health initiatives, arrange for screenings by other agencies, or develop programs for priority populations within the campus community. Program settings vary, and can include academic classrooms, residence halls, and fraternity/sorority meetings. For example, with the support of appropriate campus personnel, health education specialists may work with residence hall officials to offer educational sessions on several topics, including safer sex, alcohol and other drugs, relationship violence, stress and time management, smoking cessation, nutrition, and physical activity. Program availability must match student needs and be supported by media and activities intended to appeal to the college student. Health education specialists monitor program implementation, participant interest, and attendance, as well as request feedback to improve and direct future programming.

Key Terms

Culture involves ideas, beliefs, values, customs, and norms that are learned from family and community, and are passed down from generation to generation (Doyle et al., 2010).

Implementation is a specified set of activities designed to put into practice an activity or program. In implementation, one seeks to accomplish the setting up, management, and execution of the project, service, or program (National Implementation Research Network, 2014).

An **intervention,** or program, is a set of learning activities, delivery plan, and evaluation activities designed to achieve the desired outcomes of the program. Interventions or programs may use single or multiple strategies to accomplish objectives. An intervention is a specific component of a more comprehensive program (Green & Kreuter, 2005).

An **intervention strategy** is a specific technique or approach used in an intervention to get the desired outcome (Bartholomew et al., 2011).

Learning activities are the means used to carry out the program. These are the instructional sessions that will address the learning objectives (Simons-Morton et al., 1995). In this chapter, the phrase learning activities is used interchangeably with program activities.

Plain language is a strategy for making written and oral information easier to understand. It is one important tool for improving health literacy (Plain Language Action and Information Network, 2014).

Project management is the application of knowledge, skills, and techniques to execute projects effectively and efficiently (Project Management Institute, 2014).

A tailored message is any combination of information and behavior change strategies intended to reach one specific person or group based on characteristics unique to that person, related to the outcome of interest, and derived from an individual assessment (Krueter, Farrell, Olevitch, & Brennan, 2000).

A targeted message is intended to reach some specific subgroup of the general population, usually based on a set of demographic characteristics shared by its members (Krueter et al., 2000).

Competency 3.1: Coordinate Logistics Necessary to Implement Plan

When preparing to implement health education and promotion programs, health education specialists should first set up a project plan or work plan. The project plan or work plan is a detailed road map for how a program will achieve its goals. The plan should align with a logic model or broader strategic plan. The plan should include goals, objectives, activities, timelines, evaluation measures, and the roles and responsibilities involved in implementing the specific aspects of the plan. A separate training plan focusing on how staff and partners will assist with training might also be necessary. The Northwest Center for Public Health Practice has developed a training plan template that details how to implement such a plan. Materials created in the planning phase may help to coordinate logistics (i.e., people, facilities, supplies) for implementation.

3.1.1 Create an environment conducive to learning

Critical steps to creating an environment that is conducive to learning include: getting management or stakeholder support, identifying resources to support implementation, and obtaining buy-in from implementation staff and the audience. For a program to succeed, management or key stakeholder support from the highest level is required. This support will also help with securing financial, human, or other resources to implement the program (McKenzie et al., 2013). Health education specialists should also assess the trainees' willingness to learn. This assessment is important and may help decide the training methods to use, when and where to conduct trainings, etc. Failure to assess the willingness to learn may result in a loss of time or resources. The learning environment should be inclusive of all

KEY: no symbol - entry level; ❖ advanced 1; ■ advanced 2

learners, learner-centered, safe, and encouraging of trust and respect between the learners and the instructor (National Center on Quality Teaching and Learning, 2014; Merriam, Caffarella, Baumgartner, 2007). Additionally, the physical aspects of the learning environment can impact learning, including aspects such as temperature, adequate lighting, good acoustics, comfortable seating, room set-up, and good sightlines (Knowles et al., 2005).

3.1.2 Develop materials to implement plan

Health education specialists should develop an implementation guide, program procedural manual, project plan, or other materials to guide implementation. These "how-to" materials will ensure everyone involved understands the program and will create standards in case the program is replicated in the future (McKenzie et al., 2013). A literature review or environmental scan can help identify existing protocols, plans, or other materials available. Existing materials that have been tested and proven successful should be considered first as this may save time and money when resources are limited. See Sub-competency 6.1.2 for sources of evidence-based interventions. Another option is to consider adapting or tailoring materials for the intended audience. New materials should only be created if funds and time are available, and nothing has been successfully used before with the audience. Any materials (new, adapted, or tailored) should be pilot tested before implementation. This testing will help determine if changes are needed to ensure successful implementation.

3.1.3 Secure resources to implement plan

Implementing health education and promotion programs requires resources. A program can rarely be implemented for little to no cost. McKenzie et al. (2013) provide the following examples of resources needed for implementation of the work plan.

- **Personnel** refers to the person or people who will help with implementation
- **Curriculum and instructional resources** refer to the educational materials and curriculum
- **Space** refers to the physical space needed
- **Equipment and supplies** are the physical items needed
- **Financial resources** refer to the financial cost and how it will be covered (e.g., paid for by the agency/organization leading the work, participants, or a third-party [partner, sponsor, or grant funded])

Health education specialists should also consider questions about the number or amount of resources needed, the financial costs, and whether resources can be provided in-kind or donated, among others. Health education specialists might also consider MOUs for partners that provide in-kind or donated resources. See Competencies 5.1 and 5.6 for more information on managing resources.

3.1.4 Arrange for needed services to implement plan

Depending on the plan or program and its complexity, certain services might be required from partners, contractors, subject matter experts, or consultants. Implementation, project, or work plans should be used to identify the services needed, and health education specialists should plan for how to procure these services. Health education specialists should work through their organization, volunteers, or partners first. Services might be available at no cost or at a reduced cost. In this situation, a MOU may be needed. Another option is for health education specialists to work with contractors or consultants to provide the necessary services. In this situation, health education specialists should develop a written agreement outlining the work needed (e.g., statement of work), deliverables/products expected, a timeline to complete the work and provide deliverables/products, and a funding amount or payment.

3.1.5 Apply ethical principles to the implementation process

Health education specialists are expected to behave ethically and according to the Unified Code of Ethics approved by the CNHEO (CNHEO, 2011). Ethical dilemmas consist of issues with two sides and involving a judgment of right or wrong. Health education specialists are confronted with such dilemmas every day. The CNHEO Code of Ethics not only sets the standard for the health education specialist but also tells the public what to expect from the practitioner (Cottrell et al., 2014).

Ethics permeate all aspects of the health education specialists' various roles. Practicing within the boundaries of the profession's ethical standards is imperative. Because health education specialists are an important factor in behavioral development, professionals are expected to stay current in their knowledge of health-related content, as well as effective interventions and strategies (Plomer & Bensley, 2009). The community should also be considered if the program focuses on the community as a setting, target, resource, or agent (McLeroy et al., 2003). Health education specialists may wish to use a community advisory board or something similar to obtain community feedback and support (Newman et al., 2011).

3.1.6 Comply with legal standards that apply to implementation

Health education specialists must follow guidelines and legal standards for their organization, as well as an organization for providing funding (e.g., contract, cooperative agreement, grant). Health education specialists should always review state or local laws, rules, and regulations, as well as any funding announcements or solicitations, award notices, and/or other guidance documents. Some funding announcements place restrictions on how funds can be used (e.g., cannot be used for research, patient, or clinical care, cannot substitute for existing funds, or cannot cover pre-award costs). Examples of some administrative requirements, laws, and regulations that may apply include:

- The Paperwork Reduction Act of 1995 and information collection review helps reduce the paperwork burden and maximize information collection (USDHHS, 2014a)
- Section 508 of the Rehabilitation Act requires federal agencies to make Web sites, electronic materials, and other information technology accessible to people with disabilities (United States General Services Administration, 2014)
- The Plain Writing Act of 2010 requires federal agencies to use "clear communication that the public can understand and use" (Plain Language Action and Information Network, n.d.). **Plain language** is now expected for Web sites, print and other electronic materials, social media, and other materials (i.e., not just the informed consent)
- Cost sharing or matching funds (e.g., in-kind funds) may be required to leverage funds
- Antilobbying, smoke free worksites, and nutrition policies.
- Accounting system, security clearance, data release/sharing, and reporting requirements

KEY: no symbol - entry level;   ❖ advanced 1;   ■ advanced 2

Health education specialists might discuss questions with a supervisor, organization leadership, legal counsel, and/or the funding organization in order to determine what legal standards apply to implementation.

Competency 3.2 Train Staff Members and Volunteers Involved in Implementation of Health Education/Promotion

Depending on the magnitude of the program, health education specialists may be responsible for conducting training programs for professionals, volunteers, or stakeholders involved in delivering health education programs. Health education specialists may want to develop a train-the-trainer program that prepares staff members and volunteers to implement a specific training program (Orfaly et al., 2005). The goals of training sessions should be clearly outlined, related to the implementation of health education, and describe evidence-based strategies to deliver content. An evaluation of training sessions can provide feedback to help improve training sessions for future program personnel.

❖ 3.2.1 Develop training objectives

Objectives are focused on small steps toward the program goal or intended learning outcomes (McKenzie et al., 2013). **Training objectives** relate to both to the knowledge and skills that staff members and volunteers need to be able to implement health education/promotion interventions successfully. Objectives are worded in a way that allows a participant particular knowledge of content and the ability to apply knowledge or perform a particular task at an acceptable level by the end of the training. Implementation staff may be trained on roles during the program formation, implementation, or evaluation. Objectives for training might include that the participant can demonstrate particular learning technique (e.g., role-play), collect data for program monitoring or evaluation, provide nonjudgmental and respectful atmosphere to encourage dialogue, or dialogue with colleagues about a certain topic. As always, objectives should be Specific, Measurable, Achievable, Realistic, and Time-phased, often referred to as SMART objectives (Northwest Center for Public Health Practice, 2012; McKenzie et al., 2013). Additionally, objectives should align with goals. See Sub-competency 2.2.5 for more information on SMART objectives.

3.2.2 Recruit individuals needed for implementation

Health education specialists should think about three aspects of training when selecting individuals to deliver the program. First, the characteristics of the individual(s) who will conduct the training are critical to its success. Personal characteristics to look for in instructors include: a desire to teach, the ability to communicate, skill at getting people to participate, and being "learner-oriented" (Kirkpatrick& Kirkpatrick, 2009).

Second, participants for training sessions should be considered future intervention deliverers. By considering what the intervention requires for successful delivery, health education specialists can identify some intervention specific characteristics of participants. Examples of questions that can be asked include:

- Are specialized technology skills needed, such as working knowledge of distance learning, webinars, or blogs? Are other skills required?
- Does the intervention require multiple sessions? What does that mean about the availability of the person delivering it? Are multiple persons acceptable or should one facilitator be used throughout?
- Does the audience require a person fluent in their language?
- Would the intervention strategy benefit from a particular sort of experience helpful in using the intervention, such as experience in peer leading?

Health education specialists must take care to select individuals with skills that match those needed for the program delivery. Additionally, those individuals who implement training should know the intended audience.

Third, health education specialists should understand the organizational context where the intervention will be delivered. An intervention poorly supported or unsupported by an organization may not be delivered properly or at all, thereby making it useless regardless of its apparent efficacy. The following considerations about implementation not only assist health education specialists in selecting individuals to train but also in setting the stage for successful delivery and later maintenance of the intervention (Livet, Courser, & Wandersman, 2008).

- Will the individual delivering the intervention have the support of management or decision-makers?
- Has the organization had any experience using the particular intervention strategy?
- Is the strategy in line with the philosophy and mission of the organization?
- Does the organizational site(s) have the prerequisites for using the strategy? Prerequisites include: the essential characteristics needed in a delivery site, such as sufficient personnel, bilingual, or bicultural staff, access to meeting space, proven relationship with the intended audience, and proven fiscal responsibility. These will vary by intervention. Health education specialists can determine these from the intervention strategy, audience targeted, and setting of the intervention.

See Competency 6.2 for more information on training.

❖ 3.2.3 Identify training needs of individuals involved in implementation

In determining training needs, health education specialists must consider: intervention characteristics and requirements, the skills, knowledge, and experience of individuals involved in implementation, and the setting for the training. As stated earlier, health education specialists should understand the critical knowledge and skills necessary for implementing an intervention successfully. Before delivering training, health education specialists should conduct a needs assessment to help plan the training and ensure individual needs are met (Northwest Center for Public Health Practice, 2012; Occupational Health and Safety Administration [OSHA], 2010). A training needs assessment should determine what the desired learning outcome is, the characteristics of the participants (e.g., age, abilities such as hearing loss or visual difficulties, intellectual abilities, language, etc.), the learning context, and the content and training expertise. Health education specialists should not overlook the logistics for training when identifying training needs. For example, health education specialists might ask what type of space the training requires. A cooking demonstration, for example, needs a space with a working kitchen. The training might be best delivered in an alternative location such as a home, religious institution, community center, or other gathering place. If a location conducive to skill building is not available, health educations specialists must decide how or whether to adapt the intervention without compromising effectiveness. The Northwest Center for Public Health Practice (2012) has an example of a training needs assessment in its *Toolkit for Teaching Adults*.

❖ 3.2.4 Develop training using best practices

Health education specialists work with a wide age range of clients and participants, though training initiatives typically occur with adults. Training programs should be accurate, credible, clear, and practical (OHSA, 2010). The American Society of Training and Development (ASTD, 2014) identified five best practices of training and development. Training developers should:

- Consider the root causes of a need for training
- Conduct a systematic needs assessment and, based on that, develop a design framework
- Integrate e-learning, if appropriate
- Develop training that engages learners
- Develop an evaluation plan

The literature very clearly supports the notion that adults learn differently than children. Friere (2000), Knowles, Holten and Swanson (2005), and Merriam, Caffarella, and Baumgartner (2007) pioneered this relatively new field of study. Adult learning (andragogy) differs from children's learning (pedagogy) in several ways (Knowles et al., 2005). Bryan, Kreuter, and Brownson (2008) described ways to integrate adult learning principles in public health training:

- Actively involve adults in helping to set the curriculum, choosing training methods, or identify training goals
- Ask about adults' past experience and knowledge, and use their experiences or knowledge to avoid providing redundant content during trainings
- Use methods to help adults obtain problem solving skills rather than learning content (e.g., use problem-based learning, use broad themes that focus on a range of challenges)
- Conduct assessments to identify ways to engage adults and learn about their goals or objectives for the training
- Use a variety of methods, perspectives, and content because adults have diverse needs and learning styles

These principles are the foundation for successful trainings with adults. Health education specialists working outside of a school setting are encouraged to incorporate these principles into their training skill set. Health education specialists are also encouraged to search the literature for proven methods of training.

Agencies and organizations, such as the CDC, publicize programs and interventions that utilize best practices and that may be use in training efforts. Where no list can be considered comprehensive or exhaustive, the CDC provides a starting point for health education specialists. Recognized programs are grounded in a variety of Areas of Responsibility for health education specialists.

The health education specialist should be media literate. Health education specialists should have a basic knowledge about publication layout and design, the creation, processing, and editing of images whether printed or video, and Web site design in order to be able to create Web sites and evaluate the quality of health-related Web sites. These are especially important when reaching Limited English Proficiency audiences or low health literate audiences (United States Department of Justice, 2014; Plain Language Action and Information Network, 2014).

Instructional technology is a vital tool for reaching the intended audience and achieving program objectives. For example, the computer can be used to prepare visual aids, access the Internet for instructional resources, or conduct a virtual meeting. CD-ROMs and DVDs can be used in interactive presentations. Teleconferencing technology allows participants in different locations to attend discussions and lectures. Scanners and digital cameras can be used in the creation of print media and multimedia presentations (Fodor, Dalis, & Giarratano-Russell, 2010).

Asynchronous training is a type of distance learning in which training occurs outside of real time where the instructor and the learners communicate at different times, while synchronous training is a type of distance learning in which training in real time and the instructor and the learners communicate at the same time (Hrastinski, 2008).

❖ 3.2.5 Implement training

Health education specialists must consider the best way to instruct an intended audience while also considering available funds and expertise-levels of the individuals providing the training. Depending on cost, content, and instructional expertise required, a variety of methods should be used, such as on-the-job training, one-on-one training, in-person group work, and distance learning techniques (e.g., video conferences, computer-based training, Internet, or conference calls). A coordinator should oversee the implementation of the training.

❖ 3.2.6 Provide support and technical assistance to those implementing the plan

Support and technical assistance may be required if other people or organizations help implement the plan. Health education specialists must know (or be able to assess) the program needs and capacities, able to engage people, and build trusting relationships in order to provide quality, effective, and efficient technical assistance. These qualities are critical for health education specialists that do not live or work in geographic locations that receive technical assistance. Challenges to providing technical assistance may include inadequate funding, managing the volume of technical assistance requests, and a person or organization's readiness to receive technical assistance (West et al., 2012). See Sub-competency 6.3.3 for more information on providing technical assistance.

KEY: no symbol - entry level; ❖ advanced 1; ■ advanced 2

❖ 3.2.7 Evaluate training

Evaluation is critical to understand the factors that influence training and to make decisions to improve training. To acquire the best results from the training provided to individuals, health education specialists should evaluate the training process and content (ASTD, n.d.; OHSA, 2010). An evaluation of training can occur at the individual level, individual training workshop level, or at the curriculum level (Miner, Childers, Alperin, Cioffi, & Hunt, 2005).

In 1959, Donald Kirkpatrick developed a four-level model to evaluate training that is widely used (2009). The levels are:
- Level 1: Reaction
- Level 2: Learning
- Level 3: Behavior
- Level 4: Results

Level 1 (Reaction) evaluations measure participant satisfaction and may use a Likert scale (e.g., a scale of items used to assess agreement or disagreement) and/or open-ended questions. These evaluations are administered at the end of a learning activity (e.g., workshop, seminar, course, etc.) and can be detailed, comprehensive, and cover both individual sessions and daily activities. Participants' feedback on each session should be simple and should vary in format to address the main points covered in the course. An open-ended question requesting qualitative feedback can be helpful in planning future training activities.

Participants as well as the individual trainer or facilitator should evaluate the following course components: venue, organization, quality of presentation, and quality of participants' participation. The training presentations should be evaluated based on elements such as meeting stated objectives, clarity of presentation, interest in presentation, and responsiveness to participant's questions and concerns.

Sample questions may include:
- What will you do differently as a result of this training?
- What was the most or least useful aspect of the session?
- Were the trainee's opinions valued and how?
- What went well or did not go well in the session?

Examples of Likert scale items are:
- My learning was enhanced by the variety of teaching techniques used by the facilitator
- I will be immediately able to apply what I learned
- I was comfortable with the pace of the workshop
- I found the room setup comfortable

Such questions should be standardized so that the aggregation of results from multiple offerings can provide more reliable direction for training refinement.

Level 2 (Learning) measures the amount of knowledge gained as a result of the learning activity. In most skills-based or Competency-based training, there is an associated need for enhancement of knowledge related to the skills being developed. One way to evaluate knowledge gains is through the administration of pre- and post-tests. These may include true/false, multiple-choice questions, case-based scenarios, written essays, oral review, self-assessment of knowledge, or direct observations. It may be useful to do a before and after self-assessment rating by participants to address their perceived Competency in performing the skills described in the behavioral objectives of the course. Skills evaluations may take place through direct observation by an expert observer or by written self-assessment.

Level 3 (Behavior) evaluations measure the extent to which behavior change occurs. This evaluation is conducted sometime after the training when there has been enough time for behavior to change. Surveys and interviews are often used to measure behavior changes.

Level 4 (Results) is most often used in workforce programs to measure the longer-range results that occurred due to participation in a training session (i.e., reduced turnover or improved work quality). In this level, health education specialists can have difficulty showing that changes are directly due to a training workshop or program.

❖ 3.2.8 Use evaluation findings to plan/modify future training

Qualitative and quantitative evaluations can help to make appropriate revisions in the training. As the training is revised, health education specialists should keep in mind the stated goals and objectives of the program and the specific intervention featured in the training. For complex programs, utilizing an outside expert as a consultant may be useful. See Sub-competency 4.7.4 for more information about applying evaluation findings.

Competency 3.3 Implement Health Education/Promotion Plan

An action plan for program implementation describes how goals and objectives will be achieved, as well as identifies resources needed and how responsibilities will be assigned (Brownson, Baker, Left, Gillespie, & True, 2003). Health education specialists may consider using a project management plan or project management principles when implementing a plan. Building on the assessment and planning activities related to a particular health issue or problem, health education specialists should develop a plan of action in conjunction with members of the intended audience and those who can hinder or help implementation of the program.

Table 3.1 outlines five generic phases of the implementation process in health education and key components for effective public health program implementation.

KEY: no symbol - entry level;   ❖ advanced 1;   ■ advanced 2

Table 3.1

Phases and Components for Implementation

Five Generic Phases of Program Implementation (McKenzie et al., 2013)	Six Components for Effective Public Health Program Implementation (Frieden, 2014)
• Adopt the program • Identify and prioritize tasks to complete • Establish a management system • Put the plans into action (e.g., pilot or field testing, phasing, total implementation) • End or sustain a program or intervention	• Use innovation to develop the evidence base • Use a limited number of high priority, evidence-based interventions • Use effective program management • Use partnerships and coalitions • Communicate accurate and timely information • Obtain resources and support

A critical first step is getting the priority population to accept the **intervention** or **program** and identifying the individuals or organizations to deliver the intervention. Health education specialists should use an implementation plan, project management plan, or other process to develop a detailed list of all program activities, components, and tasks along with the relationships between and among them. Careful project management includes using a system or schedule to ensure that the program progresses as planned and in order to monitor human, financial, and other resources. Health education specialists should use pilot testing, phasing-in, or total implementation, especially when implementing an adapted or new program (McKenzie et al., 2013). Key staff and partners should communicate throughout implementation. In addition, mass communication (i.e., sharing information on a large scale) should be used to share information and support program objectives or implementation. Health education specialists should consider health impact and how to end or sustain the program before beginning implementation (Frieden, 2010; McKenzie et al., 2013).

3.3.1 Collect baseline data

Prior to program implementation, health education specialists should review available quantitative and qualitative data from national, state, and local resources. This will help assess health knowledge, beliefs, attitudes, and values of the intended audiences, as well as their psychomotor capabilities or skills related to outcomes. This baseline data is important as it will provide the beginning measure for evaluating changes in behavior, practices, or skills associated with the program goals. See Competencies 4.3 and 4.4 for more information on data collection and management.

Primary data collection may be required if health education specialists want to understand the local impact of a health issue. However, secondary data sources (i.e., data collected for another purpose) might also provide the information needed. Examples of data already available may include health data (e.g., morbidity, mortality, risk factor), open government data portals (http://www.data.gov/open-gov), or other "big data" (Kaplan, Riley, & Mabry, 2014). See Competency 1.3 for more information on primary data.

❖ 3.3.2 Apply theories and/or models of implementation

Theories are the backbone of every well-planned intervention. Although abstract in nature, theories provide a guide for to what to expect about human behavior. According to Kerlinger (1986), "a theory is a set of interrelated concepts, definitions and propositions that present a systematic view of events or situations by specifying relations among variables, in order to explain and predict the events or situations" (as cited in Glanz et al., 2008b, p. 26). Models draw upon a number of theories to help understand a specific problem in a particular setting or context.

Theories and models used in designing interventions allow health education specialists to select strategies for implementation based on known influences on human behavior. Additionally, most theories and models are laid out in a way that helps health education specialists measure change.

Health education specialists are responsible for selecting the theory or model that will be used to inform program planning and implementation based on the concepts and constructs of a theory and the program goals and objectives. Here are a few current, popular textbooks that outline the most commonly used theories of health behavior and health promotion.

- *Health Behavior and Health Education: Theory, Research, and Practice,* 4th edition (Glanz, Rimer, Viswanath, 2008a)
- *Emerging Theories in Health Promotion Practice and Research: Strategies for Improving Public Health* (DiClemente, Crosby, & Kegler, 2009)
- *Essentials of Health Behavior: Social and Behavioral Theory in Public Health* (Edberg, 2007)
- *Theoretical Foundations of Health Education and Health Promotion* (Sharma & Romas, 2010)
- *Introduction to Health Behavior Theory,* 2nd edition (Hayden, J., 2014)
- *Theory in Health Promotion Research and Practice: Thinking Outside the Box* (Goodson, 2010)

Some common theories and models used in health education are briefly described below. See Sub-competencies 2.4.1 and 7.1.1 for more information on additional theories or models.

Social Cognitive Theory. Social Cognitive Theory states that learning is an interaction between a person and his or her environment, cognitive processes, and behavior (Bandura, 1986). In this theory, this interaction is referred to as reciprocal determinism. Although different sources discuss the components in different ways, there are several major constructs associated with this theory: behavioral capability, expectations, expectancies, self-control, emotional coping responses, reciprocal determinism, and self-efficacy. Other models have adopted Social Cognitive Theory constructs to serve as an underpinning for behavior change. More specifically, self-efficacy, a person's confidence in performing a behavior and overcoming possible barriers to that behavior, has been adopted by several other models.

KEY: no symbol - entry level;   ❖ advanced 1;   ■ advanced 2

Transtheoretical Model. The Transtheoretical Model, often called the Stages of Change Model, incorporates components of many theories, thus the term "transtheoretical" (Prochaska, Redding, & Evers, 2008). This theory is particularly useful in that its planned interventions can reach people where they are in their motivation for a particular behavior. This model has several major constructs: stages of change, processes of change, decisional balance, and self-efficacy. The stages of change construct received considerable attention due to its use in determining readiness to change.

This Model proposes that change is a process, not an event, and that change occurs as people move through a series of stages to adopt a new behavior. The stages are:
- *Precontemplation:* person is not interested in addressing the problem; some people may be unaware of or in denial about the problem
- *Contemplation:* person is aware there is a problem and intends to do something in the next six months
- *Preparation:* person has taken steps and plans to address the problem in the next month
- *Action:* person has taken action (changed behavior) within the past six months
- *Maintenance:* person has maintained the behavior change for more than six months
- *Termination:* person has no temptation to return to the old behavior

(Prochaska et al., 2008)

A person can be in any stage with any behavior and move back and forth through the stages, depending on external factors affecting the individual. When using this model, health education specialists can develop materials and interventions for each stage to match individual needs for behavior change.

Health Belief Model. The Health Belief Model (Hochbaum, 1958; Rosenstock, Strecher, & Becker, 1988) is a popular behavior change model that has been extensively used and researched over the years. It is an individual-level model first developed by social psychologists in the United States Public Health Service to understand why individuals did not act on information about prevention or disease detection. In this model, there are six major constructs thought to affect behavior change:
- Perceived susceptibility: a person feels at risk for the disease
- Perceived severity: there are serious consequences to contracting the disease
- Perceived benefits: there are benefits to taking action to prevent or control the disease
- Perceived barriers: there are consequences to taking action against the disease
- Cues to action: cues or triggers that encourage a person to take action
- Self-efficacy: a person is confident in taking action against the disease

Theory of Reasoned Action and Theory of Planned Behavior. The Theory of Reasoned Action was developed first to focus on relationships between attitudes, behaviors, and intentions. The Theory of Planned Behavior was built on the Theory of Reasoned Action and added the behavioral control construct. Both theories recognize behavioral intention as key in determining behavior and assume that behavior change is influenced by a person's attitude toward the outcome and the social or subjective norms of people important in the person's life (Montaño & Kasprzyk, 2008). When using these theories, health education specialists should examine the individual's motivation to perform the behavior, determine what the individual's peers think of the behavior, and assess the difficulty the individual will have in performing the behavior.

Diffusion of Innovations Theory. The Diffusion of Innovations Theory (Rogers, 2003) is a community-level theory that describes the rate at which a new program or activity will spread throughout a group of people. According to this theory, the characteristics of those accepting the new program help to explain community readiness to change.

- *Innovators* are the first to adopt the new idea or program
- *Early Adopters* wait until after the Innovators adopt
- *Early Majority* adopts once the opinion leaders have done so
- *Late Majority* adopts once the new idea or program becomes the norm
- *Laggards* are the last to adopt or they may never adopt

Health education specialists motivate groups of people to adopt the new idea or program by demonstrating how much better it is than the status quo. The theory also incorporates constructs related to the innovation: relative advantage, compatibility, complexity, observability, and trialability. Using the Diffusion of Innovations Theory, health education specialists integrate the idea into something already accepted in the community through communication channels.

Ecological Models. Ecological models focus attention on the interaction of the individual and environment (Sallis, Owen, & Fisher, 2008). This requires that health education specialists be familiar with individual behavior change strategies as well as strategies to change the environment or physical surroundings. Several ecological models have been proposed, each with a unique way to frame this interaction. Sallis et al. (2008) propose health behavior can be affected at five levels: individual or intrapersonal, interpersonal, organizational, community, and public policy.

PRECEDE-PROCEED Model. The PRECEDE-PROCEED Model is a health program planning and evaluation framework (Green & Kreuter, 2005). PRECEDE refers to the Predisposing, Reinforcing, and Enabling Constructs in the Educational/Environmental Diagnosis and Evaluation. PROCEED refers to the Policy, Regulatory, and Organizational Constructs in Educational and Environmental Development. According to PRECEDE-PROCEED Model, multiple factors affect health, and behavioral, environmental, and social change should therefore be multidimensional and participatory (Green & Kreuter, 2005). Please refer to Sub-competency 2.3.1 for more description about this model.

Intervention Mapping. Bartholomew and colleagues first introduced intervention mapping with five steps: program objectives, theory-based intervention methods and practical strategies, designing and organizing a program, adoption and implementation plans, and program evaluation plans. Later, Bartholomew et al. (2011) made changes, such as adding a sixth step (needs assessment) and adding sustainability to program adoption and implementation. This framework can help health education specialists plan and develop interventions (i.e., the lifecycle from problem to solution).

3.3.3 Assess readiness for implementation

Health education specialists should consider readiness for implementation at the individual, organizational, and environmental levels. This readiness includes comparing program goals and objectives with the characteristics of groups, communities, or organizations that might have experience in delivering the intervention strategies. Organizational readiness for change is defined as members' commitment to change and the shared capacity to implement the change (Weiner, 2009). Identifying and contacting individuals whose professional background and experience bring skills and abilities to help groups, communities, or organizations will increase readiness to implement health education programs. Where and when necessary health education specialists should help facilitate capacity building among key stakeholders in order to increase readiness to move health education programs forward. Several methods for determining capacity exist, some using outside experts and others using only local individuals and organizations (Beaulieu, 2002).

3.3.4 Apply principles of diversity and cultural competence in implementing health education/ promotion plan

Culturally and linguistically competent health education specialists value diversity, develop the capacity for self-assessment, raise awareness of dynamics inherent when cultures interact, use organizational processes to institutionalize cultural knowledge, and strive to develop individual and organizational adaptations to diversity (Institute of Medicine, 2002). Delivering programs in a culturally sensitive manner requires conscientious attention by program planners. This may mean providing an environment in which people from diverse backgrounds feel comfortable discussing culturally derived health beliefs and sharing cultural practices.

Health information should use words and examples in the audience's primary language to ensure information is understandable (USDHHS, 2009). Literacy level, preferred language, and preferred media sources should be considered when delivering interventions. Interventions not offered in other languages should use design techniques for low-literacy audiences to improve reception of the instruction, including oral delivery (Plain Language Action and Information Network, 2014; Doak, Doak, & Root, 1996). When an audience is culturally diverse, matching the source as closely to the audience in key demographics is important to message credibility. Where languages other than English are spoken, health education specialists must take care to ensure accurate translations or develop interventions with that culture in mind to put the behavior into the proper cultural context. See Sub-competency 7.1.2 for more information about health literacy.

3.3.5 Implement marketing plan

Health education specialists have replaced a one-size-fits-all approach to program promotion with tailored and targeted promotion campaigns based on the ethnic and demographic characteristics and behaviors of the population being served. Health messages need to appeal to the audience's needs, preferences, and health concerns. **Tailored messages** are individually focused messages that appeal to a specific subpopulation, typically using information obtained from the individuals themselves. Today, computer tailoring of messages and materials can enable a program to reach a larger audience (Gilbert, Sawyer, & McNeill, 2011). By contrast, **targeting messages** focuses on subgroups, which relies on segmenting or dividing the audience into smaller groups with similar characteristics (e.g., by age, race/ethnicity, gender, geographic location, etc.) (McKenzie et al., 2013).

A **marketing plan** should identify the audience(s), message(s), and the communication methods to be used (e.g., earned media, paid media, social media, etc.) (Parvanta 2011). It is important to consider the how the audience prefers to get their information and available financial resources. The marketing plan should also support program goals and objectives. There are numerous online tools available such as CDCynergy, communication plans templates, and more.

3.3.6 Deliver health education/promotion as designed

The implementation of a program requires a variety of skills and knowledge, including the ability to use technology, execute appropriate timelines, manage program resources, and conduct an evaluation. Health education specialists seldom have unlimited resources available to them. Most successful programs are the result of the efforts and resources of a number of different people and organizations. Thus, health education specialists need to have skills to work with others who have similar interests and a stake in the outcomes of successful health education programs.

Before implementation, health education specialists should identify implementation issues such as staffing and training, intervention content, program delivery, and intervention participants (Gorman-Smith, 2006). Evidence-based interventions must be implemented as designed. Failure to implement the intervention as designed may negatively affect the intervention's success (Gorman-Smith, 2006). If the intervention is new or adapted, health education specialists should carefully follow the design and implementation plans (including any adjustments from pilot testing or phasing). The Implementation element of the Reach Effectiveness Adoption Implementation Maintenance (RE-AIM) framework may help with intervention delivery (Virginia Tech, 2015).

3.3.7 Use a variety of strategies to deliver plan

The scope and sequence of a program may contain many intervention strategies. An intervention may include single or multiple strategies and methods through which program goals and objectives are achieved. To implement an intervention, health education specialists need a variety of skills and knowledge (e.g., use of large-scale communication and technology, create appropriate timelines, manage program resources, and carry out an evaluation).

Behavior is multifaceted; therefore, multiple strategies are often needed to change behavior. Interventions or programs designed to motivate behavior change should consider strategies at various levels (e.g., individual, organizational, community, and environment). A program could include a mix of strategies focusing on socioeconomic determinants, contextual changes, protective and clinical interventions, and counseling and education (Frieden, 2010). When selecting strategies or activities, health education specialists should be sure that each strategy has evidence of efficacy. Even though the strategy may be shown to work, not all interventions using that strategy may achieve the desired outcomes. Health education specialists should look for evaluation results in the literature, program reports, or through discussion with program administrators.

KEY: no symbol - entry level;   ❖ advanced 1;   ■ advanced 2

Health education specialists should consider paid media, earned media, social media, digital media (e.g., Web sites, mobile phones and applications), online competitions (e.g., http://www.challenge.gov), and other technologies. Paid media refers to television, radio, print, billboards, transit, or digital advertising (CDC, 2014c). Earned media involves receiving free news placement (CDC, 2014c). Social media includes collaborative projects (e.g., wikis), blogs, content communities (e.g., Flickr, Slideshare, YouTube), social networking sites (e.g., Facebook), virtual game worlds, and virtual social worlds (Kaplan & Haenlein, 2010). Mobile phones offer text messaging, cameras, applications, automated sensors (e.g., Bluetooth, GPS for tracking distance), and Internet access (Klasnjal & Pratt, 2012). Health education specialists must determine the audience preference and stay abreast of continuous advances to make the best choice. See Sub-competency 7.1.7 for more information on delivering messages using media and communication.

Competency 3.4 Monitor Implementation of Health Education/Promotion

When implementing programs, health education specialists must monitor all aspects of the program, including content delivery, adherence to timelines, progress toward objectives, and use of financial resources. Data collection and record maintenance are important tasks that health education specialists must perform in order to ensure proper delivery of the program.

3.4.1 Monitor progress in accordance with timeline

Health education specialists should produce a timeline that identifies major activities and outputs, as well as monitor program implementation progress. A Gantt chart, Program Evaluation and Review Technique (PERT), Critical Path Method (CPM), work plan, a simple table, or timeline can be used (McKenzie et al., 2013). Each of these methods allows health education specialists to visually identify the progress for project management. Tools and resources are available online or in software packages (free or paid) to help develop the chart or model. Health education specialists should also hold regular meetings with stakeholders and implementation staffs in order to monitor progress, receive feedback, and report progress. It is important to know who receives progress reports (e.g., funders, leadership, stakeholders) and the preferred reporting methods (e.g., in-person, written, etc.).

3.4.2 Assess progress in achieving objectives

There are many opportunities to track progress throughout implementation. Health education specialists should use project meetings or other regular meetings to monitor progress through program management tools such as Gantt charts or work plans. Reviewing data sources or process evaluations can also help assess progress in achieving objectives. Logic models can help track whether activities are producing outputs and if the outputs lead to expected short-term outcomes. By tracking this progress, health education specialists can identify where and when something occurred that differed from the implementation plan. Tracking progress may also help health education specialists to better understand why an intervention succeeded or failed to achieve the expected results.
See Sub-competencies 4.1.3 and 4.1.4 for more information on logic models.

3.4.3 Ensure plan is implemented consistently

Health education specialists must ensure consistency and fidelity during implementation. Mowbray et al. (2012) define fidelity "as the extent to which delivery of an intervention adheres to the protocol or program model originally developed" (p.315). Activity logs, document reviews, observations, reports, surveys, or interviews can be used to measure fidelity (Mowbray et al., 2012; Substance Abuse and Mental Health Services Administration [SAMHSA], 2012). The Non-Researcher's Guide to Evidence-Based Program Evaluation, an online training from SAMHSA (2012), includes proposed questions on program delivery, dose, and quality to help measure fidelity during implementation. Failure to monitor fidelity can present numerous challenges during and after the project. Poor implementation can also lead to the program not being successful.

3.4.4 Modify plan when needed

Seldom is the perfect intervention already designed and ready to use. Typically, health education specialists must select an intervention that will work for the audience, desired outcome, and resources available. Health education specialists must have a flexible plan of action, know whom to involve when modifying the plan of action, and know when and from whom approvals are needed when modifying the plan. Health education specialists can evaluate the process and monitor the fidelity of implementation to identify when modifications may be needed.

Modifying the plan does not always mean the intervention is modified, but when the intervention is modified, primary attention should be focused on maintaining fidelity to the original intervention. Some modifications have been found to affect the efficacy of the intervention in the field. Conversely, adapting an intervention is a fundamental activity in implementation, as it allows health education specialists to create a common ground between the delivery of the intervention and the characteristics of the group using it. If adaptation to an intervention results in a form that is far from the original, tested form, it is prudent to evaluate the adapted intervention for the desired outcome.

3.4.5 Monitor use of resources

Health education specialists must recognize the importance of monitoring resources (e.g., personnel, curriculum and instructional, space, equipment and supplies, financial) used in an intervention and program as a whole. They should develop a budget to use and carefully track to monitor financial resources, especially if the program is funded by a grant or taxpayer funds. Funding agencies often require progress reports that describe expenses and revenues. Curriculum and instructional resources, space, or equipment and supplies should be monitored based on their volume, frequency of use, and relationship to the program or project plan. Human resources can be expensive and consume a large part of budgets; regular monitoring is critical to ensure successful implementation. Project plans and project management principles also help ensure resources are used properly. See Sub-competencies 5.1.6, 5.6.9, and 5.6.13 for more details regarding managing fiscal resources.

3.4.6 Evaluate sustainability of implementation

The sustainability of the intervention or program should be considered from the start. Health education specialists should create an implementation guide, use a train-the-trainer model, and document lessons learned throughout project or program monitoring. Sustainability domains or elements include leadership/political support, funding stability, collaboration/partnerships, organizational capacity, program evaluation, program adaption, communication, and strategic planning/vision (CDC, 2014b; Georgia Health Policy Center, 2011; Schell et al., 2013). Identifying partners and stakeholders who can help is necessary and should be considered at the start (not when the program or intervention is ending). These activities are critical to continue the intervention or program long-term, as well as sharing with others (CDC, 2014b).

3.4.7 Ensure compliance with legal standards

Negligence is the failure to act in a careful or reasonable manner. Negligence may result from omission (not doing something that should have been done) or commission (doing something that should not have done). To reduce the likelihood of legal improprieties:

- Be aware of legal liabilities
- Use only professionals or experts in the area being presented (when appropriate, they should be licensed, certified, or in other ways credentialed)
- When appropriate, require medical clearance for participation
- Instruct staff not to practice outside their area of expertise
- Follow building codes and regulations

(Anspaugh, Dignan, & Anspaugh, 2000)

Health education specialists should seek help from their supervisor, organization leadership or legal counsel, or partners when needed. They should ask questions and make adjustments early on rather than have to stop a program or intervention midcourse.

3.4.8 Monitor adherence to ethical principles in the implementation of health education/promotion

Health education specialists are required to comply with the Health Education Code of Ethics throughout the implementation process (http://www.cnheo.org/ethics.html). Health education specialists should maintain a high standard of conduct at all times and ensure the ethical behavior of everyone involved with implementation (CNHEO, 2011). During implementation, health education specialists are responsible to the public, the health education profession, and employers both when delivering health education and in research and evaluation. Process evaluation, project management meetings, and other regular monitoring should be used to ensure compliance with the Health Education Code of Ethics.

This page was
intentionally left blank

CHAPTER IV

Area of Responsibility IV

Conduct Evaluation and Research Related to Health Education/Promotion

4.1: Develop evaluation plan for health education/promotion
4.1.1 ❖ Determine the purpose and goals of evaluation
4.1.2 ❖ Develop questions to be answered by the evaluation
4.1.3 ❖ Create a logic model to guide the evaluation process
4.1.4 ❖ Adapt/modify a logic model to guide the evaluation process
4.1.5 ❖ Assess needed and available resources to conduct evaluation
4.1.6 ❖ Determine the types of data (for example, qualitative, quantitative) to be collected
4.1.7 ❖ Select a model for evaluation
4.1.8 ❖ Develop data collection procedures for evaluation
4.1.9 ■ Develop data analysis plan for evaluation
4.1.10 ❖ Apply ethical principles to the evaluation process

4.2 Develop a research plan for health education/promotion
4.2.1 ■ Create statement of purpose
4.2.2 ■ Assess feasibility of conducting research
4.2.3 ■ Conduct search for related literature
4.2.4 ■ Analyze and synthesize information found in the literature
4.2.5 ■ Develop research questions and/or hypotheses
4.2.6 ■ Assess the merits and limitations of qualitative and quantitative data collection
4.2.7 ■ Select research design to address the research questions
4.2.8 ■ Determine suitability of existing data collection instruments
4.2.9 ■ Identify research participants
4.2.10 ■ Develop sampling plan to select participants
4.2.11 ■ Develop data collection procedures for research
4.2.12 ■ Develop data analysis plan for research
4.2.13 ■ Develop a plan for non-respondent follow-up
4.2.14 ■ Apply ethical principles to the research process

4.3 Select, adapt and/or create instruments to collect data
4.3.1 ■ Identify existing data collection instruments
4.3.2 ■ Adapt/modify existing data collection instruments
4.3.3 ■ Create new data collection instruments
4.3.4   Identify useable items from existing instruments
4.3.5   Adapt/modify existing items
4.3.6 ■ Create new items to be used in data collection
4.3.7 ■ Pilot test data collection instrument
4.3.8 ■ Establish validity of data collection instruments
4.3.9 ■ Ensure that data collection instruments generate reliable data
4.3.10 ■ Ensure fairness of data collection instruments (for example, reduce bias, use language appropriate to priority population)

KEY: no symbol - entry level; ❖ advanced 1; ■ advanced 2

4.4 Collect and manage data

4.4.1 ■ Train data collectors involved in evaluation and/or research

4.4.2 ■ Collect data based on the evaluation or research plan

4.4.3　Monitor and manage data collection

4.4.4　Use available technology to collect, monitor and manage data

4.4.5　Comply with laws and regulations when collecting, storing, and protecting participant data

4.5 Analyze data

4.5.1 ■ Prepare data for analysis

4.5.2 ❖ Analyze data using qualitative methods

4.5.3 ■ Analyze data using descriptive statistical methods

4.5.4 ■ Analyze data using inferential statistical methods

4.5.5 ■ Use technology to analyze data

4.6 Interpret results

4.6.1 ■ Synthesize the analyzed data

4.6.2 ■ Explain how the results address the questions and/or hypotheses

4.6.3 ■ Compare findings to results from other studies or evaluations

4.6.4 ■ Propose possible explanations of findings

4.6.5 ■ Identify limitations of findings

4.6.6 ■ Address delimitations as they relate to findings

4.6.7 ■ Draw conclusions based on findings

4.6.8 ■ Develop recommendations based on findings

4.7 Apply findings

4.7.1　Communicate findings to priority populations, partners, and stakeholders

4.7.2　Solicit feedback from priority populations, partners, and stakeholders

4.7.3　Evaluate feasibility of implementing recommendations

4.7.4　Incorporate findings into program improvement and refinement

4.7.5 ■ Disseminate findings using a variety of methods

The Role. The knowledge and skill sets necessary to conduct evaluation and research related to health education/promotion have much in common. Both research and evaluation require health education specialists to be competent in developing plans to guide their work. This includes selecting, adapting, and/or creating data collection instruments, as well as collecting and managing data, analyzing collected data, interpreting results, and applying the findings. These Competencies allow health education specialists to conduct evaluations of policy, projects, and programs, as well as to plan and conduct both basic and applied research. Health education specialists with advanced-level training and several years of experience working in the field complete much of this work because of the complexity of many of these processes.

Settings. The following text is presented to describe how research and evaluation are used in different practice settings.

KEY: no symbol - entry level;　❖ advanced 1;　■ advanced 2

Community Setting. Health education specialists in a community setting must understand and interpret research findings for use in their work. Their work may include the use of epidemiological principles to explain disease outbreaks or define high-risk neighborhoods within communities that require special program emphasis. Health education specialists must master research principles and language to discuss any topic important to the community, including unintentional injuries, an outbreak of measles or food poisoning, or sexually transmitted diseases. They also must understand the importance of conducting and interpreting the results of sound evaluations. Evaluations provide necessary evidence to support programs when reviewed by local or state governments. Health education specialists working at the entry-level may be involved in data collection for both research and evaluations, as well as interpreting the results of each of these processes. Those health education specialists working at an advanced-level of practice are responsible for planning and implementing the research and evaluation processes.

School (K-12) Setting. Health education specialists practicing in the school setting may be called upon to assist in the documentation of student health knowledge, attitudes, and behaviors. Health education specialists provide data gained from a review of the literature and from qualitative and quantitative research to school boards and parents to help them understand students' needs and interests. Careful use of such research approaches helps dispel intolerant attitudes and behaviors maintained by a small but vocal population. Evaluation of curriculum goals, objectives, learning activities, and behavioral outcomes is critical to identifying, selecting, and implementing effective curricula. As accountability increases, both qualitative and quantitative research methods are increasingly being emphasized in school settings.

Health Care Setting. In a health care setting, health education specialists must be able to understand and interpret research findings for patients and their families and may be asked to participate as a member of a research team that investigates behavioral components of adherence to clinical regimens. As medical technologies and treatments advance through clinical trials, evaluative research becomes increasingly important in addressing chronic disease conditions and the reduction of health risk behaviors for primary prevention. In addition, health education specialists may be involved in quality improvement initiatives as a member of the health care team.

Business/Industry Setting. Adults spend the majority of their time in the workplace. Health education specialists in this setting need qualitative and quantitative research skills to demonstrate the efficacy of health promotion programs and the contributions of such programs to productivity and organizational goals. Health education specialists also may be asked to assist in monitoring the work environment for safety compliance and injury reduction. Additionally, using evaluative research, health education specialists may be able to help determine quality and cost-effectiveness of competing health plans to benefit employers and employees.

College/University Setting. A significant portion of the work of health education specialists in this setting deals with both evaluation and research. As faculty members, health education specialists evaluate student work and teach students to

SECTION IV

apply research and evaluation Competencies in their future professional settings. These same health education specialists may also be contracted to serve as evaluators for community projects. They are expected to engage in scholarly endeavors that include research, grant proposal writing, and dissemination of research findings via publications and presentations. These efforts each contribute to the scientific body of knowledge encompassing health behavior, disease prevention, and risk reduction strategies, as well as to the profession of health education.

College/University Health Services Setting. Health education specialists working in the campus health services setting face many of the same issues as those in the business/industry and health care settings. These health education specialists need skills in all facets of research. Evaluative research skills are necessary to determine the efficacy and cost-effectiveness of programs for students, staff members, and faculty members. Health education specialists are expected to communicate findings and solicit feedback from stakeholders. Findings and feedback are incorporated into program/intervention improvement.

Key Terms

Delimitations are decisions made by an evaluator or researcher that ought to be mentioned because they identify the parameters and boundaries set for a study. Examples of delimitations include why some literature is not reviewed, populations are not studied, and certain methods are not used (Cottrell & McKenzie, 2010).

Evaluation assesses a process or program to provide evidence and feedback for the program (Neutens & Rubinson, 2010; Simons-Morton, Greene, & Gottlieb, 1995).

Limitations are phenomena the evaluator or researcher cannot control that place restrictions on methodology and, ultimately, conclusions. Examples of possible limitations might be time, nature of data collection, instruments, sample, and analysis (Cottrell & McKenzie, 2010).

Logic models take a variety of forms but generally depict aspects of a program such as inputs, outputs, and outcomes (Healey & Zimmerman, 2010). They offer a scaled down, somewhat linear, visual depiction of programs.

Research is an organized process using the scientific method generating new knowledge (Issel, 2014).

Reliability refers to the consistency, dependability, and stability of the measurement process (McKenzie et al., 2013).

KEY: no symbol - entry level; ❖ advanced 1; ■ advanced 2

Validity is the degree to which a test or assessment measures what it is intended to measure. Using a valid instrument increases the chance of measuring what was intended (McKenzie et al., 2013).

Variables are operational forms of a construct. They designate how the construct will be measured in designated scenarios (McKenzie et al., 2013).

Unit of Analysis is what or who is being studied or evaluated (the individual, group, organization, or program, etc.) (Babbie, 2012).

Competency 4.1 Develop Evaluation Plan for Health Education/Promotion

An evaluation of health education programs determines their value or worth (McKenzie et al., 2013). Formative evaluation looks at an ongoing process of evaluation from planning through implementation (McKenzie et al., 2013). Process evaluation is any combination of measures that occurs as a program is implemented to assure or improve the quality of performance or delivery. Summative evaluation is often associated with measures or judgments that enable the investigator to draw conclusions from impact and outcome evaluations (McKenzie et al., 2013). Impact evaluation focuses on immediate and observable effects of a program leading to the desired outcomes. Outcome evaluation is focused on the ultimate goal, product, or policy and is often measured in terms of health status, morbidity, and mortality. Employing evaluation procedures that are explicit, formal, and justifiable is desirable for program improvement (McKenzie et al., 2013).

❖ 4.1.1 Determine the purpose and goals of evaluation

There are a multitude of reasons to conduct an evaluation. Ideally, the goal for program evaluation is for program or policy improvement. It is always desirable to select and use evidence-based, effective methods and strategies to plan community health promotion and education programs, so that health education specialists can expect a reasonable level of progress toward goal attainment. Using adequate and appropriate evaluation methods from the outset of any program helps to allow for and encourage improved program results. Health education specialists serving as an evaluator may need to identify or establish goals or general guidelines to explain what is desirable to achieve and then determine measureable objectives related to improved health status, program implementation, accountability to stakeholders, community support, and contribution to the scientific base for community health initiatives which inform policy and program decisions.

❖ 4.1.2 Develop questions to be answered by the evaluation

As health education specialists attempt to explore, explain, or describe ideas about some phenomena, program, or policy, they will find it necessary to develop an appropriate rationale in order to focus the evaluation and/or research (Brownson, Baker, Leet, & Gillespie, 2010) and to craft a meaningful purpose statement that is essential in the development of evaluation questions. A purpose statement (also referred to as statement of purpose) identifies in detail what health education specialists want to learn over the course of an evaluation project. The purpose statement is usually a sentence or two written with specificity and detail. The purpose statement helps to focus and guide efforts involved with data collection and analysis. Well-developed purpose statements guide the selection and/or creation of program goals. Goals are usually long-term and represent a more global vision (i.e., to reduce morbidity or mortality) whereas objectives define measureable strategies used to attain progress toward a goal.

Where program evaluation is concerned, health education specialists serve as evaluators striving to solicit answers to very specific questions that carefully align with the statement of purpose, goals, and objectives of a program. These questions follow an understanding of program operations, intentions, and stakeholders (Patton, 2014). These specially developed questions are called evaluation questions.

Evaluation questions help to establish boundaries for the evaluation by stating what aspects of the program will be addressed (Patton, 2014). Creating evaluation questions encourages stakeholders to reveal what they believe evaluation output should be. Negotiating and prioritizing questions among stakeholders further refines a viable focus. The question development phase also might expose differing stakeholder opinions regarding the best unit of analysis. Clear decisions regarding the questions and corresponding units of analysis are needed in subsequent steps of the evaluation to guide method selection and evidence gathering. Health education specialists use evaluation questions to monitor and measure processes, activities, outputs, and expected outcomes. Process questions help the evaluator understand phenomena, such as internal and external forces that affect program activities. Answers to output and short-term outcome questions help evaluators clearly understand how program activities, products, or associated services relate to or affect changes in behavior, attitudes, knowledge, skills, or the intentions of the participants of a program. Longer-term evaluation questions provide vital links between intervention activities, products and services rendered, and changes in risk factors, morbidity, or mortality. Well-developed evaluation questions provide a guide for selecting appropriate data sources, which in turn help to guide an effective analysis plan (Patton, 2014).

❖ 4.1.3 Create a logic model to guide the evaluation process

A program logic model visually outlines how program components (e.g., resources, activities, and outputs) are linked to outcomes in the form of a simple flow chart. Inputs are the resources, contributions, activities, and other investments that go into a program. Outputs are the activities, services, and products that will reach the participants of a program as a result of carefully leveraging resources through skillful planning. Outcomes are often stepwise and labeled short-term, intermediate, or long-term outcomes. Short-term outcomes – sometimes described as impact – are quantifiable changes in knowledge, skills, and access to resources that happen if planned activities are successfully carried out. Intermediate outcomes are measured in terms of changes in behaviors related to disease or health status and long-term outcomes are measured in terms of fundamental changes in conditions leading to morbidity or mortality (McKenzie et al., 2013). When logic models are used to help guide the evaluation process, they may range from simple to complex (detailed) logic models. Table 4.1 provides an example of a sample logic model template.

KEY: no symbol - entry level; ❖ advanced 1; ■ advanced 2

Table 4.1

Sample Logic Model

Inputs/ resources	Activities	Outputs	Short-term outcomes	Intermediate outcomes	Long-term outcomes
→	→	→	→	→	
Human, fiscal, physical, and intellectual resources needed to address the objectives of a program	With the resources available, the following activities will result in measurable, deliverable services and products	Activities, products and services that will influence short-term outcomes	Changes in knowledge or skills among participants of the program	Changes in behaviors or policy	Changes in morbidity or mortality

❖ 4.1.4 Adapt/modify a logic model to guide the evaluation process

Logic models can be created and used as a dynamic "living and breathing" document, subject to change as evaluators and program specialists identify areas for improvements that will likely ensure better results. When stakeholders, implementers, and evaluators revisit and modify a logic model, all parties agree to changes in processes and expected outcomes.

❖ 4.1.5 Assess needed and available resources to conduct evaluation

Evaluation of all health education programming is desirable, if not essential. Evaluation will provide health education specialists with important insights that can help improve results and outcomes. The feasibility of evaluation depends on the availability of human resources to staff and carry out relevant duties, physical resources such as a place to carry out the business required to conduct the evaluation, fiscal resources that provide the money, in-kind materials, and intellectual resources such as the expert opinions of stakeholders and conclusions from relevant literature. Evaluations conducted with sufficient resources and strong stakeholder support provide feedback on both processes and program outcomes.

Health education specialists considering evaluations should strive for the most rigorous evaluation design that is adequate in terms of observed evaluation standards, including utility, accuracy, and costs in time and resources. Evaluation plans that employ research designs such as randomized control trials, cohort studies, and case control/comparison studies provide a higher level of confidence to the evaluator and stakeholders about the validity of the investigation. Moreover, these designs provide measurable estimates of the probability that effects are due to phenomena that should or should not be attributed to the program. However, evaluation designs vary in cost, dedicated time, and outcomes, and rigorous research designs are not always feasible. Unavoidable compromises in design are often made that jeopardize the validity, accuracy, and utility of the evaluation (CDC, 1999), but are still adequate to answer evaluation questions. At times, cross-sectional, observational, and anecdotal inquiries are more feasible than more rigorous designs and can provide less expensive yet useful information.

❖ 4.1.6 Determine the types of data (for example, qualitative, quantitative) to be collected

At times, health education specialists will find secondary data, or data collected for other purposes, most feasible for answering evaluation questions. Sometimes secondary data is less intrusive to use for measuring differences in phenomena (e.g., emergency room or law enforcement records) than constructing new instruments to gather primary data on their own, especially where quantitative analysis can be used.

However, both quantitative and qualitative evaluations are used within the field of health education, and both types of evaluation have practical applications for health education specialists. Quantitative methodology focuses on quantifying, or measuring, things related to health education programs (Jack, Jr. et al., 2010) through the use of numerical data to help describe, explain, or predict phenomena (Baumgartner & Hensley, 2012). Qualitative methodology is descriptive in nature and attempts to discover meaning or interpret why phenomena are occurring (Baumgartner & Hensley, 2012). Health education specialists use both applications to obtain a deeper understanding of the program and its participants.

Often, it is advantageous to use a mixed methods approach for data collection to "tell the story" and describe classifications (e.g., how many or how much) as well as to indicate why a phenomenon is occurring within a population. Doing so helps health education specialists make sound recommendations for future programming and may help introduce new hypotheses for future evaluation and research purposes. Both advanced-level and entry-level health education specialists are responsible for assessing the merits and limitations of qualitative and quantitative data collection for evaluation.

❖ 4.1.7 Select a model for evaluation

Evaluation plans are often facilitated using concepts from discipline specific evaluation models, such as those described in Table 4.2: Attainment, Decision-Making, Goal-Free, Naturalistic, Systems Analysis, and Utilization-focused (Neutens & Rubinson, 2010; Patton, 2008). It is important to consider which models will work best for a particular situation and whether evaluation approaches should be combined or used individually. Models help evaluators make data collection and analysis decisions (Neutens & Rubinson, 2010; Patton, 2008).

KEY: no symbol - entry level; ❖ advanced 1; ■ advanced 2

Table 4.2

Evaluation Model

Attainment	focused on program objectives and the program goals; serve as standards for evaluation
Decision-making	based on four components designed to provide the user with the context, input, processes, and products with which to make decisions
Goal-free	not based on goals; evaluator searches for all outcomes including unintended positive and negative side effects
Naturalistic	focused on qualitative data and uses responsive information from participants in a program; most concerned with narrative explaining "why" behavior did or did not change
Systems analysis	based on efficiency that uses cost benefits or cost effectiveness analysis to quantify effects of a program
Utilization-focused	done for and with a specific population

In addition to evaluation models, evaluation frameworks have been developed to summarize and organize the essential elements of program evaluation. These frameworks provide a platform to perform and monitor evaluations. One such framework is the CDC's six-step framework developed to help guide program evaluation (Figure 4.1). Health education specialists should stay abreast of the availability of notable and commonly used evaluation frameworks. Evaluation standards are used as a guide to manage evaluation processes and assess existing evaluations. The standards outline the considerations that must be weighed in formulating an evaluation design (American Joint Committee on Standards for Educational Evaluation, 2008).

Figure 4.1

CDC Six Step Framework for Program Evaluation

Elements of the Framework

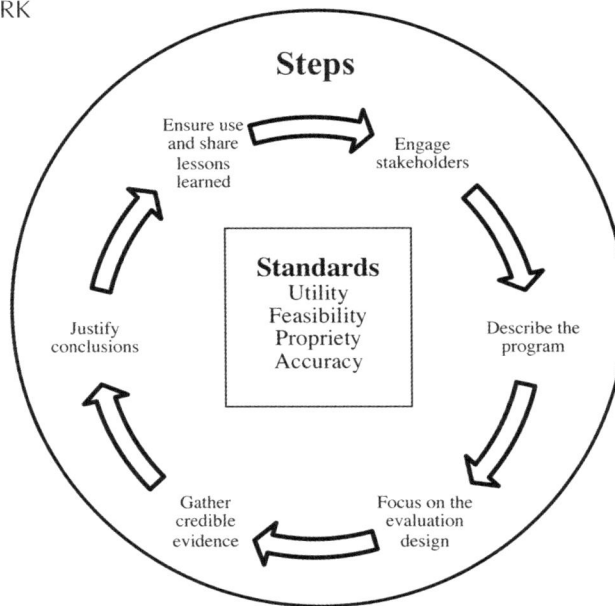

Steps

Ensure use and share lessons learned → Engage stakeholders

Standards
Utility
Feasibility
Propriety
Accuracy

Justify conclusions

Describe the program

Gather credible evidence ← Focus on the evaluation design

Steps in Evaluation Practice	Steps in Evaluation Practice
• **Engage stakeholders** Those involved, those affected, primary intended users • **Describe the program** Need, expected effects, activities, resources, stage, context, logic model • **Focus the evaluation design** Purpose, users, uses, questions, methods, agreements • **Gather credible evidence** Indicators, sources, quality, quantity, logistics • **Justify conclusions** Standards, analysis/synthesis, interpretation, judgment, recommendations • **Ensure use and share lessons learned** Design, preparation, feedback, follow-up, dissemination	• **Utility** Serve the information needs of intended users • **Feasibility** Be realistic, prudent, diplomatic, and frugal • **Propriety** Behave legally, ethically, and with due regard for the welfare of those involved and those affected • **Accuracy** Reveal and convey technically accurate information

Note. Adapted from CDC. Framework for Program Evaluation in Public Health, Centers for Disease Control and Prevention, 1999; 48 (No. RR-11).

KEY: no symbol - entry level; ❖ advanced 1; ■ advanced 2

Research studies are conducted to understand etiologies of health conditions, ascertain effectiveness of programs in terms of stated objectives, explore links between etiologies and interventions, or develop and test new research methods (Brownson et al., 2010). Researchers strive to use robust experimental designs whereby the investigator intentionally alters one or more variables or factors to study the effects of doing so. Experimental designs consist of some form of controlled trial. These trials may be randomized where all clusters or participants in the experiment have an equal chance of being allocated to each group of study. Quasi-randomized studies allocate participation in a study based on some scheme, such as an assigned number, either odd or even. Non-randomized studies do not use random allocation of participation, and groups or individuals are assigned arbitrarily. These non-randomized studies are also termed quasi-experimental studies.

In the absence of an experiment, the investigator may use one of several designs common in health education: a cohort, case control, cross-sectional, or ecological approach (Jack, Jr. et al., 2010). Most research plans include research questions and a list of variables that researchers hope to investigate. Data collection methods should be designed to ensure that they measure the effects on variables of interest and should also match data needs, sample size, and resources. Most data collection decisions are dictated by the study design and the purpose of the inquiry.

Study designs in research tend to fall into two broad categories: descriptive or analytic. Descriptive studies (i.e., cross-sectional) describe the occurrence of disease and disability in terms of person, place, and time using prevalence surveys, surveillance data, and other routinely collected data to describe the phenomena.

Analytic designs explain etiology and causal associations. Analytic studies (i.e., cohort or case control) aim to estimate the strength of a relationship between an exposure and an outcome. Table 4.3 highlights the main differences between descriptive and analytic study designs (Aday & Cornelius, 2006).

Table 4.3
Descriptive and Analytic Study Designs

Descriptive	Analytical
Describes	Explains
Is more exploratory	Is more explanatory
Profiles characteristics of group	Analyzes why a group has characteristics
Focus on *what*	Focuses on *why*
Assumes no hypothesis	Assumes a hypothesis
Requires no comparison group	Requires a comparison group

❖ 4.1.8 Develop data collection procedures for evaluation

Data should be collected in accordance with a well-developed analysis plan and with the evaluation questions and data sources in mind. Evaluation questions should be carefully considered, and decisions about type, amount, and accuracy are critical. Consideration should be given to minimize the direct or indirect burden on participants, as well as other purveyors of secondary sources. Health education specialists should consider the availability of resources, sensitivity to participants, credibility, and importance of the data with regard to stakeholders (W.K. Kellogg Foundation, 2010).

■ 4.1.9 Develop data analysis plan for evaluation

Developing a data analysis plan is a crucial step for evaluation. By creating a data analysis plan for evaluation, the data that has been collected can be integrated and structured in order to ensure understanding and the usefulness of the data to answer evaluation questions. The intended audience, often program personnel or other key stakeholders, may also influence the data analysis plan. Therefore, they may be invited to help develop or create the data analysis plan. The analysis for evaluation depends on the purpose of the evaluation as well as the availability of resources. Analysis depends on the research questions, data sources, and availability, as well as the intended audience who will use the findings. The goal of data analysis is to reduce, synthesize, organize, and summarize information to make sense of it (Fitzpatrick, Sanders, & Worthen, 2010). Analysis determines if outcomes were different than expected. Planning data analysis is a critical step in research (McKenzie et al., 2013). Research that suffers from methodological problems does not inspire confidence regarding the findings. Analysis planning proves helpful in minimizing errors due to inadequate or inappropriate statistical methods. Data analysis planning should begin with the planning of a program and guide data collection decisions. A comprehensive analysis plan identifies items or observations to be used in answering the research question. The analysis plan states the level of measurement for each survey question and states what statistical test(s) and/or descriptive data analysis will be used to answer the research questions (Baumgartener & Hensley, 2012).

❖ 4.1.10 Apply ethical principles to the evaluation process

The health education profession is dedicated to practicing and promoting individual, family, organizational, and community health. Therefore, it is necessary to conduct evaluation with human subjects central to the investigations. An institutional review board (IRB) for universities or community agencies should be consulted to help identify and avoid any possible and unforeseen risks to which participants may be subject. Regardless of job title, work setting, or population served, health education specialists are responsible to the public, the profession, and their employer. They are responsible in their delivery of all aspects of health education, research and evaluation, and professional preparation. With attention to propriety, health education specialists acknowledge the value of diversity in society and embrace a cross-cultural approach. They support the worth, dignity, potential, and uniqueness of all people, and are responsible for upholding the integrity and ethics of the profession. Respect for autonomy, promotion of social justice, active promotion of good, and avoidance of harm is the responsibility of each health education specialist (CNHEO, 2011; Bastida, Tseng, McKeever, & Jack, Jr., 2010).

KEY: no symbol - entry level;   ❖ advanced 1;   ■ advanced 2

Competency 4.2 Develop a Research Plan for Health Education/Promotion

Although there has been much discussion about the differences between evaluation and research, it is sometimes difficult to distinguish between them as methodology is often identical. A major difference between evaluation and research is that research can be conducted with the intent to generalize findings from a sample to a larger population. Research does not always aim for, or achieve, evaluative conclusions, and it is restricted to empirical (rather than evaluative) data. Research bases observed, measured, or calculated conclusions on that empirical data (Jack et al., 2010). On the other hand, the outcomes of evaluation are largely restricted to the report or to inform the population involved and are not generalized to other populations.

■ 4.2.1 Create statement of purpose

A statement of purpose clearly and succinctly defines the goal of the research project (Cottrell & McKenzie, 2010). Elements of a purpose statement include:
- research design (quantitative study) or method of inquiry (qualitative study)
- variables (quantitative study) or phenomena under investigation (qualitative study)
- the priority population
- research setting (e.g., university, worksite, etc.)

■ 4.2.2 Assess feasibility of conducting research

Important factors to consider when gauging the feasibility of a research project include funding, staffing, time constraints, recruitment potential, equipment/material needs, and site permissions.

Before undertaking a new study, the research team should determine how many participants they must recruit to address the objectives of the project or sample size calculations. For quantitative research, this will require calculating a sample size adequate to detect statistically significant effects. Depending on the timeframe of the project and intensity of participant involvement, sample size must account for participant attrition. Prior to planning a large-scale project, researchers should conduct a small scale, pilot study with a less rigorous research design. Often, pilot testing will uncover challenges the research team did not anticipate in their initial planning. Pilot testing will also aid in assessing a project's feasibility. If the research team intends to seek extramural funding, then pilot testing can help establish evidence that a particular line of research merits financial support.

■ 4.2.3 Conduct search for related literature

Conducting literature searches involves identifying a search strategy. Search strategies typically require health education specialists to identify:
- key search terms
- search sources (e.g., online, bibliographic databases such as MEDLINE, etc.)
- a period of time to conduct the search (e.g., 2005 to 2010)
- characteristics of the priority population (e.g., age, race, gender, geographic location) or intervention
- health conditions (e.g., diabetes, obesity, asthma, teenage pregnancy) of interest

In many cases, the topics being searched by health education specialists have already been evaluated or researched with a plethora of published results in the literature.

Health education specialists can avoid a duplication of effort by searching the literature specific to a criterion of interest such as study design, methods, or population. Three methods used to evaluate, critique, and report evidence are detailed below.

- *Systematic reviews*: a published qualitative review of a comprehensive synthesis of publications on particular topics. Often systematic reviews are helpful in identifying current gaps in a stream of literature that can be filled in with new, data-based health education/promotion research.
- *Meta-analyses:* a systematic statistical method of evaluating data based on numerical results of several independent studies of the same problem.
- *Pooled analyses:* a method for collecting all the individual data from a group of studies, combining them into one large set of data, and then analyzing the data as if it came from one big study.

(Brownson et al., 2010)

Given that systematic reviews, meta-analyses, and pooled analyses are not always available, it is sometimes useful to seek out other publications in the literature. In this instance, publications on the topic of interest generated since the most recent reviews or sources that were not included in the most recent reviews may serve as useful resources. Information can be found in indices, abstracts, government documents, and computerized databases. Methods for researching the literature are constantly evolving. Computer databases are widely used because they compile large amounts of information and are easily searched (Cottrell et al., 2014). Databases available today not only catalogue resources but in many cases also provide full text copies of the latest research and evaluation findings. See Sub-competency 6.1.2 for a list of databases for use in finding research.

The Internet makes available a wide array of interactive information and data that can be used by health education specialists; however, not all information found on the Internet should be considered valid and/or reliable (McKenzie et al., 2013). When using the Internet to access information, health education specialists must ensure the information provided by the resource is valid and reliable. Examples of credible sources of health information include research databases, such as MEDLINE, and secondary sources, such as the CDC and Prevention Web site.

As a literature review is conducted, it is important to understand and evaluate published information for accuracy (Cottrell et al., 2014). The eight questions that can be asked when evaluating research in the literature follow.

- Was the purpose of the study stated?
- Was the research question or hypothesis stated?
- Were the subjects in the study described? Did the literature describe participant recruitment?
- Was the design and location of the study described?
- Were the data collection instruments described?
- Did the presented results reflect the research question or hypothesis?
- Were the conclusions reflective of the research design and data analysis?
- Were the implications meaningful to the priority population?

KEY: no symbol - entry level; ❖ advanced 1; ■ advanced 2

■ 4.2.4 Analyze and synthesize information found in the literature

Research findings and results of program evaluations, including current trends and issues, are made available in published literature. Health education specialists strive to provide evidence of effective approaches to health education problems through a synthesis of professional literature. Health education specialists refer to peer-reviewed journals, which publish papers reviewed by experts in the field or in a specific content area (Cottrell et al., 2014). Published findings can provide useful information about successful study design and data collection methods, as well as data analysis and outcome sharing. While published findings and results vary in direct application and often cannot be generalized to other populations and programs, they may be useful in narrowing the breadth of possibilities for programming, policy development, and/or further inquiry. Using published literature appropriately and expeditiously enables health education specialists to conduct their work with the confidence that it is grounded in up-to-date, peer-reviewed science that will help them establish appropriate protocols for new implementations (Brownson et al., 2010).

Equally as important, using appropriate literature will help reduce the burden of unnecessary paper work or duplicate inquiry for individuals involved. Skilled health education specialists search and use literature to save considerable resources by providing guidance and baseline information to minimize duplication of measurement efforts. To that end, it is important for health education specialists to be able to find, evaluate, and explain the literature findings to their clients (Brownson et al., 2010).

■ 4.2.5 Develop research questions and/or hypotheses

A research question is an interrogative statement that reflects the central question the research intends to answer (Cottrell & McKenzie, 2010). Narrow and precisely defined research questions are more amenable to rigorous research than broadly defined research questions (Crosby, DiClemente, & Salazar, 2006). The research question will dictate implicitly whether a quantitative or qualitative research method is most appropriate. The nature of the research question will also reflect the optimal study design for addressing the research question. Quality research questions are developed in such a way that they can be translated into testable statements, called hypotheses. To translate research questions into hypotheses, it is necessary to operationally define the variables under investigation. Operationally defining a variable entails converting the variable into a measurable quantity. For example, physical activity is defined as any bodily movement produced by the skeletal muscles that results in energy expenditure; however, in health education, physical activity for adults may be operationally defined in terms of specific intensity (e.g., moderate), frequency (e.g., five or more days a week), and duration (e.g., at least 20 minutes). A sample hypothesis in this instance may be: "there will be no significant difference in the amount of physical activity participants engage in by the end of the program." In this particular instance, physical activity would be measured in terms of its operational definition of adults engaging in moderately intense physical activity five or more days a week for at least 20 minutes. This operational definition could change if the research was focused on children or the elderly. Consequently, operational definitions are tailored to the purpose of the study (Sharma & Petosa, 2012).

A key feature of a scientific hypothesis is that it must be falsifiable. The concept of falsifiability is represented through the null hypothesis. The null hypothesis is a hypothesis of skepticism, which states there is no relationship between variables. Conversely, an alternative hypothesis claims there is a relationship between variables. An alternative hypothesis may also be directional, for instance, if the research team theorizes a program may reduce or increase the quantity of a targeted behavior. In quantitative research, inferential statistical tests are used to determine if differences or relationships exist between variables. A statistical test is a procedure that when data are fed into it either rejects or fails to reject a null hypothesis.

■ 4.2.6 Assess the merits and limitations of qualitative and quantitative data collection

The primary strengths and limitations of qualitative and quantitative data collection lie within the nature of the data themselves (Sharma & Petosa, 2012). Given that qualitative and quantitative paradigms exist on opposite sides of the research spectrum, the strengths of one tend to be the limitations of the other and vice versa. For instance, a quantitative researcher may be able to identify a statistical relationship between an intervention program and an increase in the number of vegetables participants consumed, but it may not be able to contextualize the participants' experience of vegetable consumption. Major differences between quantitative and qualitative data are provided in the following Table 4.4.

Table 4.4

Differences between Quantitative and Qualitative Data

Attribute	Qualitative Paradigm	Quantitative Paradigm
View	Emic View (Reality is defined by the participants)	Etic view (Evaluator defines the reality)
Perspective	Holistic perspective (Context and values preserved)	Reductionism (Concepts reduced to context free numbers)
Role of the evaluator	Evaluator as an interactive observer	Evaluator is independent
Richness of context	Studying the rich context is encouraged	Parsimony is encouraged (ability of few variables to predict or explain)
Reality	Post positivist (Reality is multiply constructed and multiply interpreted)	Positivist (Reality can be objectively measured)
Purpose	Hypothesis generation	Hypothesis confirmation
Reasoning	Inductive (Specific to general)	Deductive (General to specific)
Design	Dynamic (No set protocol, flexible)	Fixed (Protocol once set is etched in rock)
Technology	People centered	Highly technocentric
Statistics	Not required	Required

Note. Adapted from Sharma, M., & Petosa, R., L. (2012). *Measurement and evaluation for health educators.* Burlington, MA: Jones & Bartlett Learning.

KEY: no symbol - entry level;   ❖ advanced 1;   ■ advanced 2

There are also strengths and limitations in terms of how qualitative and quantitative data are collected. Qualitative researchers, for example, must be careful not to introduce bias if they are using unstructured interviews as a data collection method. Concurrently, quantitative researchers must construct questionnaire items in such a way that the responses produce data that are reliable and valid. It is becoming more common for health education/promotion researchers to collect both qualitative and quantitative data (Perrin, 2014). This approach, called mixed methods research, is believed to produce findings that are more insightful than either approach could produce alone.

■ 4.2.7 Select research design to address the research questions

There are a variety of research designs applied in health education research (Sharma & Petosa, 2012). Often, the research questions the study is attempting to answer will dictate the optimal design. For example, if the researchers are interested in gauging the efficacy of an intervention to change behavior, they will use some variation of an experimental design. If the research team is interested in understanding the experiences of community members living with diabetes, they may want to use qualitative interviews.

In quantitative research, designs are categorized according to the amount of control they permit (Cottrell & McKenzie, 2010). They are presented in the order of least to most rigorous designs. More rigorous designs are more likely to exercise more control over the conditions and subsequently reduce or eliminate influence of extraneous factors, which helps to strengthen internal validity. If a design has high internal validity, then the researcher has more confidence that changes in dependent variables occurred because of the intervention (Crosby, DiClemente, & Salazar, 2006).

- Nonexperimental designs are cross-sectional in nature, and do no seek to manipulate any variables. Instead, these designs attempt to describe features of a priority population. These are the least rigorous designs and do not control for many threats to internal validity.
- Quasi-experimental designs also seek to manipulate at least one independent variable and they may contain a comparison group; however, due to ethical or practical reasons, random assignment of participants does not occur.
- True experimental designs manipulate at least one independent variable and the research participants are randomly assigned to either the experimental or control group arms of the trial. Due to their use of both random assignment and a control group, true experimental designs can control for most threats to internal validity.

If a qualitative design is required, the investigators may use interviews, observational research, case studies, phenomenology, content analysis, ethnography, historical document analysis, or grounded theory to answer their research questions (Perrin, 2014).

■ 4.2.8 Determine suitability of existing data collection instruments

Often health education researchers will use previously developed instruments to collect data. To determine the suitability of existing questionnaires, the researchers must determine if the questionnaire has adequate psychometric properties and if the questionnaire was developed in a population with similar demographic features (Sharma & Petosa, 2012). If not, the instrument may not be suitable.

When determining the suitability of existing data collection instruments, Kimberlin and Winterstein (2008) recommend addressing the following questions:

1. Do instruments already exist that measure a construct the same way or very similar to the one you wish to measure?
2. How well do the constructs in the instruments you have identified match the construct you have conceptually defined for your study?
3. Is the evidence of reliability and validity well established?
4. In previous research, was there variability in scores with no floor or ceiling effects?
5. If the measure is to be used to evaluate health outcomes, effects of interventions, or changes over time, are there studies that establish the instrument's responsiveness to change in the construct of interest?
6. Is the instrument in the public domain?
7. How expensive is it to use the instrument?
8. How much training is required to administer the instrument?
9. Will the instrument be acceptable to subjects?

■ 4.2.9 Identify research participants

Health education specialists/promotion researchers should consider the population and sample for their research. They must develop inclusion and exclusion criteria that will restrict participant enrollment to the population they wish to prioritize (Sharma & Petosa, 2012). For example, if the research team is seeking to study the effects of a health education/promotion tobacco cessation program, they may wish to limit enrollment in their intervention only to those adults who are current tobacco users. In such a case, the research team must determine what criteria are necessary to accurately screen participants for inclusion, as well as clearly define what constitutes a "current tobacco user." Ideally, researchers will develop inclusion criteria based on the literature and/or epidemiologically defined populations (Crosby, DiClemente, & Salazar, 2006). A variety of methods including self-report questionnaire, medical records, and physiological indices can determine if participants meet a study's inclusion criteria.

■ 4.2.10 Develop sampling plan to select participants

The goal of sampling is to select participants in such a way that research participants represent the population of interest (Cottrell & McKenzie, 2010). When this occurs, it is far more likely the values obtained from the sampled participants will be generalizable to the population of interest. When this does not occur, there is a greater risk for sampling error, which occurs when there is a difference between the observed value of a sample statistics (e.g., mean minutes of physical activity achieved by the sample) and the true value of the population parameter (e.g., actual minutes of physical activity achieved by the population of interest).

The first step in sample planning is to determine the unit of analysis the research team will target (Crosby, DiClemente, & Salazar, 2006). Units of analyses, or sampling elements, consist of either individuals or groups. Next, the research team must identify an appropriate sampling frame. A sampling frame is an accessible list of people or groups that represent the population of interest. For example, if the research team is testing a school-based health education program, they may compile a list of all

KEY: no symbol - entry level;   ❖ advanced 1;   ■ advanced 2

schools within a district from which to sample. Ideally, a sampling frame list will include all possible elements in a population; however, the existence of an exhaustive sampling frame is rarely available. For instance, if a research team wants to conduct a home-based obesity prevention research study, they may determine a telephone directory is the most exhaustive sampling frame from which to recruit participants. However, this sampling frame will not represent individuals with unlisted numbers and those who recently moved to the area (Crosby, DiClemente, & Salazar, 2006). Due to laws that protect individual privacy, it is often easier to achieve more exhaustive sampling frames when the sampling element is defined by groups rather than people (Crosby, DiClemente, & Salazar, 2006). Organizations such as churches, health agencies, schools, and neighborhood organizations often have public records of their existence or intentionally advertise their existence. If the sampling frame comprises individuals, accessibility to the sampling frame must be evaluated.

Once a sampling frame is identified, the research team must select an appropriate sampling technique. Ideally, the selected sampling technique will maximize the representativeness of the sample with respect to the sampling frame and, ultimately, the population that the sampling frame represents. As with most research methods, the more rigorous the sampling technique applied, the more resources and time are required. Thus, the research team must weigh rigidity against practicality.

There are two categories of sampling techniques: probability and non-probability sampling. Both sampling techniques have strengths and limitations (Sharma & Petosa, 2012). Probability sampling techniques are those methods in which each member of the priority population has a known chance, or probability, of being selected. Probability sampling makes use of random selection, which reduces the chance of sampling bias. Several types of probability sampling methods exist, including simple random sampling, systematic random sampling, stratified random sampling, cluster sampling, multistage cluster sampling, and stratified multistage cluster sampling. Unit of analysis and sampling frame accessibility will dictate the most appropriate probability sampling method. For example, if individuals are the unit of analysis, simple random sampling may be most appropriate. If the unit of analysis includes all public schools within the state of Nevada, multistage cluster sampling may be the optimal sampling method.

Non-probability sampling recruits sampling frames that are readily accessible to the research team (Sharma & Petosa, 2012). With non-probability samples, not all units from the priority population have an equal chance of being selected, and thus their representativeness to the population is unknown. Types of non-probability sampling techniques include convenience, purposive, quota, and network sampling. Non-probability samples are often used in health education/promotion research as they are easier and less expensive to obtain. For instance, if a health education research team is studying the health behaviors of college students, they may sample from classrooms that are readily accessible to them. An obvious limitation to such an approach is that the researchers cannot claim their findings are representative of all colleges or even to all students in their specific university. The findings are limited only to those students who were sampled.

■ 4.2.11 Develop data collection procedures for research

Developing clear and precise protocols for collecting data is an essential part of the research process (Sharma & Petosa, 2012). This is particularly true if several individuals will be responsible for collecting data. Data collection procedures often center on ensuring bias is not introduced into the study. For example, when explaining the purpose of a self-report questionnaire to participants, researchers should stay neutral as to not prompt participants to respond in a way the researchers would find favorable. In such a scenario, it is beneficial for the researchers to develop a script that all individuals involved in data collection will read to participants. As another illustration, if height and weight data are collected for calculating body mass index, the research team will want to ensure they are using consistent measurement procedures for all participants. One way to aid this process is to develop a set of standardized checklists that the research team can use as they collect data from participants. For instance, a qualitative research team may want to give precise directions for transcribing participant responses. An additional issue for consideration is how the data will be stored post collection to ensure participant privacy. The research team may state that as they collect completed questionnaires, they will be stored in a locked file cabinet for safekeeping.

An additional factor to consider is whether the data collection method is practical for the population of interest. For instance, when researching the behaviors of young children, self-report is unlikely to be accurate. Elderly individuals may not be able to read questionnaires with traditional font sizes. For such individuals, structured interviews may be more suitable. Ideally, the data collection procedures should be tested in the priority population prior to full scale implementation of the research project.

■ 4.2.12 Develop data analysis plan for research

A critical first step in developing a data analysis plan is developing a data management plan. A data management plan is a set of procedures for determining how the data will be transferred from the instruments used in the research to the data analysis software. Data entry is tedious and errors can occur (Sharma & Petosa, 2012). When dealing with large data sets, it is often helpful to have two or more people independently enter the data into separate spreadsheets. Next, a cross analysis can be conducted whereby descriptive statistics are run on the independent data sets and compared for accuracy. Another important part of the data analysis plan is specifying data cleaning procedures. For example, this might include determining how the data will be coded and how outliers and missing values will be handled (Sharma & Petosa, 2012). Next, the research team must consider how they will describe the sample. Descriptive statistics can be presented as frequency distributions (e.g., percentages), measures of central tendency (e.g., mean values), and measures of variation (e.g., range). Often, descriptive statistics are presented in tables to make the data more digestible to the consumers of the research. Next, the research team should determine which statistical tests they will use to evaluate the research hypotheses. Common inferential statistical tests include analysis of variance and multiple regression analysis. Often, the level of measurement of the variables will determine the appropriate test to apply. When planning for data analysis, it is desirable to collect data using the highest level of

KEY: no symbol - entry level;   ❖ advanced 1;   ■ advanced 2

measurement possible (Sharma & Petosa, 2012). In addition to testing statistical significance, it is becoming increasingly important to report the practical significance of findings. Practical significance is gauged by effect size. Effect sizes quantify the magnitude of the relationship between variables (Crosby, DiClemente, & Salazar, 2006). The type of statistical inferential test performed will dictate the appropriate effect size statistic to use. Interpretation of the selected effect size statistic should be guided by the literature.

■ 4.2.13 Develop a plan for non-respondent follow-up

Inevitably, some participants will drop out of the research study. This can happen for several reasons, but is more likely to occur in studies that are longer in duration. Understanding why participants drop out of a program can help determine if those who completed the full study differed in some important way from those who did not complete the full study. This is particularly important for establishing a study's validity. There are a variety of strategies for handling non-respondent follow-up. The first step is to determine how much nonresponse is allowable. Often, researchers will inflate the total sample size they require to detect statistical effects to account for assumed participant attrition (Sharma & Petosa, 2012). By convention, a 20% attrition rate is often applied in health education/promotion research; however, this standard can be higher or lower, and the literature should guide inflation rates. In addition to using inflation, the research team should develop a plan to recover participants lost to follow-up. For example, the research team may plan to contact nonresponsive participants three times before giving up. If contact is established, and the participants still cannot be recovered, then the research team should attempt to uncover why the participant dropped out as this information may provide invaluable insight into the structure of the study. For instance, if the research team is testing an online health education intervention and participants find the Web site confusing, they may become frustrated and drop out of the study. Knowing this information would be invaluable to the research team. Determining how the missing data will be analyzed is another important step for handling participants lost to follow-up. There is an assortment of statistical software packages that can attempt to model missing data. Modeling missing data is important as it can uncover patterns in the missing data. If patterns are identified, it may be possible to predict how the participants would have responded using techniques such as multiple imputation analysis.

■ 4.2.14 Apply ethical principles to the research process

The majority of ethical principles surrounding the research process will center on data integrity. Researchers must ensure participant confidentiality is maintained and that institutional guidelines are followed as approved. The planning stage is also the appropriate time to determine the level of significance that will be applied when testing the research hypotheses. By convention, a significance value of 0.05 is used in health education/promotion research (Sharma & Petosa, 2012). However, more stringent or relaxed significance values may be applied, depending on the scope of the project. Significance values must be decided a priori, or before implementation of the research, to follow ethical guidelines of research. Adjusting significance values *post hoc*, or after the fact, can be considered a violation of research ethics. Additional ethical issues that are best determined during the planning stage concern authorship and least publishable units. Prior to initiating the research process, it behooves the research team to determine how authorship will be granted, as well as the order of authorship on subsequent publications. Failing to address these issues at the outset of the research project can lead to ethical dilemmas. Specifying how to present the findings of the research is another issue that should be determined during the initial stages of research planning. Researchers must carefully consider if they will publish in least publishable units, or the minimal amount of information that can generate a peer-reviewed publication. This type of publishing occurs when data are published incrementally as opposed to simultaneously (Karlsson & Beaufils, 2013). There are instances in which this practice may be beneficial; however, "salami publishing," as it is frequently called, can fragment the literature and compromise the legitimacy of significance testing (Karlsson & Beaufils, 2013).

Competency 4.3 Select, Adapt and/or Create Instruments to Collect Data

Data gathering instruments are used for both quantitative and qualitative data collection methods. Prior to developing data gathering instruments, researchers consider the type of data collection that is going to occur. Common data collection strategies include face-to-face surveys, telephone surveys, self-administered surveys, traditional mail-in surveys, and electronic platforms (e.g., Survey Monkey) (Johnson & Turner, 2010). Data collection instruments are designed to answer questions that are being asked by the evaluator or researcher (McDermott & Sarvela, 1999). Each of the various data collection instruments available has advantages and disadvantages, and the choice of an instrument depends on priority, the population under investigation, and the resources of those trying to collect data (McDermott & Sarvela, 1999).

■ 4.3.1 Identify existing data collection instruments

An important initial step in data collection is to identify types and sources of data that will be useful in answering research/evaluation questions. Depending on the goals and objectives set by health education specialists, a variety of methods can be used to gather data (Cottrell et al., 2009). Health education specialists may choose to use existing data collection tools. Once the evaluation/research questions are established, the evaluator or researcher should consider relevant existing data and use instruments already in existence, when appropriate. A myriad of data collection instruments exists for both qualitative and qualitative inquiry. Many instruments have been validated and tested for reliability and used repeatedly by national, state, and local health surveillance programs as well as some parallel ongoing programs or inquiries. Health education specialists should be familiar with the existing instruments commonly used in the field. Table 4.5 below provides basic information about these surveys.

KEY: no symbol - entry level; ❖ advanced 1; ■ advanced 2

Table 4.5

Health Surveillance Programs

Behavioral Risk Factor Surveillance Survey (BRFSS) http://www.cdc.gov/brfss/index.htm	Telephone surveys that collect state data from United States adults regarding their health-related risk behaviors, chronic health conditions, and use of preventive services. BRFSS collects data in all 50 states, as well as the District of Columbia and three United States territories.
Youth Risk Behavioral Surveillance System (YRBSS) http://www.cdc.gov/healthyyouth/yrbs/index.htm	Telephone survey of youth and young adults about behaviors leading to violence, tobacco use, alcohol and other drug use, inadequate physical activity, unhealthy diet, and sexual behavior.
National Youth Tobacco Survey (NYTS) http://www.cdc.gov/tobacco/data_statistics/surveys/nyts/index.htm	National survey of middle and high school youth's tobacco-related beliefs, attitudes, behaviors, and exposure to pro- and anti-tobacco influences.
National Health and Nutrition Examination Survey (NHANES) http://www.cdc.gov/nchs/nhanes.htm	A series of studies that assess the health and nutritional status of adults and children in the United States. The survey collects both interviews and physical examinations.
National Health Interview Survey http://www.cdc.gov/nchs/nhis.htm	The survey monitors the health of the United States population through the collection and analysis of data on a broad range of health topics.

Program evaluation often focuses on an internal situation, such as collecting data about specific programs, with no intent to generalize the results to other settings and situations. Program evaluations are often conducted using existing data collection instruments. However, using an instrument that has been developed by someone else for among different populations in different places and at different times can introduce a level of internal bias that may be problematic. The evaluator should review existing instruments thoroughly and be sure that each item is appropriate and adequately examines **variables** of interest. Evaluators should be certain there are no extraneous items on instruments that are not relevant to the intent of the evaluation. They should be sure that the language is clear and appropriate for the population to which the instrument will be administered, as well as sure that the instrument has been tested for validity and **reliability**. Finally, existing instruments should be pilot tested with a sample population before use for evaluation purposes (Trochim & Donnelly, 2008).

■ 4.3.2 Adapt/modify existing data collection instruments

Developing data collection instruments can be arduous and time consuming. In many social service sectors existing data collection instruments may be used or adapted to suit the needs of the evaluator/researcher. Depending on the respondent and method of data, collection instruments should be tested for literacy reading level. A Simple Measure of Goobledygook (SMOG) test should be performed to ensure validity of responses (Journal of the National Area Health Education Center [AHEC] Organization, 2010).

It can be advantageous to adapt or modify existing data collection instruments to be used effectively with new scenarios. Some advantages include previously tested reliability, direct comparison measures, reduced costs as compared to the creation of new instruments, and user familiarity. One caveat to using previously developed instruments is that while the items on the instrument may have been extensively tested for reliability, there still exists the potential for unreliable measures given different population demographics and situations.

It is common for health education specialists to create new items, and therefore instruments to be used for data collection, especially with regard to program activities, outputs, and short-term outcomes. These may include survey questions, behavior assessment items, and interview questions/guides for face-to-face interviews or focus groups, among others (Baker, Crawford, & Swineheart, 2004; Saris, van der Veld, & Gallhofer, 2004). Regardless of the method selected, it is the role of health education specialists to ensure the reliability and validity of the data collection instrument (Jack, Jr. et al., 2010).

■ 4.3.3 Create new data collection instruments

When preparing a new data collection instrument for research or evaluation, the developer should do the following:

- Write an easy to understand and complete introduction to the instrument
- Ask only questions that provide useful information in accordance with a well-developed analysis plan
- Ask the most important questions first (demographic questions last)
- Organize the questions in logical order
- Use plain, easy-to-understand language
- Avoid technical terms, jargon and acronyms
- Use an even number of responses
- Randomize the order of the response choices;
- Avoid unnecessary graphics
- Be sensitive to the feelings of respondents
- Thank respondents
- Keep it as short as possible

KEY: no symbol - entry level;   ❖ advanced 1;   ■ advanced 2

4.3.4 Identify useable items from existing instruments

Existing instruments are useful for investigating similar variables in contextually different investigations. It is not always appropriate to use the entire instrument; however, it may make sense to use previously tested, reliable items selected from them. It is imperative that scales and other aspects of the item be retained to maintain validity, especially for research studies. The developer of the instrument can provide information to help ascertain validity and reliability information. Before using items from an existing instrument, it is important to consider:

- If the item is appropriate for the intended purpose
- If the language appropriate for the population
- Whether a test has been performed using a sample from the intended population
- To whom you should give credit for using the item

4.3.5 Adapt/modify existing items

At times, it is appropriate to make modifications to the content, format, or presentation of any part of a question, questionnaire, or instrument. The purpose of adaptation is to better fit the needs of a new population, location, or language (Harkness, 2008). Often questions are modified that have been used for other evaluations, and then these modified versions are used. Changes are often associated with adapting to data needs and often result in a more versatile, useful instrument (Hyman, Lamb, & Bulmer 2006).

At times, items and survey instruments are deliberately modified. As with longitudinal inquiry, wording might be adapted/updated to reflect current nomenclature, for instance "American Indian" may have been replaced with "Native American." Word choice might also be changed to reflect current social realities, such as adding "Facebook" as an information source in media usage questions. Modifications might also be made to accommodate new populations. Modifications might include vocabulary, updates in evidence or science, presentation style, and instructions to suit a child population rather than an adult one. Regarding multicultural projects, modification and adaptation is often related to the need to translate a questionnaire into another language in order to study new populations.

■ 4.3.6 Create new items to be used in data collection

Evaluators must decide whether items developed for quantitative methods, qualitative methods, or mixed methods will be appropriate and adequate to answer the evaluation or research questions for the program. When quantitative, closed-ended items are indicated, respondents make selections that represent their knowledge, attitude, or self-reported behavior from predetermined lists, scales, or categories. It is good practice for the evaluator to acknowledge that survey recipients may have a variety of backgrounds. Respondents should be able to clearly understand the purpose of the question items; therefore, it is best to use simple language. When the question requires respondents to use a rating scale, it is best to mediate the scale so there is room for both extremes. At times it may be helpful to relax grammatical standards if the questions sound too formal. There are several phenomena to avoid:

- Assumptions that everyone has a common basis of knowledge
- Abbreviations

- Leading questions that demand a specific response
- Questions that use two negative words
- Long lists of choices
- Recall questions over extended time frames

(Saris et al., 2004)

By contrast, open-ended items solicit written or verbal responses to items that cannot be adequately answered with a single word or phrase. Careful composition of qualitative items is as important as with the preparation of quantitative items. Evaluators ask fewer carefully crafted items that require people to respond freely. When composing qualitative items, the same rules apply as with quantitative items, but evaluators must also be sure the questions provoke respondents to provide insightful information. As with quantitative item development, there are several phenomena to avoid:

- Asking a "yes/no" question or those that invite a specific (and often brief) answer
- Being too broad to capture useful information
- Being too specific with probing items
- Asking too many questions

(Saris et al., 2004)

Investigators use the findings from research to test hypotheses concerning specific variables established in the planning phases for research plans. They will have determined why they intend to ask the question in accordance with the purpose of the study and research questions. In general, the same rules apply to the development of instrument items for evaluation as for research. Researchers should use language familiar to their audience. Education level, age, and other relevant cultural characteristics should be taken into account. Items will vary according to the type of information solicited. As with evaluation, there are two basic types of instrument items: open-ended and closed-ended. Open-ended items provide qualitative information that participants offer in their own words and provide descriptive information. Closed-ended items require participants to choose a response predetermined by the researcher; these responses may be multiple choice, categorical, Likert-scale, ordinal, or numerical.

■ 4.3.7 Pilot test data collection instrument

The pilot test seeks to answer the question: does the instrument consistently measure whatever it should measure? Reliability can be established using a pilot test by collecting data from sample subjects not included in intervention. With the pilot study complete, researchers and evaluators can be assured that the data they collect will provide consistent measures and give credibility to the validity of outcomes.

■ 4.3.8 Establish validity of data collection instruments

Data collection instruments gather data that will describe, explain, and explore a priority population in a uniform or standardized fashion. When considering an instrument's validity, the researcher should consider content, criterion, and construct validity (Jack, Jr. et al., 2010). Content, or face, validity considers the instrument's items of measurement for the relevant areas of interest. Review of an instrument by topical experts or researchers could be a method to assess content validity. Criterion validity refers to a measure's correlation to another measure of a variable. Construct validity ensures

KEY: no symbol - entry level; ❖ advanced 1; ■ advanced 2

that the concepts of an instrument relate to the concepts of a particular theory (Jack, Jr. et al., 2010). Data gathering processes and instruments should be pilot tested to ensure they are correctly measuring the concepts under investigation (Brownson et al., 2010).

■ 4.3.9 Ensure that data collection instruments generate reliable data

It is desirable to for researchers and evaluators to know that the data gathering tools they use are reliable. The reliability of a data collection instrument can be assured by carrying out a pilot test. Reliability indicates the accuracy or precision of the measuring instrument. Reliability is an issue of concern for observational data collection, as well as with data gathering instruments (Simons-Morton et al., 1995). Specific procedures are performed to estimate instrument reliability among data gathering instruments. Internal consistency considers intercorrelations among items within an instrument. Selecting a reliability test such as internal consistency, test-retest, split half, and alternate form depends on the nature of data (i.e., nominal, ordinal, interval/ratio). To assess the reliability of questions measured on an interval/ratio scale, researchers should use internal consistency. To assess reliability of knowledge questions, researchers should use test-retest or split-half.

Data from the pilot test is analyzed with statistical software (i.e., Statistical Package for Social Science [SPSS], Statistical Analysis System [SAS]), which can provide two important pieces of reliability information: "correlation matrix" and "view alpha if item deleted" column. Analysts can delete items that substantially improve reliability and still preserve content, as long as they delete no more than 20% of the items. The reliability coefficient (alpha) can range from 0 to 1, with 0 representing an instrument with full of error and 1 representing total absence of error. A reliability coefficient (alpha) of .70 or higher is considered acceptable reliability.

Test-retest reliability considers evidence of stability over time. Rater reliability considers differences among scorers of items and controls for variation due to error introduced by rater perceptions (McKenzie et al., 2013).

■ 4.3.10 Ensure fairness of data collection instruments (for example, reduce bias, use language appropriate to priority population)

Existing data collection instruments should be reviewed thoroughly, and each item should appropriately and adequately examine variables of interest. Researchers should be certain to exclude extraneous items that are not associated with the intent of the research. As with critiquing instruments for evaluation, evaluators should be sure that the language is clear and appropriate for the population to whom the instrument will be administered. This could be assessed in the piloting of instruments. In addition, health education specialists should be sure that the instrument has been tested for validity and reliability, and that it has been pilot tested with a similar sample population before being used (Baumgartener & Hensley, 2006; Jack et al., 2010).

Competency 4.4: Collect and Manage Data

Once the data gathering instruments have been developed and reviewed, health education specialists carry out the evaluation or research plan. The plan may be simple or advanced, depending on intended uses and the needs of the program, as well as the expectations of the program planners, funding agencies, and end users (Cottrell et al., 2014). It is usually desirable to utilize the most rigorous evaluation model or research design available. However, ethics, cost, and political and resource realities sometimes indicate a lesser approach to evaluation and research designs. Fortunately, these less rigorous approaches and designs are feasible and adequate to answer some evaluation/research questions when precision might not be as valuable. The evaluator is always professionally and ethically bound to provide the most rigorous design and scientifically sound data information to the audience of interest.

■ 4.4.1 Train data collectors involved in evaluation and/or research

Data that has been collected is subject to a variety of bias and error. Controlling for researcher bias can be accomplished in part by making sure that trained specialists collect all data. Health education specialists should provide data collectors with clear instructions on how to use instruments and to conduct interviews, focus groups, and other data collection activities. The following steps help reduce error in findings that may be due to issues regarding inter-rater reliability.

1. Walk through the instrument with data collectors to point out specific instructions.
2. Provide an example of a completed instrument or interview transcript for data collectors.
3. Provide clear instructions and/or a script (for phone surveys or interviews) for data collectors to follow.
4. Allow data collectors to practice with a "standard" data set or example to make sure everyone is getting the same answers, when consistency is desirable.
5. Allow interviewers and focus group facilitators to practice in a "role play."
6. Give feedback to them or offer fidelity checks to improve their methods.

■ 4.4.2 Collect data based on the evaluation or research plan

It is important to formally map each piece of data collected to the analytic plan or reporting requirements and make sure that the data collection will supply everything needed. At times, it seems reasonable to collect as much data as possible, but more is not usually better. When searching for intriguing new discoveries unrelated to the research or evaluation questions, researchers focusing on extraneous data find it is extra work to extract and manage that data, and that ultimately the extraneous data produces spurious, undesirable results and associations. Yet another reason to avoid collecting too much data is that trying to manage too many data elements makes it easy to overlook tiny critical errors in the most important data.

4.4.3 Monitor and manage data collection

Data are used to investigate or track progress toward one or more program objectives. Data can also be used to assess the effectiveness of organizations, services, programs, and policy. Data collection must be carefully monitored and managed to ensure optimal utility. Prior to the administration of data collection instruments, health education specialists should decide about incentives for participants, respondents as proxies for other people, acceptable response rates, and what documentation or

KEY: no symbol - entry level;   ❖ advanced 1;   ■ advanced 2

information should be provided to the respondent. Field procedures for carrying out data collection include protocols for scheduling initial contacts with respondents, introducing the instrument to the respondent, keeping track of individuals contacted, and following up with non-respondents when appropriate. Data should be organized in such a manner that they may be analyzed to interpret findings. It often requires statistical understanding and extensive training in order to get optimal use from the collected data. Data collectors should follow all protocols and engage quality control measures when necessary to assure usability of the data collected. Computer assisted data collection requires up-front effort, but can greatly expedite data collection, monitoring, and quality control. It is important that all data are carefully coded and organized into a useable format (McKenzie et al., 2013). Research and evaluation data can help not only to record what changes have occurred, but also to identify what led to those changes (Aday & Cornelius, 2006).

4.4.4 Use available technology to collect, monitor, and manage data

Managing data is an integral part of the research/evaluation process. How the data are managed depends on the type of data, how the data are collected, and how the data are used throughout the project lifecycle? Effective data management helps the researcher/evaluator organize files and data for access and analysis. It helps ensure the quality of research and supports the published results of said research. It is common today to use Web-based computer platforms and programs to collect data.

It is becoming increasingly popular to use online survey platforms to collect and manage evaluation and research data. Electronic data collection is a relatively new technique that has both strengths and limitations. Two strengths of this method are its cost-effectiveness and reach potential (Cottrell & McKenzie, 2010). Web-based data collection also offers convenience to participants as they can complete the survey at a time that is best for them. From a monitoring perspective, most survey software will allow the evaluators to download the responses and import them directly into statistical software. In doing so, the risk of data entry errors from transcribing data from paper-and-pencil surveys into statistical software is dramatically reduced.

Despite its strengths, electronic data collection has several shortcomings. In general, online surveys are known to have lower response rates compared to other survey delivery systems (Cottrell & McKenzie, 2010). This is likely due to the perception that participants view e-mails from unknown sources as spam, or "junk" e-mail. For example, if the research team is using online surveys to collect data from a sampling frame (e.g., electronic mailing lists) that has no knowledge of the importance of the topic, then the evaluation team should expect a low response rate.

Due to the reach potential of this vehicle, people are becoming inundated with requests to complete surveys. Subsequently, unless respondents perceive value in the survey, they are unlikely to complete it. Online surveys generally work better for participants that are already recruited into a study and have been trained to use the software.

When determining whether or not to use online surveys, the evaluation team should also consider the audience's computer literacy and accessibility to high-speed Internet. If participants are not familiar with how to use a computer, online surveys may not be the optimal way to collect data. This may also be an issue if researchers are collecting data in communities that have limited access to the Internet or only have dial-up Internet.

In terms of managing electronic data, it should be noted that online platforms are susceptible to server crashes, as well as hackers. Hackers are individuals that "break into" servers to steal data. It would behoove evaluators using commercial survey companies to investigate the security of the vendor of the platform they are considering. Additionally, the evaluation team should routinely check and download the data to ensure its integrity.

4.4.5 Comply with laws and regulations when collecting, storing, and protecting participant data

When planning and conducting research or evaluation, health education specialists do so in accordance with federal and state laws and regulations, organizational and institutional policies, and professional standards. The CNHEO provides health education specialists engaged in research or evaluation guidelines for ethical behavior in Article V of the Code of Ethics for the Health Education Profession. Article V outlines health education specialists' responsibility in research and evaluation (CNHEO, 1999). See Sections 1-7 of the CNHEO Article V below:

Section 1: Health Educators support the right of individuals to make informed decisions regarding their health, as long as such decisions pose no risk to the health of others.

Section 2: Health Educators encourage actions and social policies that promote maximizing health benefits and eliminating or minimizing preventable risks and disparities for all affected parties.

Section 3: Health Educators accurately communicate the potential benefits, risks and/or consequences associated with the services and programs that they provide.

Section 4: Health Educators accept the responsibility to act on issues that can affect the health of individuals, families, groups and communities.

Section 5: Health Educators are truthful about their qualifications and the limitations of their education, expertise and experience in providing services consistent with their respective level of professional competence.

Section 6: Health Educators are ethically bound to respect, assure, and protect the privacy, confidentiality, and dignity of individuals.

Section 7: Health Educators actively involve individuals, groups, and communities in the entire educational process in an effort to maximize the understanding and personal responsibilities of those who may be affected.

Section 8: Health Educators respect and acknowledge the rights of others to hold diverse values, attitudes, and opinions.

(CNHEO, 2011)

Human subjects' protection establishes a standard for ethics, and details can be found in the Belmont Report (National Commission for the Protection of Human Subjects of Biomedical and Behavioral Research, 1979). This report summarizes the basic ethical principles and guidelines for the protection

KEY: no symbol - entry level;   ❖ advanced 1;   ■ advanced 2

of human subjects of research. Not all health education specialists will conduct research, but all health education specialists should recognize the fundamental concepts for human subjects' protection: respect for persons, beneficence, and justice.

Health education specialists conducting research will be required to obtain informed consent. The informed consent is designed to allow participants to choose what will or will not happen to them, and the informed consent is signed by participants to indicate their choice. Informed consent includes the following information:

- Nature and purpose of the program
- Any inherent risks or dangers associated with participation in the program
- Any possible discomfort that may be experienced from participation in the program
- Expected benefits of participation
- Alternative programs or procedures that would accomplish the same results
- Option of discontinuing participation at any time
  (National Commission for the Protection of Human Subjects of Biomedical and Behavioral Research, 1979)

Furthermore, in accordance with the Paperwork Reduction Act of 1980, it is unethical for health education specialists and any federal agency to seek information from populations irrelevant to a specific research or evaluation program. Health education specialists should focus all data collection on carefully designed research/evaluation questions. They also should refrain from collecting data at intervals too close together to show meaningful measures and all quantitative data involving dichotomous or ordinal data should not be gathered in qualitative format.

Institutions, such as universities and hospitals, involved in conducting research that includes human subjects are required to establish an IRB. The IRB functions to protect human subjects involved in research (Neutens & Rubinson, 2010). Since evaluations may have similar ethical considerations, an IRB review and approval is often desired or required prior to data collection (McKenzie et al., 2013). An IRB is at times referred to as an independent ethics committee, or a committee that has been formally designated to approve, monitor, and review biomedical and behavioral research involving humans. This type of monitoring and oversight is designed to protect the rights and welfare of the research participants. An IRB performs critical oversight functions for research conducted on human subjects that are scientific, ethical, and regulatory.

Special attention should be given to legal issues that will affect data sharing with regard to Health Insurance Portability and Accountability Act (HIPAA) laws (PL 104-102), informed consent, and commitments to confidentiality (McKenzie et al., 2013). The HIPAA "Privacy Rule" establishes conditions when protected health information may be used for research or program evaluation. Under the Privacy Rule, investigators are permitted information for research with individual authorization or for limited circumstances without individual authorization (CDC, 2003b).

SECTION IV

Competency 4.5: Analyze Data

Health education specialists with advanced degrees often collect, analyze, and interpret data. The research/ evaluation questions and the level of measurement of the data, whether for evaluation or research purposes, should guide data analysis. Expert consultants in qualitative or quantitative data analysis can guide the process if the research/evaluation questions are complex, or if the health education specialist is unfamiliar with the specific analysis tool or software.

■ 4.5.1 Prepare data for analysis

Preparing data for analysis will primarily involve adhering to the data management plan developed during the data analysis planning stage. The data management plan should include procedures for transferring data from the instruments to the data analysis software. The data analysis plan should also detail how data will be scored and coded, how missing data will be managed, and how outliers will be handled. For questionnaires, a scoring guide will tell the research team how to code the variables. The scoring guide will also detail if any items are filler items that should not be included in the scoring calculations, as well as provide scores for any items that need to be reverse coded.

Another important part of the data analysis plan is data screening. Data screening may include assessing the accuracy of data entry, how outliers and missing values will be handled, and if statistical assumptions are met (Sharma & Petosa, 2012). Outliers can be either univariate or multivariate in nature. Statistical software can identify outliers; however, the research team often decides how to handle outliers. Problematic outliers are outliers that are not representative of the population. These outliers can arrive from implausible data or biased data. Beneficial outliers are outliers that are representative of the population. Interpretation of whether outliers are beneficial or problematic is often based on the expertise of the research team. It should be noted that many inferential tests are sensitive to outliers, especially multivariate outliers. Multivariate outliers are unusual combinations of scores on different variables. Multivariate outliers are difficult to detect without the aid of statistical tests. Prior to deleting outliers, the research team should double check to make sure the data are accurately entered. Researchers will also have to deal with missing data (Sharma & Petosa, 2012). Missing data are observations that were intended to be made, but were not made. Handling missing data depends largely on how much is missing and if there are patterns to the missing data.

Parametric tests rest upon many assumptions, which, if not met, can compromise the integrity of the study results. The research team should determine which assumptions they will need to test and how they will be tested during the data analysis planning phase. During the preparation phase, the research team should test the assumptions of the statistical tests they will use. For example, most parametric tests assume linearity between the independent and dependent variables, absence of multicollinearity, and normality of the variables. Ungrouped inferential tests, such as regression analysis, assume homoscedasticity while grouped inferential tests, such as analysis of variance, assume homogeneity of variance.

KEY: no symbol - entry level; ❖ advanced 1; ■ advanced 2

❖ 4.5.2 Analyze data using qualitative methods

Qualitative research methods include a wide range of data collection strategies (Patton, 2014). The type of qualitative method the researchers use depends on the purpose of the evaluation, resources, and use of other techniques. Following are qualitative approaches often used in health education:

- Observation/audit
- Participant observation
- Document study
- Interviews
- Focus groups

(Patton, 2014)

Analyzing data using qualitative methods helps evaluators or researchers become more experienced with the variables or phenomenon of interest. Hence, evaluators or researchers use qualitative analysis methods to achieve a deep understanding of the issues surrounding items or variables of interest. Qualitative research has special value for investigating complex and sensitive issues. It is extremely useful to achieve a deep understanding of how people think about specific topics and can be especially helpful when the researcher is willing to trade generalizability for contextual detail. Qualitative analysis enables the researcher to describe the phenomena of interest in great detail and in the original language of the research participants (Brownson et al., 2003).

Sample sizes in qualitative data are generally small. Sound qualitative research and evaluation is controlled and systematic. Most analyses involve systematically analyzing the content of the data, breaking it into meaningful pieces, and organizing pieces in a way that allows the characteristics and meaning to be better understood. There are several steps involved in qualitative data analysis.

1. *Data reduction*: This step involves selecting, focusing, condensing, and transforming data. The process should be guided by thinking about which data best answer the evaluation questions.
2. *Data display:* This involves creating an organized, compressed way of arranging data (i.e., through a diagram, chart, matrix, or text). Display helps to facilitate identifying themes, patterns, and connections that help answer evaluation questions. This step usually involves coding, or marking passages in text (or parts of images, sections of a video, etc.) that have the same message or are connected in some way. An accompanying explanation of what the selected passages have in common is created.
3. *Conclusion drawing and verification:* During this last step, the data is revisited multiple times to verify, test, or confirm the themes and patterns identified (Miles, Huberman, & Saldana, 2013).

(Jeanfreau & Jack, 2010)

Qualitative analysis is a cyclical and iterative process with many rounds of investigating evidence, modifying hypotheses, and revisiting the data from a new light. Evaluators and researchers reexamine data repeatedly as new questions, themes, and connections emerge. Evaluators and researchers examine qualitative data to identify:

- Patterns, recurring themes, similarities, and differences
- Ways in which patterns (or lack thereof) help answer evaluation questions
- Deviations from patterns and possible explanations for divergence

SECTION IV

- Interesting or particularly insightful stories
- Specific language people use to describe phenomena
- The extent to which patterns are supported by past studies or other evaluations (and if not, what might explain the differences)
- The extent to which patterns suggest that additional data needs to be collected

(Malterud, 2012)

■ 4.5.3 Analyze data using descriptive statistical methods

Data can be analyzed using descriptive analysis that aims to summarize characteristics of the group of people or the program being studied (Aday & Cornelius, 2006). Descriptive analysis is exploratory in nature and designed to describe phenomenon specific to a population using descriptive statistics such as raw numbers, percentages, and ratios. Descriptive statistics describe what the data reveals, as well as provide simple summaries about the samples' measures. There are a variety of ways to represent descriptive data numerically. Two such classifications include continuous data that have the potential for infinite values for variables, or discrete data that are limited to a specific number of values to represent variables. Descriptive data may also be classified as nominal, ordinal, interval, and ratio. Nominal scores cannot be ordered hierarchically, but are mutually exclusive (i.e., male and female). Ordinal scores do not have a common unit of measurement between them but are hierarchical. Interval scores have common units of measurement between scores, but no true zero. Ratio scores represent data with common measurements between each score and a true zero (Last, 2001). Mean, median, and mode are measures of central tendency that can be used depending on the type of data collected. Variance, range, and standard deviation can describe dispersion of the data.

■ 4.5.4 Analyze data using inferential statistical methods

Analytic analysis is explanatory in nature and may use both descriptive statistics and inferential statistics to explain phenomenon. Inferential statistics, such as t-test, analysis of variance (ANOVA), analysis of covariance (ANCOVA), regression analysis, and many of the multivariate methods like factor analysis, multidimensional scaling, cluster analysis, discriminant function analysis, and so on are used when researchers or evaluators wish to draw conclusions about a population from a sample (Neutens & Rubinson, 2010). This involves inferences about central tendency such as mean, median, mode, or any of a number of other aspects of a sample distribution of a population. A variety of sampling methods is common to research and program evaluations to a lesser degree. Health education specialists are responsible for knowing terms that relate to using inferential and other statistical methods.

■ 4.5.5 Use technology to analyze data

A variety of computer software technologies are available to analyze data. Some data analysis software is open source software. Open source software is in the public domain and may be used free of charge. The majority of data analysis software is commercial, meaning it is designed to meet the needs of a specific customer base. Consequently, commercial software may vary in the types of statistical analyses packages they offer. If the research team would like to perform specialized analyses, they should consult with the vendor prior to purchasing a software license. Software learning curves can range from easy to very difficult. Many software companies provide training and tutorials on how to use their

KEY: no symbol - entry level;   ❖ advanced 1;   ■ advanced 2

software, and some offer certification programs. Depending on the sophistication of the analyses, the research project may need to hire a statistical consultant to perform data analysis.

Popular software for analyzing quantitative data include:
- *Microsoft Excel* for comprehensive statistical analysis
- *SPSS* for comprehensive statistical analysis
- *SAS* for comprehensive statistical analysis
- *Stata* for comprehensive statistical analysis
- *R* open source software containing a variety of statistical packages

Popular software for analyzing qualitative data include:
- *ATLAS.ti* for visual analysis of data
- *Ethnograph* for analysis of textual data
- *HyperRESEARCh* for analysis of textual and multimedia data
- *QSR Nvivo* for assisting in code-based theorizing
- *MAXQDA* for analysis of text-based data from focus groups, unstructured interviews, case histories, field notes, observation protocols, and document letters

(Sharma, & Petosa, 2012)

Competency 4.6: Interpret Results

Health education specialists' ability to interpret results from their own and others' evaluations/research is essential. Uncovering facts regarding a program's performance is not sufficient to draw evaluative conclusions. Interpretation is the effort of figuring out what the findings mean and is part of the overall effort to understand the evidence gathered (CDC, 1999). Ideally, health education specialists incorporate evaluation/research findings and scientific evidence into decision-making, policy development, and the implementation of programs. The evidence comes from carefully planned reviews of research and evaluation processes (Brownson et al., 2003). Programs steeped in the principles of evidence-based practice have gained favor among professionals practicing health education. Evidence-based practice uses epidemiological insight while studying and applying research, clinical and public health experience, practice, programs, and policies (Anderson et al., 2005). Whatever the source or format, evidence must be interpreted to determine the practical significance of what has been learned. Interpretations draw on information and perspectives that stakeholders bring to evaluation inquiry and can be strengthened through active participation or interaction (CDC, 1999).

■ 4.6.1 Synthesize the analyzed data

In evaluations using multiple methods, health education specialists detect evidence patterns by isolating important findings (analysis) and combining different sources of information to reach a larger understanding (synthesis). When agencies, communities, and other stakeholders agree with the synthesis of analyzed data, they are more inclined to use the evaluation results for the program. The five steps in data analysis and synthesis are straightforward:

1. *Enter the data into a database and check for errors:* If the health education specialists are using a surveillance system, such as BRFSS or PRAMS, the data have already been checked, entered,

and tabulated by those conducting the survey. If the health education specialists are collecting data with their own instruments, they will need to select a computer program to enter and analyze the data, as well as determine who will enter, check, tabulate, and analyze the data.

2. *Tabulate the data:* The data need to be tabulated to provide information, such as a number or percentage, for each indicator. Some basic calculations include determining the number of participants achieving the desired outcome or the percentage of participants achieving the desired outcome.

3. *Analyze and stratify the data:* Health education specialists analyze and stratify the data by various demographic variables of interest, such as participants' race, sex, age, income level, or geographic location.

4. *Make comparisons:* When examination of health education specialists' program includes research as well as evaluation studies, they should use statistical tests to show differences between comparison and intervention groups, geographic areas, or the pre-intervention and post-intervention status of the priority population. They should present data in a clear and understandable form. Data can be presented in tables, bar charts, pie charts, line graphs, and maps.

■ 4.6.2 Explain how the results address the questions and/or hypotheses

Health education specialists conducting research or evaluation should compare the results of their investigations against previously developed research/evaluation questions. The questions asked reflect the values held by stakeholders, and those values provide a basis for forming judgments concerning program performance. In practice, when stakeholders articulate and negotiate their values, these negotiations become the standards for judging whether a given program's performance will be considered successful, adequate, or unsuccessful. The evaluation and research questions generated early in the process reflect the stakeholders' values. When operationalized, these standards establish a comparison by which the program can be judged. Data collection methods and analyses determine the probability that findings are not due to chance. The results of the evaluation/research can provide a narrative of experiences, as well as the strengths and weaknesses of the investigations. Properly interpreting results will put valuable information in perspective, enabling evaluators and/or researchers to compare results and findings to the expected outcomes of stakeholders.

■ 4.6.3 Compare findings to results from other studies or evaluations

Health education specialists serving as researchers/evaluators should describe the results of data analyses clearly in writing, so that they can be compared to other programs or studies. Results and statistical data that are appropriately presented provide health education specialists with comparable findings. Findings might be compared to previous reports on the same priority population or with similar programs through parallel studies, surveillance data, online databases, and investigations reported in peer-reviewed articles. A variety of techniques can be used to compare data from different sources (Neutens & Rubinson, 2010). Data comparisons can be presented graphically in tables, figures, bar or line graphs, and pie charts. Comparing findings with other published literature creates useful information for stakeholders and evaluators to consider.

KEY: no symbol - entry level;   ❖ advanced 1;   ■ advanced 2

■ 4.6.4 Propose possible explanations of findings

Lessons learned throughout the course of an evaluation or research do not automatically translate into informed decision-making and appropriate action. Deliberate effort is needed to ensure that the processes and findings are used and disseminated appropriately. Understanding and being able to clearly articulate the findings of an evaluation/research investigation provides stakeholders the perspective necessary to make judgments concerning its merit, worth, or significance. Five elements are critical for ensuring use of an evaluation. They are:

- *Design*, which refers to how the questions, methods, and overall processes are constructed
- *Preparation,* which refers to the steps taken to rehearse eventual use of the findings
- *Feedback*, which is the communication that occurs among all parties
- *Follow-up*, which refers to the technical and emotional support that users need during the evaluation and after they receive evaluation findings
- *Dissemination,* which is the process of communicating either the procedures or the lessons learned from an evaluation to relevant audiences in a timely, unbiased, and consistent fashion (CDC, 2010)

■ 4.6.5 Identify limitations of findings

Even under the best of circumstances, the findings from evaluation and research are subject to systematic error in the sampling, design, implementation, or analysis that compromises the results to some degree. Often this error is referred to as bias. Confounding variables (or factors) are extraneous variables outside the scope of the intervention that can impact the results (Jack, Jr. et al., 2013). In other words, there are variables that affect results and are not accounted for in the study design. Health education specialists need to be able to evaluate sources of error in evaluation or research critically in order to make sense of scientific reports, as well as popular media. Health education specialists should be able to identify research errors such as sampling errors, lack of precision, and variability in measurement. They should also be able to spot systematic errors such as selection bias, instrumentation bias, and other internal threats to validity (Friis & Sellars, 2013).

■ 4.6.6 Address delimitations as they relate to findings

In research, delimitations are parameters or boundaries placed on the study by the researchers that help to manage the scope of a study (Cottrell & McKenzie, 2010). Delimitations differ from limitations in that limitations are boundaries placed on a study by factors or people other than the researchers (Cottrell & McKenzie, 2010). Delimitations often involve narrowing a study by geographic location, time, and population traits. Subsequently, findings must be analyzed within the context of the study's specific delimitations.

■ 4.6.7 Draw conclusions based on findings

After analyzing the data, the research team is in a position to draw conclusions from the study. Conclusions should be derived from the study findings. Keeping conclusions grounded in the research questions and hypotheses will prevent unwarranted extrapolation. Furthermore, conclusions should be constrained by a study's delimitations and limitations (e.g. the sampling technique used). The research team must be careful to interpret conclusions in light of the specific delimitations and limitations of their study.

■ 4.6.8 Develop recommendations based on findings

Recommendations are actions for consideration resulting from evaluation or research. They help program staff improve programs, make decisions about program operations, and move toward program goals. Forming recommendations is a distinct element of program evaluation that requires information beyond what is necessary to form judgments regarding program performance. Recommendations for continuing, expanding, redesigning, or terminating a program are separate from judgments regarding a program's effectiveness. In order to make recommendations, information concerning the context, particularly organizational context in which programmatic decisions will be made, should guide the process. Recommendations that lack sufficient evidence or those that are not aligned with stakeholders' values can undermine an evaluation's credibility. By contrast, an evaluation can be strengthened by recommendations that anticipate political sensitivities of intended users and highlight areas that users can control or influence. Sharing draft recommendations, soliciting reactions from multiple stakeholders, and presenting options instead of directive advice increase the likelihood that recommendations will be relevant and well received (CDC, 2010).

Competency 4.7: Apply Findings

Findings from evaluation and research can be applied based on the intention of the user. Evaluators should make certain stakeholders have an opportunity to carefully review and discuss findings before applying recommendations to programs or policy. Evaluators translate recommendations to action plans, including who is going to do what about the program and by when. Stakeholders will likely require various reports that may include an executive summary with an explanation of the evaluation goals, methods, and analysis procedures, listing of conclusions and recommendations, and any relevant attachments, including evaluation questionnaires, interview guides, etc. Evaluators may deliver the results in the form of a presentation accompanied by an overview of the report. Evaluators should be sure to record details of the evaluation plan that can be referenced as needed in the future.

4.7.1 Communicate findings to priority populations, partners, and stakeholders

Reporting or communicating research involves detailed documentation. Research is often prepared with the intention of publishing findings in professional peer-reviewed literature for use by other investigators. Although a report may be developed to meet the needs of stakeholders, typically the first part of the report includes an introduction (Neutens & Rubinson, 2010). This may include the front matter (such as the title of the program, names of the evaluators or researchers, and date of the report) and the executive summary. It should also include an explanation of the program's background and the health-related and/or other problems addressed by the program (Neutens & Rubinson, 2010).

The second part of the report, the literature review, may include an explanation of relevant studies and an understanding of the background for the study. The literature review will also relate to the purpose of the study, research questions, hypotheses, and the priority population. It will provide a theoretical orientation, which may also provide the framework for the review (Neutens & Rubinson, 2010).

KEY: no symbol - entry level; ❖ advanced 1; ■ advanced 2

The **methodology** section describes how the evaluation or research plan was carried out. It includes an overview of the procedures, subjects, and data gathering instruments used in the study (Neutens & Rubinson, 2010). The data analysis plan is often described within the methodology section.

The **results** section presents evidence tested against the stated hypotheses or research questions, presents the statistical findings, and also includes a discussion of what the findings mean. Findings should be presented in factual and descriptive terms to meet the needs of the intended audience. The results are often communicated in words, numbers, and statistics. The discussion of the data findings typically provides interpretation, implications, and applications to practice (Neutens & Rubinson, 2010).

The final portion of the written report may include **conclusions, recommendations**, or a **summary** (Neutens & Rubinson, 2010). This section is the part of the report most likely to be read by the stakeholders (Jack, Jr. et al., 2010). The conclusions indicate whether the analysis supports the hypothesis and often includes recommendations for future research and new research questions. The summary briefly restates the problems, procedures and principal findings (Neutens & Rubinson, 2010).

4.7.2 Solicit feedback from priority populations, partners, and stakeholders

Current trends indicate that the profession of health education is moving towards a greater involvement in policy and environmental change. As health education specialists engage in the work of policy analysis and program development, they need to come armed with evaluative findings. Policy analysis is defined as the use of any evaluative research to improve or legitimate the practical implications of a policy-oriented program. Among policy-makers, program evaluation is performed when the policy is fixed or unchangeable. However, policy analysis is carried out when there is still a chance that the policy can be revised.

Health impact assessments (HIAs) are used to objectively evaluate the potential health effects of a project or policy before it is developed or implemented. HIAs can provide recommendations to increase positive health outcomes and minimize adverse health outcomes. The HIA framework is used to bring potential public health impacts and considerations to the decision-making process for plans, projects, and policies that fall outside traditional public health arenas, such as transportation and land use.

The major steps in conducting an HIA include:
- Screening to identify projects or policies for which an HIA would be useful
- Scoping to identify which health effects to consider
- Assessing risks and benefits to identify which people may be affected and how they may be affected
- Developing recommendations to suggest changes to proposals to promote positive or mitigate adverse health effects
- Presenting results to decision-makers
- Evaluating to determine the effect of the HIA on the decision

(Kemm, Parry, & Palmer, 2004)

4.7.3 Evaluate feasibility of implementing recommendations

Robust evaluation designs that utilize randomized control trials, cohort studies, and case control/comparison studies provide evaluators and stakeholders with confidence in the validity of the evaluation. These designs can provide recommendations that may be generalized to other similar scenarios. However, most recommendations derived from program evaluation will be specific to the program itself and directed at program planners and stakeholders either involved in the effort or affected by it. The feasibility of implementing recommendations from evaluations depends on cost, resources, time, politics, and other contextual factors. Programs planned with an evaluation plan and developed with provisions for flexibility allow for early adjustments in programming that may have the potential to maximize desired effects or minimize costs. With sufficient time and strong stakeholder support, feedback on program processes and impacts can serve to improve programming and the feasibility of implementing recommendations.

4.7.4 Incorporate findings into program improvement and refinement

Program evaluation and research provide important information for the incorporation of recommendations that will help improve programs based on their results. Forming recommendations requires information beyond just what is necessary to form judgments. For example, knowing that a program is able to increase the services available to battered women does not necessarily translate into a recommendation to continue the effort, particularly when there are competing priorities or other effective alternatives. Thus, recommendations about what to do with a given intervention go beyond judgments about a specific program's effectiveness.

If enough evidence does not support recommendations or if they are not in keeping with stakeholders' values, they can undermine an evaluation's credibility. By contrast, an evaluation can be strengthened by recommendations that anticipate and react to what users will want to know.

■ 4.7.5 Disseminate findings using a variety of methods

Health education specialists contribute to the profession and to the professional development of other health education specialists by sharing their research/evaluation findings. A common way to disseminate research findings is through presentations at local, state, national, and international health-related conferences. Presentations encourage dialogue about the processes and outcomes related to evaluation/research. Often, the abstracts and objectives of the presentations are required to facilitate a peer-reviewed process for selecting the presentations that appear in conference programs. Conference sessions may include poster sessions, breakout sessions (i.e., session time shared with other speakers), concurrent sessions (i.e., session time dedicated to one presentation), and keynote sessions. If a research/evaluation study will have a major impact in health education, the investigator may be asked to be a keynote speaker.

An evaluation or research report is the typical form of communication used to disseminate the outcome of the plan set forth by the evaluation or research planners (Neutens & Rubinson, 2010). Although reports take on different styles, it is important for these documents to provide user friendly information to the stakeholders involved (CDC, 2010).

KEY: no symbol - entry level; ❖ advanced 1; ■ advanced 2

Dissemination is the process of communicating procedures, findings, or lessons learned from an evaluation to relevant audiences in a timely, unbiased, and consistent fashion. Like other elements of the evaluation, the reporting strategy should be discussed in advance with intended users and other stakeholders. Such consultation ensures that the information needs of relevant audiences will be met. Planning effective communication also requires considering the timing, style, tone, message source, vehicle, and format of information products. Regardless of how reports are constructed, the goal for dissemination is to achieve full disclosure and impartial reporting. Developing a checklist of items to consider in creating a tailored evaluation report may help to direct the report content for the audience by explaining the focus of the evaluation, its limitations, strengths, and weaknesses (Issel, 2013).

SECTION IV

This page was
intentionally left blank

CHAPTER V

Area of Responsibility V
Administer and Mange Health Education/Promotion

5.1: Manage financial resources for health education/promotion programs
5.1.1 ❖ Develop financial plan
5.1.2 ❖ Evaluate financial needs and resources
5.1.3 ❖ Identify internal and/or external funding sources
5.1.4 ❖ Prepare budget requests
5.1.5 ❖ Develop program budgets
5.1.6 ❖ Manage program budgets
5.1.7 ❖ Conduct cost analysis for programs
5.1.8 ❖ Prepare budget reports
5.1.9 ❖ Monitor financial plan
5.1.10 ❖ Create requests for funding proposals
5.1.11 ❖ Write grant proposals
5.1.12 ❖ Conduct reviews of funding proposals
5.1.13 ❖ Apply ethical principles when managing financial resources

5.2: Manage technology resources
5.2.1 Assess technology needs to support health education/promotion
5.2.2 Use technology to collect, store, and retrieve program management data
5.2.3 Apply ethical principles in managing technology resources
5.2.4 Evaluate emerging technologies for applicability to health education/promotion

5.3: Manage relationships with partners and other stakeholders
5.3.1 Assess capacity of partners and other stakeholders to meet program goals
5.3.2 ❖ Facilitate discussions with partners and other stakeholders regarding program resource needs
5.3.3 Create agreements (for example, memoranda of understanding) with partners and other stakeholders
5.3.4 Monitor relationships with partners and other stakeholders
5.3.5 ❖ Elicit feedback from partners and other stakeholders
5.3.6 Evaluate relationships with partners and other stakeholders

5.4: Gain acceptance and support for health education/promotion programs
5.4.1 Demonstrate how programs align with organizational structure, mission, and goals
5.4.2 Identify evidence to justify programs
5.4.3 Create a rationale to gain or maintain program support
5.4.4 Use various communication strategies to present rationale

SECTION V

KEY: no symbol - entry level; ❖ advanced 1; ■ advanced 2

5.5: Demonstrate leadership

5.5.1 ❖ Facilitate efforts to achieve organizational mission

5.5.2 Analyze an organization's culture to determine the extent to which it supports health education/promotion

5.5.3 Develop strategies to reinforce or change organizational culture to support health education/promotion

5.5.4 ❖ Facilitate needed changes to organizational culture

5.5.5 ❖ Conduct strategic planning

5.5.6 ❖ Implement strategic plan

5.5.7 ❖ Monitor strategic plan

5.5.8 Conduct program quality assurance/process improvement

5.5.9 Comply with existing laws and regulations

5.5.10 Adhere to ethical principles of the profession

5.6: Manage human resources for health education/promotion programs

5.6.1 ❖ Assess staffing needs

5.6.2 ❖ Develop job descriptions

5.6.3 ❖ Apply human resource policies consistent with laws and regulations

5.6.4 ❖ Evaluate qualifications of staff members and volunteers needed for programs

5.6.5 Recruit staff members and volunteers for programs

5.6.6 ❖ Determine staff member and volunteer professional development needs

5.6.7 ❖ Develop strategies to enhance staff member and volunteer professional development

5.6.8 ❖ Implement strategies to enhance the professional development of staff members and volunteers

5.6.9 ❖ Develop and implement strategies to retain staff members and volunteers

5.6.10 ❖ Employ conflict resolution techniques

5.6.11 ❖ Facilitate team development

5.6.12 ❖ Evaluate performance of staff members and volunteers

5.6.13 ❖ Monitor performance and/or compliance of funding recipients

5.6.14 ❖ Apply ethical principles when managing human resources

The Role. Health education/promotion programs must not only be planned and implemented well but also administered and managed well once launched. While some administrative (i.e., gaining program support) and managerial (i.e., managing technological resources) functions may fall to the entry-level health education specialist, administration and management is generally a function of the more advanced-level practitioner. Health education specialists often become program managers or supervisors of other health education specialists and/or teams of allied health professionals. Good management incorporates effective leadership skills with managing financial, technological, and human resources. Successful managers maintain relationships with partners and other stakeholders, assign tasks, and conduct performance evaluations. Supervisors facilitate discussions with both internal and external stakeholders such as advanced-level management as well as funding agencies in

KEY: no symbol - entry level; ❖ advanced 1; ■ advanced 2

regards to program resource needs. This role requires effective communication skills, organizational knowledge, and objectivity. Because of their broad training and their understanding of individuals and communities, health education specialists can be effective managers who consider potential partnerships in the larger context of their institution and environment.

Settings. The following text is presented to describe how administering programs is used in different practice settings.

Community Setting. Health education specialists in a community setting, especially those working at an advanced-level, may be responsible for managing and administering health education/promotion programs. Such work includes gaining acceptance for programs and managing the financial, technological, and human resources associated with programs. These tasks require health education specialists to create and monitor a program budget, hire and evaluate personnel, and work with both internal and external partners, as well as stakeholders, to ensure a program's success. In addition, health education specialists are responsible for managing the relationships with program partners and other stakeholders.

School (K-12) Setting. In addition to managing students in the classroom, health education specialists in the school setting must identify and secure financial resources to support program and policy changes that help improve students' learning and health. Health education specialists serve as curriculum coordinators or project directors, manage curricular and budgetary issues for the school health program, and work with school health advisory councils to obtain acceptance and support for content areas

addressed in the curriculum. Health education specialists also frequently supervise pre-service interns (student teachers). As curriculum specialists or program heads, they serve as team leaders to promote health education in their school, throughout the school district, and at the state level.

Health Care Settings. Health education specialists may manage professional development programs in medical complexes, nursing homes, or transitional facilities. The ability to communicate and facilitate partnerships with a variety of medical professionals, aides, volunteers, patients, family, or community members is very important in this setting. Planning programs that contribute to institutional maintenance of accreditation and compliance with government regulations also may be the task of health education specialists. These health education specialists may supervise institutional service learning activities that augment staff efforts.

Business/Industry Setting. In this setting, health education specialists may lead or be part of a team as either a coordinator for an employee assistance program or director of a health promotion effort. As employees, health education specialists also may supervise or provide support for employed staff members, contracted staff members, vendors, or volunteers in health promotion programs (e.g., smoking cessation, stress management, substance misuse, and weight loss).

College/University Setting. Health education specialists in the college/university setting may be involved in a variety of administrative responsibilities, including coordinating professional preparation programs and chairing academic departments. In this role, health education specialists must develop and manage program budgets, supervise part-time faculty members, and be responsible for the annual evaluations of those employed in the department. They also must align their professional preparation program goals with the goals and mission of college/university. In addition, health education specialists may coordinate and supervise student internships, analyze the program's curriculum for appropriate goals and objectives, and chair or facilitate committees. In this setting, health education specialists also must teach administration and management Competencies to students in their professional preparation program.

College/University Health Services Setting.

Health education specialists in a campus health services setting may coordinate special events, develop health initiatives, arrange for health screenings by other agencies, or develop health education programs for priority populations within the community. These same health education specialists also may administer health education/promotion programs, as well as health, counseling, or fitness/wellness services centers. In this role, they must demonstrate leadership, plan strategically, and organize the center. Health education specialists also must hire, administer, train, manage, and evaluate personnel, as well as secure funds and manage financial, technological, and other resources. In addition, they advocate for support and acceptance of health education/promotion programs, conduct quality assurance, process improvement studies, facilitate organizational change, and manage stakeholder relationships.

Key Terms

Coalitions are groups of individuals in an alliance who represent various organizations from within the community who agree to work together toward a common goal (McKenzie et al., 2013).

Conflict resolution is a strategy utilized for resolving issues or problems between two or more individuals (Rowitz, 2014).

Culture is the patterned ways of thought and behavior that characterize a social group and are learned through socialization processes (McKenzie, Neiger, & Thackeray, 2013).

Cultural competency is the organization's or individual's capacity to engage effectively within the cultural context of the priority population (USDHHS, 2014).

Goals can be defined as broad statements of intent that provide directions related to where the organization or program should direct its efforts (McKenzie et al., 2013).

KEY: no symbol - entry level; ❖ advanced 1; ■ advanced 2

Ecological approaches utilize the various dimensions, (e.g., physical, social, and cultural) to affect behavior change. Ecological perspectives take into consideration five levels of influence on health behavior: intrapersonal (individual), interpersonal (group), institutional, community, and public policy (Cottrell et al., 2014).

Mission statements are concrete, outcome-oriented statements that provide information about the overarching goals of an organization in a broad context (University of Wisconsin, 2010).

Negotiation is the utilization of a third party to aid in conflict resolution (Rowitz, 2014).

Organizational Development (OD) is a term that encompasses strategies and interventions that focus on building capacities and well-being within groups and organizations to achieve maximum effectiveness and efficiency. It includes team building, organizational design, fostering strong and ethical organizational cultures, intergroup relations, group problem solving, and managing organizational change (Robbins & Judge, 2015).

Strategic planning consists of the process of developing strategies to reach a defined set of objectives designed to fulfill the mission of an organization (Kreuter et al., 2003).

Competency 5.1: Manage Financial Resources for Health Education/Promotion Programs

Health education specialists often have to secure and manage fiscal resources. Health education specialists work in many different settings often requiring skills such as completing funding searches, writing and submitting grants, budgeting, and managing resources.

❖ 5.1.1 Develop financial plan

A broad plan for financial sustainability can help organizations or initiatives reach both short- and long-term goals. Similar to other planning documents, the financial plan should include specific objectives, strategies, and action steps. Components of the plan may include a review of the current operating budget, plans for expansion, fundraising goals, and a timeline of action steps. Health education specialists should check with those stakeholders who oversee their organization (e.g., Board of Directors) to confirm which components may be required for their plan.

Ideally, a team should be assembled to lead financial plan development (e.g., a standing financial committee or a temporary working group). The group should make time to circulate an initial draft of the plan to stakeholders such as funders, clients, and staff members. Their comments can help guide revision of the financial plan before implementation (University of Kansas, 2014a).

SECTION V

❖ 5.1.2 Evaluate financial needs and resources

An important part of your financial plan is evaluating the financial needs and resources necessary to reach the goals set forth by your organization. This evaluation may include reviewing:

- A list of all items and needs of the project
- The amount required to sustain each item
- Current resources
- Required resources
- Potential matching and funding organizations or individuals
  - Amount that will be requested from each organization, individual, or funding source
  - How it will be requested, by whom, and when

(University of Kansas, 2014a)

❖ 5.1.3 Identify internal and/or external funding sources

Health education specialists, especially at advanced-levels, may have the responsibility of securing resources for program activities. Resources may be procured through participant fees, third-party support, cost sharing, organizational sponsorship, grants, gifts, and a combination of the various sources (McKenzie et al., 2013). Each source may apply different rules to obtaining and using funds. Therefore, health education specialists must understand the policies, rules, and laws that govern these processes.

Health education specialists must also be aware of possible sources of funding that are likely to support their initiatives. Some funding sources can be found internally (e.g., general organizational funds, specific program/intervention funds, and cost sharing from other departments). Potential external sources may include foundations, governmental agencies, corporations, local businesses, and civic organizations.

In addition to consulting with colleagues and mentors about opportunities, health education specialists can also access many electronic resources to help identify external funding sources:

1. *Searchable funding databases.* For example, the Grants.gov Web site (http://www.grants.gov/web/grants/home.html) managed by the United States Department of Health and Human Services centralizes more than 1,000 different grant programs across 26 federal grant-making agencies.
2. *Searchable foundation directories.* For example, the Foundation Directory online (https://fconline.foundationcenter.org/) provides access to over 120,000 foundations and corporate donors.
3. *Alerts from potential funders.* For instance, health education specialists can sign up for electronic funding alerts from the Robert Wood Johnson Foundation (http://www.rwjf.org/en/grants/funding-opportunities.html).

❖ 5.1.4 Prepare budget requests

With the broader financial plan of the organization in mind, health education specialists and program managers will need to prepare specific budgets. A budget lays out a plan for how funds will be used (Fallon & Zgodzinski, 2011).

KEY: no symbol - entry level; ❖ advanced 1; ■ advanced 2

Fallon and Zgodzinski (2011) outline five components of complete budget:

- *Statistics budget:* includes items that can be accurately predicted (e.g., service utilization and staffing levels)
- *Expense budget:* includes a calculation of the total expenses needed to do business (e.g., staff wages and office space)
- *Revenue budget:* includes a prediction of the amount of income that will be generated through various streams and sources (e.g., grants and donations)
- *Cash budget:* includes a summary of the anticipated cash receipts and payments for an agency
- *Capital budget:* includes a plan for purchasing or upgrading long-term assets with significant purchase prices (e.g., property and technology infrastructure)

Chenoweth (2011) delineates key factors that should be considered when preparing budgets. Preparers should be aware of how others in the organization view the project/program. It is important to also be aware of how recent programs/projects and budgets have performed. Health education specialists should be aware of available program analysis outcomes and utilize input from all staff members when making any decisions about the budget. Finally, health education specialists should be flexible and keep everything regarding any actual or potential budget changes in perspective.

❖ 5.1.5 Develop program budgets

Health education specialists should finalize the development of their budget based on their approved request. The complexity of the actual budget document will vary from organization to organization. It is dependent on factors such as the size of the budget, amount of funders (and their requirements), and the breadth of programs or services. Regardless of the complexity of the budget, it should include the following components:

1. Projected expenses: This section should be broken down into specific categories (e.g., salaries).
2. Projected income: This section should be broken down by sources (e.g., fundraising).
3. The interaction of expenses and income: This section explicitly states which funding sources will fund each program activity or item.
4. Adjustments: As the fiscal year progresses, estimates will be updated or replaced by actual costs to keep the budget as accurate as possible.

(University of Kansas, 2014)

❖ 5.1.6 Manage program budgets

In conjunction with securing fiscal resources and developing budgets, health education specialists are often responsible for continual management of the budget. Ongoing monitoring is essential since fiscal viability is related to program evaluation performance and overall well-being of the organization, program, or project (Longest, 2011). The primary method for using a budget as a monitoring tool is tracking the budget variance (Issel, 2013). The budget variance is defined as the difference between the projected and actual expenditures.

According to Issel (2013), program managers should review the budget variance on an ongoing and regular basis, typically monthly. One reason that it is important for organizations to maintain updated and accurate budgets is so they can communicate to funders exactly how their investment is being used (University of Kansas, 2014a).

❖ 5.1.7 Conduct cost analysis for programs

There are several types of analyses that can be completed to evaluate the costs of health programs. The selection of analysis methods is based on whether one or more programs are being compared, and whether program outcomes are being assessed in addition to cost (Issel, 2013). The primary types of analyses are:

- *Cost description:* This is the simplest form of economic analysis and is appropriate when only one program is being considered. It merely presents the expenses related to the delivery of a program.
- *Cost analysis:* When a cost description examines expenses by more specific factors (e.g., time periods), it becomes a cost analysis.
- *Cost minimization:* This analysis is used to determine the most effective ways to deliver the program at the lowest cost.
- *Cost comparison*: This analysis compares the costs to deliver two or more programs. However, it does not take into account the programs' outcomes or impacts.
- *Cost effectiveness:* This analysis compares the costs of two programs alongside one type of impact that is identically measured in both programs.
- *Cost benefit:* This analysis also compares the costs of two programs; however, the programs do not need to measure the same impact or focus on the same health problem. Instead, larger societal impacts are considered.
- *Cost utility:* This analysis is the most complex and measures the impact of health programs in terms of the prospective participants' inclination for the health outcome.

❖ 5.1.8 Prepare budget reports

Reports related to project/program budgets are typically prepared and distributed to funding agencies and other key stakeholders on a monthly, quarterly, and/or annual basis. Routinely, reports include information related to fiscal activity during the time period for which it was prepared, as well as total income and expenditures for the budget year (McKenzie et al., 2013).

Budget reports serve several purposes. Internally, program managers and other organizational leaders utilize accurate and updated budget information in order to make appropriate decisions about organizational operations. External stakeholders, such as funding agencies, may use the information to assess program feasibility and to assure fiscal and programmatic accountability.

❖ 5.1.9 Monitor financial plan

Financial planning should be seen as an ongoing process. Sub-competency 5.1.1 recommends that a group be convened to develop a financial plan. This group should also be involved with monitoring and reviewing/revising of the plan. Procedures should be put in place that not only allow for monitoring but also communicate the findings of each review to relevant stakeholders (e.g., staff, board of directors, funders, etc.).

KEY: no symbol - entry level; ❖ advanced 1; ■ advanced 2

❖ 5.1.10 Create requests for funding proposals

Funding sustainability may be the primary responsibility of advanced-level health education specialists, which means that they must be forward thinking with a broad knowledge of fundraising and other methods of securing fiscal resources. When searching for external funding, health education specialists will come across announcements for Requests for Proposals (RFPs) or Requests for Applications (RFAs). These requests come from agencies that invite organizations to submit proposals. Miner and Miner (2013) recommend that organizations keep three issues in mind when reviewing an RFP to determine if it is a good match:

- Relevance: Do we want to do this?
- Feasibility: Can we do this?
- Probability: Will we be competitive?

If an organization decides to pursue an RFP or RFA, then the health education specialists involved should review the instructions carefully and follow them exactly in order to have their proposal considered. The instructions provide guidance regarding topics such as:

- Letter of intent (if required)
- Deadlines
- Formatting and page limits
- Checklists of required components
- Section scoring
- Grant requirements for funded grantees (e.g., reporting requirements)

(University of Kansas, 2014a)

❖ 5.1.11 Write grant proposals

After reviewing available RFPs/RFAs and determining the best fit, health education specialists must be prepared to respond in an appropriate and timely manner. In addition to the activities discussed in Sub-competency 5.1.10, they must be ready to develop a full grant proposal.

Grant proposals typically contain, at a minimum, the following elements:

- Cover letter: identifies the program to which the proposal is being submitted and an overview of the proposal
- Abstract or executive summary: a summary of the entire proposal
- Table of contents: the basic layout of the submission
- Proposal narrative broken down into key sections:
  - Introduction/background: a description of the problem, its magnitude, and the purpose of the funding request
  - Significance of the proposed project: a justification for the request (e.g., literature, data, evidence, and information about the issue for which funds are requested), and information about the requesting organization's experience with the issue
  - Proposed program description: goals, objectives, priority population, activities that are to be performed, expected outcomes, an evaluation plan, and a timeline for when the objectives and activities are to be accomplished

SECTION V

- Dissemination plan: detailed strategy to circulate project results (e.g., through peer-reviewed publications and professional conferences)
- Sustainability plan: detailed strategy to continue some or all of the project activities beyond the grant period
- Resources: facilities, equipment, supplies, personnel, etc.
- Key Personnel: resumes and job descriptions of personnel associated with the program
- Budget and budget narrative: The budget should include all expenditures for the project (e.g., salaries, employee benefits, travel, equipment, materials/supplies, consultants, contracts, etc.) The narrative should justify every line item in the budget and describe (a) the specific item, (b) the item's relevance to the project, and (c) the basis of cost calculations for that item.

- References: list of cited sources
- Appendices: supportive secondary information (e.g., letters of support and consortia agreements)

(Miner & Miner, 2013; University of Kansas, 2014a)

❖ 5.1.12 Conduct reviews of funding proposals

Health education specialists are often called upon to provide service to the field by serving as a reviewer of grant proposals. This offers many benefits to the participating health education specialist including: having the opportunity to improve their own grant writing by reviewing/evaluating those written by others and obtaining firsthand knowledge about the funder and their priorities (University of Northern Iowa, n.d.).

The review process can vary by funder. For instance, some agencies may ask reviewers to review the proposals independently and communicate their recommendations directly to the funding agency coordinator. Other agencies may convene a review panel where recommendations will be discussed as a group. In general, reviewers are asked to evaluate proposals based on specific criteria (e.g., how closely the proposal aligns with the RFP instructions, the strength of the budget justification, inclusion of clear and evidence-based research/evaluation methods, etc.)

❖ 5.1.13 Apply ethical principles when managing financial resources

Health education specialists have an obligation to manage fiscal resources in an ethical manner. However, the demonstration of ethics relative to fiscal management is a complex process that encompasses considerations that are more expansive than the legality of specific actions. Part of managing fiscal resources in an ethical manner is being able to understand which programs offer the best value. Therefore, it is important that health education specialists understand and are able to utilize the various types of economic analysis described in Sub-competency 5.1.7. Health education specialists have an obligation to apply and utilize findings from these various types of analyses to make informed, responsible, and timely programmatic decisions. The ethical guidelines in Appendix A should be reviewed as they are relevant to managing financial resources (specifically Article 3, Section 4).

Competency 5.2: Manage Technology Resources

Technology can be integrated into all aspects of health education/promotion, from needs assessment to evaluation. Technology needs can vary from basic office support to advanced program delivery using cutting edge technology. Therefore, health education specialists must be prepared to broadly assess their technology needs and consider the unique ethical and planning considerations that accompany its integration in their programs.

5.2.1 Assess technology needs to support health education/promotion

When assessing technology needs, health education specialists should consider both organization-level needs and program specific needs. These assessments are also relevant to Sub-competencies 5.1.2, 5.1.4, and 5.1.5, since technology capacity and needs should be integrated into financial planning and budgeting conversations.

Organization-level assessments may include:
- Infrastructure/Supplies: When organizational inputs are assessed, computer hardware and software costs are included in the budget, typically categorized as physical resources (Issel, 2013). Examples of relevant supplies in this category also include computers, phones, mobile devices, Web sites, and data storage and back-up systems.
- Human resources/knowledge: Issel (2013) notes that knowledge can be considered a resource that managers should consider. Therefore, a technology assessment should include a review of the technology knowledge required to deliver the program. Does the program manager need to hire additional technology professionals and/or provide technology professional development for staff?

Program specific assessments may include:
- *Technology needs for intervention delivery and evaluation:* For example, during program development for a technology-based intervention, the unique benefits and challenges of possible delivery modalities should be reviewed. Relevant considerations can include cost, reach, complexity, accessibility, and portability (Bull, 2011).
- *Technology needs for team collaboration:* Leadership may want to consider project management software, document sharing resources, and Web meeting or videoconference resources depending on the location and size of the project team. Examples of team collaboration technology options include Dropbox, Google Docs, and Skype.
- *Technology capacity/comfort of your priority audience:* It is important to know the primary audience and what modalities they use. Bull (2011) encourages program planners to ask if their audience currently has access to (and uses) the planners' modality of choice.

5.2.2 Use technology to collect, store and retrieve program management data

As discussed in Sub-competency 5.2.1, technology can be used to assist the project team in managing program data and collaboration efforts. In addition, it can assist with the collection, storage, and retrieval of data collected from program participants. For example, electronic surveys can be used to enroll participants in an intervention and collect demographic data and responses that can be accessed later for follow-up and/or evaluation. Program planners can also use database software like Microsoft Access to develop a participant tracking system and run queries on a variety of variables (Bull, 2011).

5.2.3 Apply ethical principles in managing technology resources

According to Bull (2011), there are several unique ethical issues related to technology-based health promotion:

- *Beneficence:* Program planners need to justify why the chosen technology modality is best for participants (not the health promoter).
- *Transparency:* Informed consent processes and information provided by both participants and health promoters must be clear and accurate.
- *Equity:* Given health disparities data, special attention should be paid to who has access to the technological modality.
- *Confidentiality:* Data security protocols must be employed to protect private participant data.
- *Special populations:* Additional standards to verify participant identity must be employed and regulations for protecting special populations must be followed if participants are members of included categories such as pregnant women.

Health education specialists should also consider the Health Information Technology for Economic and Clinical Health (HITECH) Act when managing technology resources. HITECH proposes the meaningful use of interoperable electronic health records throughout the United States health care delivery system as a critical national goal. The HITECH Act addresses the privacy and security concerns associated with the electronic transmission of health information (USDHHS, 2014a).

Please refer to Appendix A to review relevant Health Education Codes of Ethics for managing technology resources. These include Article V, Section 3 and Section 4.

5.2.4 Evaluate emerging technologies for applicability to health education/promotion

Health education specialists should keep up with emerging technology that holds promise for intervention development. Since technology can be trendy and fleeting, it is important to be selective about the methods incorporated into programs. There are several ways to research potential technologies:

- Review guidance from trusted public health agencies: For example, the CDC has released several guides that acknowledge the value of social media and discuss strategies for effectively integrating the technology into health communication programs (CDC, 2011; CDC, 2012).
- Review the evidence presented in peer-reviewed literature: For example, in 2014 the Journal of Medical Internet Research published an e-collection focused on "Web-based and Mobile Health Interventions" (http://www.jmir.org/themes/50).
- Review national trends regarding technology use: For example, the Pew Research Internet Project (http://www.pewresearch.org) regularly publishes data on the demographics of social media users and which platforms are most popular.

KEY: no symbol - entry level;   ❖ advanced 1;   ■ advanced 2

Competency 5.3: Manage Relationships with Partners and other Stakeholders

Since many health challenges experienced by individuals and communities are associated with multiple risks and causations, the ecological systems approach is one of the most effective models for leveraging the complexity of managing relationships with partners and other stakeholders (Healey & Lesneski, 2011). Therefore, multilevel, multisectorial, and multidisciplinary partnerships are necessary for health education specialists to be competent in creating, sustaining, monitoring, and managing partnerships, coalitions, and collaborations (Schiavo, 2014; Healey & Lesneski, 2011; Butterfoss, 2007).

With increasing numbers of organizations and institutions incorporating partner relationships through "community engagement" administering partnerships may be facilitated through:
- Creating community-based participatory research
- Developing partnerships, coalitions, and networks
- Interfacing with community-based, nonprofit, and/or voluntary organizations that have common agendas
- Working with special interest groups to expand the reach of the initiative
- Providing critical links between community members and institutions/organizations to assure coordination, congruence, and sustainability

5.3.1 Assess capacity of partners and other stakeholders to meet program goals

When developing partnerships, leaders must assess the appropriateness of potential partners. As part of the assessment, an examination of the potential partner's history, capabilities, resources, and vision/mission needs to be undertaken to determine if they are a good fit for the partnership (Healey and Zimmerman, 2010).

Frameworks such as the social determinants of health and the ecological systems model can serve as invaluable tools for identifying partners that can provide the leverage and insight necessary to address community needs (Healey and Lesneski, 2011). Several factors that can contribute to the success of these partnerships include: (a) determining the needs, capacity, and resources of the organizations as early as possible, (b) raising awareness of policy requirements and regulations that are critical to the mutual interests and goals of the potential partners, and (c) developing alliances through positive relationships with constituency groups (Schiavo, 2013).

In this role, health education specialists' responsibilities may include conducting assessments, selecting appropriate evidence-based strategies and interventions, and using assessment information to adapt the selected interventions to respond to the priority population's or organization's needs.

❖ 5.3.2 Facilitate discussions with partners and other stakeholders regarding program resource needs

Coalitions, partnerships, committees, subcommittees, advisory boards, consortia, and other organizational structures can be used to facilitate intra- and inter-organizational cooperation to meet the needs of the program and achieve mutual goals (University of Kansas, 2014a).

After identifying partners with mutual and/or supporting interests, the following are critical to establishing viable working relationships:

- Develop trust and credibility
- Arrange a meeting with leaders from various organizations who have the ability to make decisions
- Have the leaders identify where coordination is required or beneficial and where various resources can be utilized
- Identify common interests
- Develop memorandums of agreement or understanding (MOUs) after trust and other issues have been resolved

(Fallon and Zgodzinski, 2011; Burke and Friedman, 2011)

Effective leadership skills, including team building, conflict resolution, and the ability to communicate effectively, are key to facilitating discussions with and among partners and other stakeholders. As such, advanced-level health education specialists may play a key role as facilitators of community dialogues by conducting assessments, translating technical information, and undertaking other processes that enhance community participation within the broader context of programs and operations.

5.3.3 Create agreements (for example, memoranda of understanding) with partners and other stakeholders

Cooperative agreements with other agencies and organizations are critical to having effective relationships and partnerships. This is best achieved by having clear and documented goals, objectives, and expected outcomes. A MOU is not an enforceable or legal document (unless it indicates an exchange of money), but it is a means of facilitating interagency cooperation.

5.3.4 Monitor relationships with partners and other stakeholders

A successful program is often indicative of successful relationships. Therefore, establishing clear mission statements, goals, and agreed upon outcomes are essential first steps for monitoring relationships with internal and external stakeholders (Longest, 2014; Shi and Johnson, 2013).

A social network analysis tool that can be used to measure and monitor relationships between and among people and organizations is The Program to Analyze, Record, and Track Networks to Enhance Relationships (PARTNER). As a tool, it can be used to collect data and monitor the extent to which partnerships are engaged, resources are effective/efficiently used, and the benefits are being attained (Shi and Johnson, 2014). The Community Engagement Continuum is another tool that can be used to guide and monitor the evaluation of relationships among partners and other stakeholders through (a) outreach, (b) consultation, (c) involvement, (d) collaboration, and (e) shared leaderships (http://www.atsdr.cdc.gov/communityengagement/pdf/PCE_Report_508_FINAL.pdf; Shi and Johnson, 2014).

KEY: no symbol - entry level; ❖ advanced 1; ■ advanced 2

❖ 5.3.5 Elicit feedback from partners and other stakeholders

Constituency relations through bidirectional communication are important to the viability of an organization that values cooperation (Schiavo, 2013). Whether partnerships are translated into organizational structures, such as internal/external advisory boards, committees, coalitions, or collaboratives, effective communication is critical for identifying and addressing program resource needs. Furthermore, community concerns and needs should be addressed in ways that are consistent with the values and expectations of their constituencies (Shi and Johnson, 2013; Schiavo, 2013).

Communication with internal and external stakeholders is essential, and, optimally, the process includes a feedback loop through which intentions, ideas, and information can be exchanged (Longest, 2014). This information can be used as a part of process evaluations in order to guide and inform the actions of a program, project, or organization. The structures through which feedback can be elicited can include coalitions, coordinating councils, committees, and other partnering organizations. Specific vehicles for sending, eliciting, and capturing the feedback include face-to-face meetings, phone calls, Web-based conferences, e-mails, memoranda, policy statements, reports, and letters (Longest, 2014).

Additional tools include surveys, questionnaires, checklists, key informant interviews, focus groups, and community conversations. However, it is most important to establish feedback loops, so that adjustments can be made when needed to improve the program (Johnson & Brekton, 2007).

5.3.6 Evaluate relationships with partners and other stakeholders

Just as health education programs are evaluated, partnerships and collaborations should be evaluated to determine their effectiveness. A plan should be established to evaluate partnership or collaboration activities before they begin. A determination needs to be made about what will be measured, when measurements will occur, and who will do the measurements. Healey and Zimmerman (2010) provide the following as a guide for evaluating partnerships and collaborations:

- Develop an evaluation plan
- Evaluate progress toward goal and objective achievement
- Record and track data based on established timeline
- Report the results
- Determine the levels of goal, objective and other achievements
- Use the findings for program improvement
- Prepare evaluation reports
- Broadly share achievements as a mechanism for partnership promotion

After partnerships have been evaluated, health education specialists have to decide if the partnership should be sustained. Health education specialists can make informed decisions regarding the utility of continued partnerships by weighing the results of the evaluation against resources used or saved in the partnership, as well as a reevaluation of the mission and goals of each organization.

SECTION V

Competency 5.4: Gain Acceptance and Support for Health Education/ Promotion Programs

Obtaining acceptance and support for programs has increasingly become a critical role for health education specialists. Programs require acceptance and support in order to ensure stakeholder involvement from beginning to end. Having acceptance and support from key stakeholders will also help ensure that necessary human and fiscal resources are available in order to maintain program strengths and, if necessary, to address program weaknesses. Health education specialists must work closely with supporters in order to identify ways to sustain programs beyond the project period. Recommended strategies in order to obtain, increase, and sustain program acceptance and support are discussed below.

5.4.1 Demonstrate how programs align with organizational structure, mission, and goals

The goals of the program and organization should be consistent with the organizational mission. Furthermore, organizational structure, roles, and functions should assure that the goals of the organization are achieved. A common tool used for portraying this alignment is a logic model. A logic model cannot only provide a graphic representation of the program but can also include the organizational mission, the context in which the program operates, and external variables that can influence outcomes (McKenzie et al., 2013). Please refer to Sub-competency 4.1.3 for more information on logic models.

5.4.2 Identify evidence to justify programs

Accessing, using, and understanding information to justify programs and identify the capacities, assets, and needs of a community/constituency and/or program require proficiency in conducting targeted searches for information.

Evidence to substantiate the status of or extent to which an issue exists can be accessed through: primary (e.g., surveys, interviews) and secondary data sources (e.g., national, regional, and local databases (e.g., clearinghouses, registries and surveillance data). Geographic information systems (GIS) and data mapping can be used to aggregate information from many sources to create a visual representation of the evidence in order to justify or support a program (Shi and Johnson, 2013).

Healthy People 2020 is an excellent resource that provides objectives, baseline data, targets, and supporting evidence and data sources. The Community Guide (http://www.thecommunityguide.org) is also an invaluable resource that provides evidence to substantiate and justify interventions and strategies that have been selected by a program or partnership.

Local needs assessments with information prioritized and compared with benchmarks or national/regional standards can be used to justify programs. Data from the following can be used to substantiate the initiation and/or continuation of a program or intervention (Hodges and Videtto, 2011).

KEY: no symbol - entry level;   ❖ advanced 1;   ■ advanced 2

Table 5.1

Examples of Sources of Evidence

Sources of Evidence		
Surveys	Activity Logs	Maps
Interviews	Observations	GIS
Community forums	Archives	Asset mapping
Public records	Photographs	Story telling
Newspaper articles	Videos	National strategy reports
Nominal group processes	Journals/diaries	Psychological tests
Morbidity/mortality data	Census reports	Focus groups
Reports from advocacy organizations	Community health indicators	Funding agencies requests for proposals

Online sources of evidence to justify and support programs can include:
- National Center for Health Statistics and its surveys and databases (http://www.cdc.gov/nchs/)
- CDC Wonder Online Databases(http://wonder.cdc.gov)
- The National Library of Medicine (PubMed/MEDLINE) which provides full text articles, citations, and summaries of research from journals and online books (http://www.ncbi.nlm.nih.gov/pubmed)
- The Cochrane Library which provides systematic reviews that can facilitate decision-making (http://www.thecochranelibrary.com/)
- AHRQ which provides research findings, reports, publications, data, and statistical tools (http://www.ahrq.gov)

(Hodges and Videtto, 2011)

5.4.3 Create a rationale to gain or maintain program support

Identifying partners that are knowledgeable and committed to the effort, forming viable coalitions, and working with the community to identify and/or validate issues that are important to them is critical in gaining and maintaining program support. Furthermore, establishing clear relationships between the program's goals and the assets, capacities, and values of the community are critical (Butterfoss, 2007).

5.4.4 Use various communication strategies to present rationale

Organizations that address health education are commonly funded by private donations, contracts, and grants from foundations and/or government agencies. As a result, health education specialists may be responsible for lobbying, attending hearings, managing fundraising, and participating in grant writing activities. Competency in this area requires skills in effective communication among individuals, groups, and organizations through written, oral, and nonverbal means (Longest, 2014; Robbins & Judge, 2015).

Key to program and organizational success is the acceptance and support for programs among internal and external stakeholders/partners. The ability to clearly articulate the aims, goals, and ambitions of the initiative is critical. Effective communication includes developing and selecting appropriate content, formats, and vehicles for formal and informal communications, such as the Internet, telephone calls, meetings, and MOUs.

Competency 5.5: Demonstrate Leadership

There are various definitions and principles of "leadership" that are applicable to the practice of health education. Fallon and Zgodzinski (2011) define leadership as the skills needed to incorporate local rules and policies to allow an organization to be successful in a particular setting. Johnson and Breckon (2007) define it more in terms of influence, where leadership aims to achieve goals and objectives by influencing people in the organization. Healy and Lesneski (2011) indicate that the ability of an individual to influence others to accomplish a predetermined goal is a tenet of leadership. A combination of these various definitions and tenets provides a good perspective of leadership and offers a framework for health education specialists.

Health education specialists are called upon to exercise leadership within a variety of contexts, situations, and environments to address health-related behaviors and systems change within and throughout groups, organizations, and communities. Health education specialists design strategies, lead projects, make decisions, and communicate program inputs and outcomes in order to ensure programs are administered effectively and efficiently (Longest, 2011).

Although advanced-level health education specialists perform more administrative functions than entry-level, all health education specialists are expected to exemplify the ideals of organizational leadership and conduct themselves in accordance with The Code of Ethics for Health Educators (CNHEO, 2011).

❖ 5.5.1 Facilitate efforts to achieve organizational mission

Health education specialists can contribute to the achievement of organizational missions and visions in several ways. They can provide technical assistance, advocacy, strategic planning, and aid in building and supporting teams that plan and implement interventions or strategies. Each task or set of tasks is associated with specific knowledge, skills, and abilities.

5.5.2 Analyze an organization's culture to determine the extent to which it supports health education/promotion

Culture is the patterned ways of thought and behavior that characterize a social group and are learned through socialization processes (McKenzie et al., 2013). Social groups include organizational groups and groups of individuals within organizations. Health education specialists have to be aware of an organization's culture because it impacts how individuals that make up the organization will respond to health education/promotion efforts and programs. When considering the implementation of a health education/promotion program, an analysis or assessment, also referred to as cultural audit and health cultural audit, should be conducted to gain an understanding of the assumptions, values, and other factors that may impact program implementation. There are various Web-based resources, including checklists, available to aid in the accomplishment of this task (McKenzie et al., 2013).

KEY: no symbol - entry level;   ❖ advanced 1;   ■ advanced 2

5.5.3 Develop strategies to reinforce or change organizational culture to support health education/promotion

Health education specialists must consider organizational culture in their efforts, as well as develop and implement effective strategies to manage or change it, as appropriate. Rowitz (2013), Johnson and Breckon (2007), and others present various methods or strategies that may be utilized to reinforce or change organizational culture.

Rowitz (2013) presents a systems approach to organizational change that includes various stages linked to the development of a strategic plan, business plan, work plan, and evaluation plan. The stages include:

- Values clarification
- Mission and vision construction or revision
- Goals and objectives identification
- Action plan development
- Action plan implementation
- Evaluation

There are evolutionary and revolutionary approaches to organizational change. The revolutionary approach is often utilized when there is new leadership, during a crisis, or when an organization may fail if things are not done differently; the evolutionary approach is often utilized when there is stable leadership and long-range program planning and execution is an option (Johnson & Breckon, 2007).

❖ 5.5.4 Facilitate needed changes to organizational culture

Health education specialists may often find themselves in situations in which they are required to facilitate needed organizational cultural changes. In this role, health education specialists may be an organization's staff member (i.e., internal change agent) or work in a consulting capacity (i.e., external change agent). In order to be successful change agents, health education specialists must develop strategies to reinforce or change organizational culture to achieve health education goals. Sub-competency 5.5.3 presents techniques that may be utilized to facilitate change.

❖ 5.5.5 Conduct strategic planning

Strategic planning should assist the administrative process by analyzing availability of resources in an organization, as well as barriers to implementation of the organizational mission (Kreuter et al., 2003).

Strategic planning is a process that encompasses individual, group, community, environment, policy, and other systems-level factors that support or impinge upon the successful implementation of an organizational mission. The strategic planning process captures the course of managing the constant change that affects almost any organization.

The term strategic planning is often misused to refer to a specific document, the strategic plan. A strategic plan document is a product of the strategic planning process. The document serves as a road map that can be referred to over time to serve as reminder, check assumptions, and measure progress (Kreuter et al., 2003). Within various strategic planning models, there are four common questions:

1. What is the current status of the organization?
2. What is the desired direction of the organization?
3. What steps are necessary to move the organization towards its desired future?
4. What progress is being made?

Kreuter et al. (2003) specified tools and actions that may be used to implement a comprehensive strategic planning process using the first three questions, with Longest (2004) adding a fourth question that makes the connection between program performance, evaluation, fiscal viability, and the overall well-being of the organization, program, or project. A more detailed discussion of the questions follows.

- *What is the current status of the organization?*
  The answer to this question provides a baseline measure of where the organization stands at the current time. Internal and external relationships are examined in order to assess how well the organization can meet its goals. An internal assessment generally focuses on the strengths and weaknesses of the organization. An external assessment looks at the opportunities and threats outside the organization. One useful tool in assessing the baseline is a stakeholder analysis. This takes into account the following considerations:
    - Who are the key stakeholders for the organization?
    - What do they think of the organization's performance?
    - What criteria do they use in judging the organization's performance?

- *What is the desired direction of the organization?*
  The answer to this question provides a measure of organizational direction. It should consist of short- and long-term timeframes, such as one year and four to five years or more into the future. This is designed to capture where the organization should be at the end of the time frame in a perfect world without real world constraints.

- *What steps are necessary to move the organization towards the desired future?*
  The answer to this question identifies specific steps by the organization could take to get to its perfect world ideal, which are described in question two above. It addresses questions such as:
    - What resources are required (e.g., money, people, skills, and training)?
    - What alternative routes exist if some or all of these resources are not available?
    - What kinds of new or reinforced collaborations may be required?
    - Who will be responsible for implementation of the steps, and when will they be implemented?

- *What progress is being made?*
  Each of the preceding questions has various dimensions, such as funding levels, staff skill sets, new programs, collaborative relationships, and the use of resources tied to effective outcomes. The nature and complexity of maintaining quality while monitoring costs, requires attention to fiscal and human resources, program standards, desired outcomes, and planning with the end in mind. When tracked over time, each of the factors offers insights into how programs are managed, as well as their performance, strengths, weaknesses, and areas for improvement.

Kreuter et al. (2003) present a ten step strategic planning process (See Table 5.2).

KEY: no symbol - entry level;   ❖ advanced 1;   ■ advanced 2

Table 5.2

Ten Strategic Planning Steps

Step	Activities Performed
1. Initiate and agree on a planning process	• Identify key decision-makers • Determine who should be involved
2. Clarify organizational mandates	• List mandates and sources of mandates • Determine implications of mandates • Determine if mandates should be changed
3a. Identify and understand stakeholders	• Identify internal and external stakeholders • Determine criteria stakeholders use to judge performance • Determine how stakeholders would rate performance
3b. Develop/refine mission statement and values	• Clarify organizational purpose • Respond to key stakeholders • Define philosophy/core values • Identify distinct/unique contributions • List current values and additional values to guide conduct in the future
4. Assess the environment	• List internal strengths and weaknesses • List external opportunities and threats • Identify options for building on strengths and opportunities, and minimizing weaknesses and threats
5. Identify/frame strategic issues	• Identify challenges that require immediate action, monitoring, or action in the near future • Identify consequences of not addressing issues
6. Formulate tactics to manage strategic issues	• Determine strategies, barriers, and actions • Develop a draft strategic plan
7. Review and adopt the plan	• Include key internal and external stakeholders
8. Establish an effective organizational vision for the future	• Describe the "vision of success" based on the mission statement, values, and strategies
9. Develop an implementation process	• List existing programs and services • Set priorities • Determine actions, results, and milestones • Decide who is responsible • Assign dates and resources
10. Reassess the process	• Identify strengths and weaknesses • Suggest modifications • Decide what should be maintained, revised, or terminated

SECTION V

KEY: no symbol - entry level; ❖ advanced 1; ■ advanced 2

Rowitz (2013) outlines J.M. Bryson's 10-step strategic planning model and links it to public health's core functions, organizational practices, essential services, and system activities. The model's steps with public health core function linkages include:

1. Initiation and agreement on a planning process which is linked to policy development
2. Identification and clarification of mandates, which is linked to policy development and assurance
3. Mission and values clarification which is linked to policy development
4. Organization strength, weakness, opportunity, and threat (SWOT) analysis which is linked to assessment
5. Organization strategic issues identification which is linked to policy development as assessment
6. Strategy formulation for addressing identified issues which is linked to policy development
7. Strategic plan(s) review and adoption which is linked to policy development
8. Vision establishment which is linked to policy development
9. Implementation process development which is linked to assurance
10. Strategy and planning reassessment, which is linked to assessment, policy development, and assurance

❖ 5.5.6 Implement strategic plan

Implementation of the strategic planning process is ninth step of the processes presented by Kreuter et al. (2003) and Rowitz (2013). The implementation process involves:

1. Listing programs and services
2. Setting priorities
3. Determining actions, results, and milestones
4. Deciding who will be responsible for specific tasks
5. Assigning dates for the completion of tasks
6. Assigning resources

Specific implementation processes presented by others may be different, but should lead to similar results.

❖ 5.5.7 Monitor strategic plan

The tenth step of the strategic planning processes presented by Kreuter et al. (2003) and Rowitz (2013) involves monitoring or reassessing/revisiting strategies, as well as making changes as appropriate. The process includes identifying of strengths and weaknesses, making suggestions for modifications, and making decisions about what should be maintained, revised, or discontinued. Specific monitoring processes presented by others may be different, but should lead to similar results.

5.5.8 Conduct program quality assurance/process improvement

Consumers of health education and public health services should receive the highest quality of services possible. There are various techniques that may be used to ensure high quality services including, but not limited to: Continuous Quality Improvement (CQI), Total Quality Management (TQM), and Six Sigma (Rowitz, 2013). CQI is a performance management approach that monitors program and service

KEY: no symbol - entry level; ❖ advanced 1; ■ advanced 2

effectiveness with a focus on positive results over times. TQM focuses on customer satisfaction through continuous improvements of organization processes. Six Sigma is a management approach that focuses on objectives and data collection, as well as analysis as mechanisms for reducing or eliminating errors (Rowitz, 2014). Each technique has positive and negative factors and should be examined in detail before an organization selects a specific one to utilize as a mechanism for quality assurance/process improvement.

5.5.9 Comply with existing laws and regulations

Health education specialists must comply with all laws and regulations that apply to the profession in the context in which they practice. The laws and regulations may be at the federal, state, or local level, and they may be in a broad range of categories and specific to a setting (i.e., laws related to employment practices or laws related to business operations). For example, health education specialists within a health care setting must be familiar with the policies related to confidentiality, compliance, and government regulations related to institutional accreditation. Further, health education specialists in school settings may have responsibilities that include the implementation of obesity prevention activities, which may have federal, state, and local regulations related to food services, student exposure to nutrition education, and time allocations for physical activities to which they must be taken consider and adhered.

5.5.10 Adhere to ethical principles of the profession

Professional ethics guide health education specialists in the performance of their duties. The Code of Ethics for the Health Education Profession (2011) includes the following articles:

1. Responsibility to the Public
2. Responsibility to the Profession
3. Responsibility to Employers
4. Responsibility in the Delivery of Health Education
5. Responsibility in Research and Evaluation
6. Responsibility in Professional Preparation

The complete Code of Ethics is provided in Appendix A.

Competency 5.6: Manage Human Resources for Health Education/Promotion Programs

The management of human resources is integral to working with any health agency, association, or organization. Health education specialists have to be aware of the division of work to be accomplished within the context of designated roles and functions. Entry-level health education specialists may be responsible for building, leading, and sustaining teams or work groups within and between organizations. Advanced-level health education specialists are likely to be placed in the unique position of developing job descriptions, selecting staff for program or organizational roles and functions, forming teams, and guiding other leaders. Both the entry- and advanced-level health education specialists may be responsible for facilitating and supporting the work of people both internal and external to their direct line of operations. For example, human resources responsibilities may include managing coalitions, facilitating community-based initiatives, and forming or sustaining interagency collaborations. Effectively managing human resources requires familiarity with participatory forms of leadership that consider diverse work styles, respect the talents of group members, and incorporate the strengths of team members to achieve organizational and programmatic mission.

❖ 5.6.1 Assess staffing needs

In order to ensure appropriate staff is available to meet the needs of the organization, human resource assessments must be conducted. The assessments should be based on strategic and other appropriate plans to ensure current and future human resource needs are taken into consideration. An assessment may begin by conducting an inventory of current employees to determine the knowledge and skills they possess and then determining what will be needed in the future. In some cases, current employees may have the knowledge and skills needed for future endeavors, or they may be trained for the endeavors in lieu of procuring new or additional employees. There are electronic resources available that can aid in this process of assessment, such as online survey systems or task appraisals (DeCenzo & Robbins, 2013).

❖ 5.6.2 Develop job descriptions

Job descriptions present information on the duties of a job and the attributes the individual filling the job should possess. The content and style of job descriptions may vary, but they typically include the following elements:

1. Date of development
2. Job status – exempt/nonexempt
3. Title
4. Identification – position number/code, department
5. Position objectives
6. Supervisor's position
7. Summary of responsibilities
8. Education, experience, licensure, and other requirements
9. Essential functions of the position
10. Disclaimers
11. Signatures or appropriate individuals

(DeCenzo & Robbins, 2013)

❖ 5.6.3 Apply human resource policies consistent with laws and regulations

Federal, state, and local laws, regulations, and policies govern human resources, and it is essential that program managers be familiar with them. Laws, regulations, and policies are updated periodically, and state and local laws, regulations, and policies vary. This variance makes periodic review and familiarization essential. Major federal laws, regulations, and policies that apply to human resource management include, but are not limited to, the following:

- Statutes Prohibiting Discrimination in Employment
  - *Civil Rights Act of 1964/1991*
  - *Age Discrimination in Employment Act (1967)*
  - *American with Disabilities Act (1990)*
  - *Rehabilitation Act (1973)*

KEY: no symbol - entry level; ❖ advanced 1; ■ advanced 2

- *Pregnancy Discrimination Act (1978)*
- *Fair Credit Reporting and Disclosure Act (1970)*
- *Immigration Reform and Control Act (1986)*
- Employment Rights
  - *Family Medical Leave Act (1993)*
- Employee Benefits and Compensation
  - *Fair Labor Standards Act (1938)*
  - *Employee Retirement Income Security Act (1974)*
  - *Consolidated Omnibus Budget Reconciliation Act (COBRA)(1986)*
  - *Federal Unemployment Compensation Act (1939)*
  - *Equal Pay Act (1963)*
  - *Lily Ledbetter Fair Pay Act (2009)*
- Other Federal Laws
  - *Social Security Act (1935)*
  - *National Labor Relations Act (1935)*
  - *Labor-Management Relations Act (1947)*
  - *Occupational Safety and Health Act (1970)*
  - *Health Insurance Portability and Accountability Act (HIPAA)(1996)*
  - *Employee Polygraph Protection Act (1988)*
  - *Pension Protection Act (1987)*
  - *Drug Free Workplace Act (1988)*
  - *Genetic Information Nondiscrimination Act (2008)*
  - *Sarbanes-Oxley Act (2002)*
  - *Privacy Act (1974)*
  - *Uniformed Services Employment and Reemployment Act (1994)*
  - *The Affordable Care Act (2010)*

(Fallon & Zgodzinski, 2011; DeCenzo & Robbins, 2013)

❖ 5.6.4 Evaluate qualifications of staff members and volunteers needed for programs

In order to have successful programs, managers must select appropriate individuals to fill positions within an organization/program. There are a number of instruments available to aid managers in the evaluation of staff and volunteer qualifications. Instruments commonly used by health organizations include: tests, interviews, reference checks, job simulation, work sampling, credentialing, licensing, application forms, resumes, and assessment centers (DeCenzo & Robbins, 2012). Each of the methods or instruments that are available for use has strengths and weaknesses. Therefore, each method should be carefully examined to determine which is most appropriate for the category of personnel being sought for a particular position and the organization that is seeking to fill a position.

5.6.5 Recruit staff members and volunteers for programs

The recruitment of volunteers and staff is essential to the successful achievement of goals and objectives. Individuals filling positions within an organization can come from within the organization or from outside of the organization if they have the required knowledge and skills (Fallon & Zgodzinski, 2011). Recruiting individuals that will successfully fill positions within organizations consists of a process of planning, implementation, and evaluation. During the process the following questions must be answered (Hernadez & Conner, 2009).

- Planning Phase
  - Why is a position required?
  - What are the qualifications required of the individual(s) needed to fill the position(s)?
  - When are the services of these individuals required?
  - Who will be responsible for recruiting for the position?
- Implementation Phase
  - Where will potential volunteers/staff be recruited?
  - Who in the organization will attract potential individuals to fill the positions?
  - Who will be the appropriate individuals to fill the positions?
- Evaluation Phase
  - Determine if the strategy resulted in the selection of appropriate personnel.

❖ 5.6.6 Determine staff member and volunteer professional development needs

Maintaining and improving the abilities of staff should be an ongoing effort, and it should be an important part of a manager's job. In order to accomplish the maintenance and improvement of staff, abilities assessments are necessary. Information for completing assessments and determining needs may be gathered from employee and manager questionnaires and interviews, focus groups, and exit interviews (Fallon & Zgodzinski 2011). In addition, the self-assessment in the beginning and the practice questions at the end of this publication can be used to identify health education Areas of Responsibility that require further training. The gathered information should be utilized to determine professional development needs.

❖ 5.6.7 Develop strategies to enhance staff member and volunteer professional development

Employee and volunteer training and development, and career development are among the myriad of tasks that health education specialists must manage. Training and development are important tasks because they:

- May provide employees with essential knowledge and skills
- Improve employee performance and learning culture of an organization
- Increase sense of usefulness and belonging to an organization
- Help an organization achieve its strategic objectives
- Offer opportunities for employees
- Can serve as a mechanism for the orientation of new employees

(Saks, Hoccoun, & Belcourt, 2010)

Employee/volunteer training focuses on assisting the individuals with acquiring or improving knowledge, skills, attitudes, and/or behaviors necessary to perform in their current position. Development is designed to assist the organization and the employee with preparing for future needs within the organization. Strategies to accomplish this task may include: job rotations, acting as an assistant to the individual filling the position, committee assignments, lectures/seminars, and simulations (DeCenzo, Robbins, & Verhulst, 2013). Career development is designed to assist employees

KEY: no symbol - entry level; ❖ advanced 1; ■ advanced 2

with advancement in their career, but it focuses on the long-term career effectiveness and success of an individual versus the more immediate/intermediate effectiveness that is the focus of training and development programs (DeCenzo, Robbins, & Verhulst, 2013).

Fallon and Zgodzinski (2012) provide the following as methods for employee training and development: (a) new employee orientation, (b) training to correct performance issues, (c) training within departments, (d) cross-training for efficiency, (e) on-the-job training, and (f) mentorship. Health education specialists should also join professional associations and organizations, attend meetings and conferences, and read the latest periodicals sponsored or endorsed by those organizations in order to ensure they stay abreast of information and developments in the field.

❖ 5.6.8 Implement strategies to enhance the professional development of staff members and volunteers

A variety of strategies may be utilized to enhance the training and professional development of staff members and volunteers. Training focuses on current jobs and the enhancement of skills necessary to perform the current job; development focuses on future jobs (DeCenzo, Robbins, & Verhulst, 2013). Training strategies may include on-the-job training or off-the-job training methods. On-the-job training methods include: job rotation, apprenticeships, and internships. Off- the-job training methods include: lectures, multimedia learning, simulations, and vestibule training. Community practices can gather people with a common interest to share knowledge and expertise with each other and identify new approaches for problem solving (Saks, Hoccoun, & Belcourt, 2010).

❖ 5.6.9 Develop and implement strategies to retain staff members and volunteers

The retention of good staff members is linked to making work a positive experience and motivating employees (Rowitz, 2013). Knowledge, skills, and abilities enhancement are factors in motivating employees and making work a positive experience, and they should be included in any retention strategy. Methods for motivating employees include: (a) coaching and mentoring, (b) rewards and recognition, (c) training and conference opportunities, (d) career opportunities, (e) employee benefits, and (f) good communications (Rowitz, 2013).

❖ 5.6.10 Employ conflict resolution techniques

Organizations can be affected by intra- or inter-personal, intra- or inter-group, and inter-organizational conflict. Effective leadership includes negotiating, mediating, planning proactively, designing programs, and communicating effectively to prevent or minimize its effect on the organization's climate and performance (Hellriegel & Slocum, 2013).

Conflict resolution directs individuals and organizations to see the similarities and differences that exist between them and then leads them to focus on reducing or eliminating differences in order to accomplish goals and objectives. Rowitz (2013) presents an eight step process for conflict resolution that can be applied in most situations:

1. Create an atmosphere that is effective for goal or objective accomplishment
2. Clarify the perceptions of all parties involved

3. Focus on the needs of the individuals and organizations as separate entities, as well as the needs of collective individuals and organizations
4. Build shared positive power
5. Work toward and with a future orientation, but learn from past activities
6. Create options
7. Develop goals, objectives, and activities that can be accomplished
8. Make sure there are benefits for all involved parties

Negotiation between two or more individuals or organizations may be part of the conflict resolution process. Among the models for negotiation, a 14-step model developed by Schoenfield and Schoenfield (1991) incorporates many of the strategies from other models (Rowitz, 2013). The steps of this model include:

Pre-negotiation:
1. Information gathering
2. Goal determination
3. Issues identification
4. Analysis
5. Assessment of strengths and weaknesses
6. Estimation of the parties' positions
7. Consideration of outcomes that present wins for both/all parties

Negotiation:
8. Setting the opening position
9. Setting the bottom line
10. Selection of strategies
11. Concession consideration
12. Agenda determination
13. Timing analysis
14. Selection of communication modes

❖ 5.6.11 Facilitate team development

Teams of individuals or groups from different departments or organizations may be brought together to accomplish specific goals and objectives. In order for the individuals and groups to work together effectively, activities to enhance members' trust and openness may have to be undertaken. Activities to help build individuals and groups into effective teams involve:

- Goal setting
- Interpersonal relationship development
- Role and responsibility clarification
- Process analysis

(DeCenzo & Robbins 2013)

KEY: no symbol - entry level;   ❖ advanced 1;   ■ advanced 2

❖ 5.6.12 Evaluate performance of staff members and volunteers

Evaluating the performance of staff and volunteers is an essential aspect of management and provides organizational leadership with important information. The benefits of performance evaluations include:

- Reinforcing open communication and rapport-building
- Provision of two-way performance feedback
- Recognition or motivating employees
- Opportunity to reinforce and note personnel feedback and decisions
- Goal-setting for the next review period in the context of organizational needs

(Armstrong, 2010)

There are various methods for conducting performance appraisals including:

- Critical incidents which focus on key behaviors related to accomplishing the job
- Checklist which utilizes a list of behaviors
- Graphic rating scale which accesses where an individual is on a scale based on a list of factors such as job knowledge, cooperation, and attendance
- Forced-choice, which requires the rater to choose between two or more statements
- Behaviorally anchored rating scales which combine critical incident and graphic rating scales
- Group ordered ranking requires employees to be placed in a classification (i.e., top ten percent of organization's health education specialists)
- Individual ranking, which requires employees be ranked from highest performers to lowest performers
- Paired comparison, which requires an employee trait be selected and all employees in a group be compared based on that trait

(DeCenzo & Robbins, 2013)

Program managers must understand the method or methods their organization prescribes and evaluate their staff accordingly.

In addition to being aware of the evaluation process, program managers also need to be aware of and avoid distorted evaluations/appraisals. Distortions can occur in the following forms: (a) leniency errors, (b) halo errors, (c) similarity errors, (d) low appraisal motivation, (e) central tendency, (f) inflationary pressures, and (g) using something other than actual job performance to provide the evaluation (DeCenzo & Robbins, 2013).

❖ 5.6.13 Monitor performance and/or compliance of funding recipients

The methods utilized for performance monitoring or evaluation may be based on absolute standards, relative standards, or outcomes (DeCenzo & Robbins, 2013). The absolute standards methods consist of comparison to a standard. These include techniques such as critical incident, checklist, graphic rating scale, forced choice, and behaviorally anchored rating scale appraisals. Relative standards methods consist of comparing an individual to other individuals, and these include methods such as group order ranking, individual ranking, and paired comparisons. Outcomes methods, or management by objectives (MBO), are based on the achievement of established objectives or outcomes (DeCenzo & Robbins, 2013).

The following are steps in an appraisal process: 1) establish performance standards, 2) communicate expectations, 3) measure actual performance, 4) compare actual performance with established standards, 5) discuss the appraisal or findings with employee (funding recipient), and 6) initiate corrective action, if necessary (DeCenzo & Robbins, 2013). Other individuals present different steps, but the underlying process is basically the same: establish and communicate standards, monitor performance based on established standards, and communicate and correct failures to perform to established standards.

❖ 5.6.14 Apply ethical principles when managing human resources

Ethics are principles or rules which provide guidance for behaviors that may be classified as right or wrong (DeCenzo & Robbins, 2013; Fallon & Zgodzinski, 2011). Ethics are often delineated in Codes of Ethics, which various organizations and professions utilize to govern its members. (It must be noted, the concepts of right and wrong may not equate to legal or illegal.) The Code of Ethics for health education specialist is presented in appendix A.

Issues that may not be clearly defined as right or wrong, legal or illegal, that ethical principles may be applied to and managers may have to respond to include:

- Electronic surveillance of employees (i.e., monitoring Internet usage, telephone usage, and email)
- Monitoring employees access to records and documents (i.e., employees looking at electronic records on clients that they may not need to know information about in the direct performance of their job)
- Monitoring employees personal behaviors that may not be directly related to job performance (i.e., smoking or tobacco usage)

(DeCenzo & Robbins, 2013)

KEY: no symbol - entry level;   ❖ advanced 1;   ■ advanced 2

CHAPTER VI

Area of Responsibility VI

Serve as a Health Education/Promotion Resource Person

6.1 Obtain and disseminate health-related information

6.1.1   Assess needs for health-related information
6.1.2   Identify valid information resources
6.1.3   Evaluate resource materials for accuracy, relevance, and timeliness
6.1.4   Adapt information for consumer
6.1.5   Convey health-related information to consumer

6.2 Train others to use health education/promotion skills

6.2.1   ❖ Assess training needs of potential participants
6.2.2   ❖ Develop a plan for conducting training
6.2.3   ❖ Identify resources needed to conduct training
6.2.4   ❖ Implement planned training
6.2.5   ❖ Conduct formative and summative evaluations of training
6.2.6   ❖ Use evaluative feedback to create future trainings

6.3 Provide advice and consultation on health education/promotion issues

6.3.1   ❖ Assess and prioritize requests for advice/consultation
6.3.2   ❖ Establish advisory/consultative relationships
6.3.3   ❖ Provide expert assistance and guidance
6.3.4   ❖ Evaluate the effectiveness of the expert assistance provided
6.3.5   ❖ Apply ethical principles in consultative relationships

SECTION VI

The Role. The setting in which health education specialists function largely determines the nature of the resources provided for a program. When requested, health education specialists need to serve as a resource for valid health information and materials. They must be aware of a variety of community resources at the local, state, and national levels as well as familiar with online databases and able to evaluate the accuracy, relevance, and timeliness of resource materials. In addition, health education specialists must be able to adapt health related information for, and to, those in the priority population. Finally, health education specialists practicing at the advanced-level need to train others to use health education/promotion skills, assess and prioritize requests for advice and consultation, and establish advisory and consultative relationships, as well as provide and evaluate the effects of expert assistance and guidance.

Settings. The following text is presented to describe how acting as a resource is used in different practice settings.

Community Setting. Health education specialists serving as resource persons in a community setting may be asked to assist community-based organizations, local voluntary health organizations, churches, civic organizations, neighborhood associations, and other nonprofits. In this capacity, health education specialists might be asked to provide current health information (i.e., suggestions on relevant literature findings, audiovisual materials, educational pamphlets, and posters for distribution) and serve on various community-wide coalitions to help identify and implement strategies to improve health. They also may be called on to train others to better plan, implement, and evaluate health education/promotion programs. Those health education specialists practicing at an advanced-level may serve as advisors or consultants for new community organizations just beginning to offer health education/promotion programs.

School (K-12) Setting. Health education specialists in the school setting may participate in the work of a curriculum committee formed to identify and select educational materials in compliance with state legislative mandates and school district policies. Health education specialists provide expert assistance to committee members in examining state laws and codes, establishing criteria for the evaluation of instructional materials, and recommending placement of the topic in the overall curriculum scope and sequence plan. After selecting the material, health education specialists arrange preview sessions for interested parents and community members.

Health Care Setting. Health care settings may include hospitals, medical centers, clinics, and satellite clinics. Health education specialists in these health care settings serve as consultants to

a community group by developing chronic disease prevention and control education programs. Health education specialists provide information on successful or evidence-based programs, help identify culturally and linguistically appropriate materials, conduct focus groups to assist in planning interventions, identify expert speakers, and help identify media and other communication channels for disseminating information about the program to the community. These health education specialists also may facilitate use of community services by providing links to health care services and the community.

Business/Industry Setting. Physical fitness, stress management, and nutrition programs are frequently featured in worksite health education/promotion programming. As resource persons, health education specialists are responsible for disseminating information to employers and employees about these programs in a timely manner. Health education specialists identify and organize resources needed for the implementation and continuation of health education/promotion programs and policy changes at the worksite to promote health. They also identify data to present to key personnel and monitor the plans of those responsible for conducting the program in order to ensure that activities match the stated goals, objectives, and budget. In addition, health education specialists identify and/or develop relevant health promotion materials about specific topics to display and distribute to employees at the worksite.

College/University Setting. Health education specialists often serve as consultants to

KEY: no symbol - entry level;   ❖ advanced 1;   ■ advanced 2

community agencies and local school districts. In that role, they often provide and share health education/promotion resources and information. Health education specialists must be able to teach students how and where to obtain valid and reliable health information so that students may serve as resource persons in their future professional endeavors.

College/University Health Services Setting. Health education specialists in the campus health services setting serve as health education/promotion resources for the campus community. This role includes assessing needs for health information, evaluating resources, and adapting materials for the campus community. Some health education specialists may train others to use health education/promotion skills, as well as consult and advise on campus health issues.

Key Terms

Adaptation is making changes to health education messages, materials, or programs to make them more suitable for a population of interest (Moore, Bumbarger, & Cooper, 2013).

Consultation is the process by which the knowledge of one person is used to help another make better decisions (Dickert & Sugarman, 2005).

Informal consulting does not require a written agreement or formal contract. This type of consulting consists of acting as a resource person responsible for organizing health education materials and responding to requests for health education information and literature/materials (Dickert & Sugarman, 2005).

Formal consulting requires a contract or written agreement between two parties, the client and consultant. Formal consultants are hired for their expertise in a particular area for which the client needs assistance, advice, direction, etc. Formal consulting follows the steps of diagnosis, recommendation, action, evaluation, and termination (Dickert & Sugarman, 2005).

Evidence-based public health refers to application of observation-, theory-, and science-based experiments (evidence) to improve the health of populations (Brownson et al., 2011).

Online database refers to any systematically organized information accessible on the Internet, which may be used by health education specialists to obtain health knowledge and/or resources for the health education process. An online database may include text documents, citations, abstracts, images, audios, videos, and/or Web links (McKenzie et al., 2012).

SECTION VI

Technical Assistance is a dynamic, capacity building process for designing or improving the quality, effectiveness, and efficiency of specific programs, research, services, products, or systems (West, Clapp, Averill, & Cates, 2012).

Competency 6.1: Obtain and Disseminate Health-Related Information

Health resources are critical to health promotion, and health education specialists are often gatekeepers to them for other professionals and the community. Health information can be obtained from a variety of sources, including professional journals, textbooks, government publications (e.g., local, state, and federal publications), colleges/universities, medical centers, professional conferences, public health agencies, associations, and the Internet. Health information may be converted into electronic documents and images including digital audio, video, and multimedia formats.

6.1.1 Assess needs for health-related information

Health education specialists should start by defining the information needs of a population, which may include statistics for community assessment or formative research, educational materials, evidence-based programs or strategies for program planning, survey tools for data collection or evaluation, or topic-specific health information. They can use a variety of software and/or Web applications to save and retrieve data and/or literature necessary for program planning, assessment, implementation, or evaluation.

Health education specialists need to know where to obtain the resources and materials needed to effectively implement programming. Resource materials can increase awareness and enhance learning. Health education specialists should select the most appropriate materials and resources from credible, reliable sources that match audience needs.

Regardless of where health information originates, the following are steps for identifying the information needed for dissemination:
1. Identify the need
2. Match the need to likely source
3. Pursue lead
4. Judge the quality and quantity of the information found
5. Organize the available material in a format most useful to the user

6.1.2 Identify valid information resources

As resource persons, health education specialists should be able to locate a variety of credible health information resources and interpret the findings. Valid information resources may include governmental agencies, quasigovernmental agencies, and nongovernmental agencies (i.e., voluntary, philanthropic, service, religious, and professional) (Cottrell et al., 2014). Several categories and examples of useful

KEY: no symbol - entry level; ❖ advanced 1; ■ advanced 2

resources are provided below including governmental sources, professional organizations, clinical health care organizations, resources for evidence-based approaches, and social networking tools, among others. These examples are a starting point and are not meant to be exhaustive. Health education specialists are also tasked with staying current on emerging public health priorities and evolving resources that arise in the field.

Population and Heath Statistics. Two primary sources for population and health statistics are the United States Census and the National Center for Health Statistics (NCHS). The United States Census offers quality data about the people and economy in the United States. It has tables of data, searchable queries, and maps of data. The data include the results from the Population and Housing Census, Economic Census, American Community Survey, and Economic Indicators (http://www.census.gov/). The NCHS is a rich source of information about the health status of the population and monitors trends in health status and health care delivery (http://www.cdc.gov/nchs/). Health education specialists can access data and also health questionnaires for NCHS' major surveys.

Governmental Sources. Government health agencies are part of national, state, or local structures (McKenzie et al., 2012). Leading government health agencies provide information about health topics and access to electronic or printable health promotion materials, campaigns, or reports. Some examples of these are the following:

- United States Government's Web site (http://www.firstgov.gov/)
- United States Department of Health and Human Services (http://www.dhhs.gov/)
- Healthy People 2020 (http://www.healthypeople.gov/)
- Centers for Disease Control and Prevention (http://www.cdc.gov/)
- National Institutes of Health (http://www.nih.gov/)
- Government Printing Office (GPO) Access (http://www.gpoaccess.gov/)
- Health Resources and Services Administration (http://www.hrsa.gov)
- Agency for Healthcare Research and Quality (http://www.ahrq.gov)
- Environmental Protection Agency (http://www.epa.gov)
- Food and Drug Administration (http://www.fda.gov/)
- United States Department of Agriculture (http://www.usda.gov/wps/portal/usda)

Community Organizations and Local Resources. Community organizations can also be good sources of health statistics and information. Health education specialists can search for local resources in their community, including telephone and online directories, public libraries, wellness councils (group of businesses interested in health promotion), health coalitions/partnerships, city and county health departments, neighborhood health centers, colleges and universities, and community organizations (McKenzie et al., 2012).

Public Health and Professional Organizations. Health education specialists can also employ professional associations/organizations, such as the Society for Public Health Education (SOPHE) or American School Health Association (ASHA), and their Web sites or electronic mailing lists to acquire recommendations and information sources from colleagues in the field. Professional associations are effective channels to reach experts on topical issues. They may have a directory that is searchable by members' areas of interest. Below are examples of public health professional health organizations that provide an array of resources and linkages:

- American Public Health Association, Public Health Education and Health Promotion (PHEHP) Section (https://www.apha.org/)
- Association of State and Territorial Health Officials (http://www.astho.org/)
- Directors of Health Promotion and Education (http://www.dhpe.org/)
- National Association of Chronic Disease Directors (http://www.chronicdisease.org/)
- National Association of County and City Health Officials (http://www.naccho.org/)
- National Association of Local Boards of Health (http://www.nalboh.org)
- SOPHE (http://www.sophe.org/)

The Public Health Accreditation Board (PHAB) (http://www.phaboard.org/) also offers useful background and resources for health education specialists that may be involved with state, local, and tribal health departments pursuing or maintaining accreditation.

Health Care Financing Resources. Health care financing is an important resource for health organizations and consumers. They need to know how health care is covered and options for paying for their health care. Community members receive health insurance from a range of sources, including:

- Self-funded insurance programs (e.g., employers, union, trade)
- Managed care plans
- Government provided
    - Medicare (http://www.medicare.gov/) – insurance for those 65 and older and younger people with disabilities
    - Medicaid (http://medicaid.gov/) – jointly funded federal and state insurance for people with low income
    - Children's Health Insurance Program (https://www.healthcare.gov/medicaid-chip/childrens-health-insurance-program/) – insurance coverage for children who are low income and uninsured and not covered by Medicaid
- Affordable Care Act health exchanges (http://www.healthcare.gov)

(McKenzie et al., 2013)

Clinical Health Care Organizations and Agencies. Several resources promote public health and clinical linkages such as the Institute of Medicine (http://www.iom.edu) and The Practical Playbook (https://practicalplaybook.org/).

Health education specialists can serve as a linkage to connect clinical practice with public health. Other clinical resources that could be useful to public health practice include:

- 2014 Guide to Clinical Preventive Services (http://www.ahrq.gov/professionals/clinicians-providers/guidelines-recommendations/guide/)
- Affordable Care Act (https://www.healthcare.gov/)

KEY: no symbol - entry level; ❖ advanced 1; ■ advanced 2

- Healthcare Effectiveness Data and Information Set (HEDIS) & Performance Measurement (http://www.ncqa.org/HEDISQualityMeasurement.aspx)
- Health Information Technology (HIT), Electronic Health Records (EHRs), & Meaningful Use (http://www.healthit.gov)
- Centers for Medicare & Medicaid Services (http://cms.hhs.gov/)

Voluntary Organizations and Foundations. Voluntary health agencies are organizations that deal with health needs and may rely heavily on donations or volunteers to function (Cottrell et al., 2014). The World Health Organization, located in Geneva, Switzerland, is the most recognized international health organization, and provides a variety of health information and data on their Web site (http://www.who.int/en/). Some other sources of information are voluntary health agencies and foundations. Examples of voluntary health organizations are the:

- American Cancer Society (http://www.cancer.org/)
- American Heart Association (http://www.heart.org)
- American Lung Association (http://www.lung.org/)
- American Red Cross (http://www.redcross.org/)
- American Diabetes Association (http://www.diabetes.org/)

Foundations are charitable organizations that donate funds or assets for a specific purpose. The Foundation Center provides program details for thousands of foundations (http://fconline.fdncenter.org/). For example, the Robert Wood Johnson Foundation (http://www.rwjf.org/) publishes reports and other documents from its funded public health projects. Other education and policy Web sites contain useful resources such as the:

- Aspen Institute (http://www.aspeninstitute.org/)
- California Endowment (http://www.calendow.org/)
- Partnership for Prevention (http://www.prevent.org/)
- Policy Link (http://www.policylink.org/)

Networks of Universities and Research Institutions. Multiple academic institutions provide applied research data, resources, training, community assessment, and evaluation content useful across public health topics and regions. Below are a few of these networks:

- Association of Schools and Programs of Public Health (http://www.aspph.org/)
- National Network of Public Health Institutes (http://www.nnphi.org/) – CDC/RWJF
- Prevention Research Centers (http://www.cdc.gov/prc/) - CDC
- Public Health Services and Systems Research (PHSSR) Practice-Based Research Networks (http://www.publichealthsystems.org/) - RWJF
- Public Health Training Center Network (http://www.publichealthtrainingcenters.org/) - HRSA

Internet Consumer Information Sites. In addition, the Internet is a source for many excellent health education resources that are both accurate and current. Several authoritative sources of consumer health information exist, including MedlinePlus, Healthfinder, Health on the Net (HON), and WebMD.

SECTION VI

A description of each source follows.

- MedlinePlus is the National Library of Medicine's Web site (in both English and Spanish) for consumer health information. It includes health topics, a medical encyclopedia, interactive health tutorials, and health news. (http://medlineplus.gov).

- Healthfinder is a Department of Health and Human Services Web site for consumer access to information from governmental agencies and their partners. It offers links to online journals, medical dictionaries, and prevention and self-care. (http://www.healthfinder.gov).

- HON is a nonprofit medical information portal that links to reliable and trustworthy medical sites on the Internet (http://www.hon.ch/HONcode/).

- WebMD is a health information Web site for the public that provides updated content on a variety of health issues, health news, reference materials, and tools for managing health. (http://www.webmd.com/)

Resources to find Evidence-based Approaches. Evidence-based public health refers to application of observation-, theory-, and science-based experiments (evidence) to improve the health of populations (Brownson et al., 2010). Examples of evidence-based interventions that have been proven to work can be found at several Web sites. These provide information about evidence-based strategies (e.g., one-on-one education for cancer screening) programs or policies and also may have the packaged materials available or a link to the program developer's site. Some of these sites include:

- The Guide to Community Preventive Services (http://thecommunityguide.org)
- Cochrane Reviews | The Cochrane Collaboration (http://www.cochrane.org)
- AHRQ Innovations Exchange (https://innovations.ahrq.gov/)
- National Cancer Institute's (NCI) Research-tested Intervention Programs (RTIPs) (http://rtips.cancer.gov/rtips)
- Diffusion of Effective Behavioral Interventions (DEBIs) for HIV programs (http://www.effectiveinterventions.org/)
- SAMSHA's Guide to Evidence-based Practices (EBP) (http://www.samhsa.gov/ebpwebguide)
- National Registry of Evidence-based Programs and Practices (NREPP) (http://nrepp.samhsa.gov)
- Partnership for Prevention (http://www.prevent.org/)
- Center for Training and Research Translation (https://www.center-trt.org)

Social Networking Resources. Health education specialists are increasingly using social media such as Facebook, Twitter, LinkedIn, You Tube, Pinterest, Web feeds, podcasts, and other social networking sites to efficiently reach communities with which to network and communicate (Capurro et al., 2014; Heldman & Schindelar, 2013). Many of the Web sites listed in this chapter have multiple social media communication outlets that can provide rapidly changing information. The CDC has a Social Media Web site and toolkit (http://www.cdc.gov/socialmedia/). The United States Department of Health and Human Services links to Resources for social media use in public health and a Social Hub of related agencies (http://www.hhs.gov/web/socialmedia/). New social networking capabilities and applications are continually under development and rapidly evolving to allow health education specialists to follow

KEY: no symbol - entry level;   ❖ advanced 1;   ■ advanced 2

the priorities and trends. Health education specialists can use electronic mailing lists to broadcast messages and questions to other health education specialists via e-mail. One example is the International Electronic Mail Directory of Health Education specialists (HEDIR) (http://hedir.org).

Health education specialists can use online resources to locate educational materials for a variety of populations. Some materials are free to health education specialists, while some are available at minimal charge. The following Web sites readily provide health education materials:

- *CDC.* Their Web site has health promotion materials for the public and health professionals. It is located at http://www.cdc.gov/.
- *Health Resources and Services Administration (HRSA)* of USDHHS provides a wide variety of health education materials free of charge. Its public health page is accessible at http://www.hrsa.gov/publichealth.
- *National Health Information Center* offers a referral source for health information and has a Health Information Resource Database. It is located at http://www.health.gov/nhic/.

Health education specialists can also proactively subscribe to tailored topic-specific updates with desired frequency settings (i.e., daily, weekly, etc.) by signing up for PubMed search alerts or e-mail updates from health and government sites such as http://www.firstgov.gov/ and http://www.thecommunityguide.org.

Journals and Print Materials. Online health information, such as journals, other documents, and databases can be accessed using indexed retrieval systems at libraries. Web browsers access search engines to review relevant records in response to a query for a key word, title, or phrase. The following bibliographic databases offer access to health information in published journals.

- *MEDLINE*: Although this database contains primarily medical journals, many health education journals are also indexed. PubMed is its online searchable interface through the Web site of the National Library of Medicine (NLM). It offers free access to citations from MEDLINE and other journals. Users can search health information by keywords in title, author, abstract, source, and other search fields. The results are provided in the form of article sources, abstracts, and, sometimes, Web links to retrieve full text documents. This database is free and can be accessed at http://www.ncbi.nlm.nih.gov/PubMed. Full-text articles may require a fee from the publisher.

- *Education Resource Information Center (ERIC):* This database contains journals related to school health, school-aged children, and education in its broadest sense. Often, ERIC includes articles from professional journals and documents, which are available online in full text or on microfiche in large libraries, especially at colleges or universities. ERIC documents are materials that are not found in journal literature, such as proceedings from conferences or policies. This database is free and can be accessed at http://www.eric.ed.gov/.

- *Cumulative Index for Nursing and Allied Health Literature (CINAHL):* This is a database for health education information indices, major health education journals, and journals from nursing and many other disciplines. The use of CINAHL may involve a fee for subscription. This database can be accessed at http://www.cinahl.com/.

KEY: no symbol - entry level; ❖ advanced 1; ■ advanced 2

- *Evidence-based Medicine Reviews (EBMR):* This is a collection of databases that offer evidence-based strategies, programs, and medicine, such as Cochrane Database of Systematic Reviews, The Database of Abstracts of Reviews of Effectiveness (DARE), Health Technology Assessments (HTA), methods, and article reviews. Each database from the EBMR collection is a separate file and must be browsed separately. For example, the Cochrane Library offers full reports that provide the evidence for and against the effectiveness and appropriateness of treatments, such as education and medication. It is located at http://www.ovid.com.

- *Health and Psychosocial Instruments (HaPI):* This database collects rating scales, questionnaires, checklists, tests, interview schedules, and coding schemes/manuals for health and social sciences. Health and psychosocial instruments in this database are used and/or published in literature and often recognize reliability and validity concerns. Health education specialists may use these instruments for assessment and/or evaluation purposes. The use of HaPI may involve a fee for subscription. This database can be accessed via the search feature at http://www.ovid.com.

- *PsycInfo*: This database includes a summary of journal articles, books, dissertations, and technical reports from professional and academic literature in psychology. The search is free, and single articles or book chapters can be purchased. There is also an option to purchase a 24-hour pass. The database can be found at http://psycnet.apa.org/.

Health education research or practice articles can be found in some leading journals in the field: *Health Education & Behavior, Health Promotion Practice, American Journal of Health Education, American Journal of Health Promotion, American Journal of Health Behavior, Pedagogy in Health Promotion, Health Education Research, Journal of School Health, Journal of Community Health, Journal of American College Health, and Patient Education and Counseling*, among others. Along with information collected regularly by government agencies, these are good sources of health information.

6.1.3 Evaluate resource materials for accuracy, relevance, and timeliness

To determine if the health information source is credible and reliable, health education specialists should be mindful of the following: purpose of the source, scientific methodology, qualifications of the author, standing of the publication or organization in the profession, and the quality of references and sources (Cottrell et al., 2014).

Health education specialists need to be aware of the types of electronic health-related resources available and how to make decisions about when each is appropriate to use based on the information needed. Whether the resource is a bibliographic database or a Web-based information source, health education specialists need to analyze and evaluate the worthiness of the information retrieved, as some information on the Web is inaccurate, untruthful, or outdated. Health education specialists should look for Web sites hosted by reputable sources, consider biases reflected in the information, and determine if the information is outdated or misleading.

Accuracy. It is important to evaluate the accuracy, quality, and significance of the information in relation to the needs of the priority audience. When assessing online information, consider the following:

- Who is responsible for managing the site?
- What is the site's funding source?
- What is the purpose of the site?
- Does it cite evidence-based references?
- What are the credentials of the reviewers/editors that proof the accuracy of content?
- How is personal user information utilized and protected?

(NCI, 2015)

For electronic apps and devices, ask:

- Do they address user needs as described?
- Are the tools or resources easy to use to find the specific information you need?
- Does it work compatibly with other tools and resources you need to connect to (e.g., options to export data)?

(USDHHS, 2014)

Critically evaluating the reliability of information is key, especially given the emergence of more Web content generated by end-users ("Web 2.0"). On blogs, comment fields, wikis, and online community boards, contributors may not clearly self-disclose identity, credentials, expertise, or distinguish opinion from fact. Interactive information sharing and personal experiences can enhance resource sharing as long as health education specialists can clarify how this information may complement evidence-based and accurate sources (Adams, 2012).

Relevance. In addition to knowing where to find and how to access health information, health education specialists must be able to evaluate the relevance, appropriateness, and effectiveness of materials for the priority population, group, or client. Resource materials for any program, such as handouts, brochures, fact sheets, talking points, and Frequently Asked Questions (FAQs), should be carefully reviewed to make sure they enhance message appeal.

Resources and materials should be selected based on the client/community's needs and the program objectives. When evaluating resources, consider the following:

- Does the resource contain the information that the client/community wants to know?
- Does the material address needs and priorities identified in the community assessment?
- Is the information compatible with the community context and culture?
- Can the client/community understand the information contained in the resource?
- Is the format appropriate and the information culturally appropriate?
- Will the resource meet program objectives?
  What is the reading level of the materials?

(Doak, Doak, Gordon, & Lorig, 2001; Doak, Doak, & Root, 2002)

When reviewing written resource materials, consider the following questions:

- Does the material have audience appeal?
- Is it complete? Is there sufficient, too much, or too little information?
- Is it written in a logical, clearly developed, easy to follow format?
- Is the message supportive, positive, and personal?
- Does it attract and keep the reader's attention?
- Is the physical appearance (color, layout, print, illustrations) appropriate for the audience?
- Are the graphics simple, clear, and compatible with the text?
- Is the vocabulary appropriate for the audience? Are new terms defined, and has jargon been avoided?
- Is the reading level appropriate for the audience?

(Plomer & Bensley, 2009)

The materials should be compiled and evaluated through a quick review process. An Educational Materials Review Form (Wurzbach, 2004) or a modified version may have health education specialists inventory the materials and determine which is most relevant and appropriate for your community group. The form assesses these aspects of the materials:

- Form
- Length
- Topic
- Mode of delivery
- Setting
- Intended audience
- Language
- Readability
- Scope of the material (national to local)
- Pretest or evaluated
- Availability
- Language

Timeliness. Health education specialists are also tasked with evaluating if the information and resources are accurate, current, updated, and timely (NCI, 2014; Plomer & Bensley, 2009). Recommendations may change over time. For example, fruit and vegetable intake changed from the Five-A-Day Campaign to More Matters (http://www.fruitsandveggiesmorematters.org/) based on enhanced USDA guidelines. Public health goals and objectives may change periodically over time, such as Healthy People 2020 may soon be planning for the next iteration of emerging issues (http://www.healthypeople.gov/). The evidence-base is continually evolving as research and evaluation fill the evidence gaps. Health education specialists should stay abreast of new evidence and updated findings in their areas of expertise.

As resource persons, health education specialists may need to share that in a timely and rapid manner, especially when health issues are time sensitive, such as in crisis and emergency situations. The CDC's

KEY: no symbol - entry level;   ❖ advanced 1;   ■ advanced 2

Office of Public Health Preparedness and Response (OPHPR) hosts a Web site with tools for Crisis & Emergency Risk Communication (CERC) (http://www.bt.cdc.gov/cerc/). The CERC manual offers tools to help develop communication messages that are timely, correct, and credible.

Timeliness may also consider whether a message is being delivered at the appropriate timing given contextual circumstances and priorities. For example, if food insecurity is a top priority for a population, addressing chronic disease prevention may not be the timely priority to address right away. However, the less urgent issue could still be woven into a message that addresses the more pressing one. In this case, food insecurity could be addressed by initiatives to bring local healthy produce to increase access in food deserts, which in turn could contribute to chronic disease prevention via healthier options.

Evaluating Online Resources. While assessing resource materials from the Internet, health education specialists can consider elements such as the Web site purpose, domain name, appropriateness, readability, and affiliations. Then, they can gauge if those elements are applicable to those that need those resources. Considerations for evaluating the quality of online resources are summarized in the Table 6.1 below.

Table 6.1

Considerations for Evaluating Quality of Online Resources

Element	Application of Element
Web site purpose	Intention of the site consistent with the institutional affiliation and author credentials (NCI, 2014)
Domain name	The URL ends in .org, .gov, or .edu. A Web site's domain name and extension may offer information about the credibility of the source. Those sites ending in .org (organization) or .gov (government) likely offer more unbiased information than those with a .com (commercial) extension
Priority population	Content of the Web site is appropriate for the audience whether consumer, professional or both (Cottrell et al., 2014)
Web site's appropriateness	Review of sources and timeliness of information (NCI, 2014; Plomer & Bensley, 2009).

Element	Application of Element
Web site's accuracy	Content of the site is backed by empirical research or facts and verified by expert opinion. References are available for statistics and information. (Eysenbach et al., 2002; Dreier et al., 2013)
Web site's adequacy	Determine if Web site's research was conducted independently (Doyle et al., 2010)
Web site's currency	Health information changes constantly; data updated regularly (National Library of Medicine, 2009)
Readability	Reading level of the content of the Web site is acceptable to audience (Dreier et al., 2013)
Reputable affiliations	Type of organizations sponsoring the Web site; Materials being published consistent with the agency's mission
Author/administrative names	Qualified people writing the information posted (professional credentials) (NCI, 2014)
Author contact information	A mailing address, telephone, fax or E-mail information available on the site (Cottrell et al., 2014)

6.1.4 Adapt information for consumer

Adaptation is making changes to health education messages, materials, or programs to make them more suitable for a population of interest or an organization. Common reasons for adaptation are: differences between the intended population and the audience for which the program/materials were designed, limited resources (e.g., money, time), resistance of implementers or priority population, or competing demands (Moore, Bumbarger, & Cooper, 2013). Before adapting information, it is helpful to consider what elements to adapt, the reason for that change, and to what extent that modification changes the original product. Health education specialists should not try to change the core behavior or organizational theory, behavior, environmental factors, risk factors, or strategy employed without advice from the original developer or content experts. Some types of adaptations include changes to content (e.g., adding or substituting), participants (e.g., priority population), cultural relevance (e.g., beliefs, customs, practices), dosage (e.g., number or length of materials/sessions), and logistics/procedures (e.g., time, location, deliverer) (Moore, Bumbarger, & Cooper, 2013).

For most materials, changes to materials that increase the fit with the age, culture, or context of the population served are encouraged. Safe changes to materials or program activities to better fit are modifications for the age (e.g., games, font sizes), culture (e.g., beliefs, attitudes), and context of the population served (e.g., setting). These changes may include substituting statistics for another racial population or tailoring instruction or activities (e.g., different knowledge game for youth). If health

KEY: no symbol - entry level; ❖ advanced 1; ■ advanced 2

SECTION VI

education specialists are choosing a packaged program, they do not want to change the core elements or key components that make the program effective, such as dropping a core activity or shortening a program (Castro, Barrera, & Holleran Steiker, 2010).

If health education specialists have to undertake a more formal adaptation process of materials or health programs, then they might consider a staged process. The steps are outlined below.

Table 6.2

Steps for Adapting Materials or Programs

Gather information	Review the literature and/or community assessment data to understand the risk factors and health issue for that population
Select best health education material	Select from materials or programs based on your goals/objectives, and needs of the intended population
Make changes	Modify materials content (e.g., statistics, cultural aspects), logistics or delivery based on information found in the needs assessment
Preliminary test or review	Have experts or small group of similar to final intended audience to review materials and make any necessary modifications
Pilot testing	Pilot test the adapted intervention and make refinements

Note. Adapted from Castro, Barrera, & Holleran Steiker, 2010

6.1.5 Convey health-related information to consumer

Priority populations. Health education specialists have to present health information to priority populations or communities across different settings. It is important to consider communication objectives and best strategies for the presentation of the data. Some examples are presentations, discussions, lectures, demonstrations, printed educational materials, or posters. For statistical health data, it may be more effective to present graphical data instead of tabulations of numbers in tables for the lay audience. It is helpful to ask people knowledgeable about the population for the presentation style that would be best received by the audience. Remember that simplicity is best to increase the understanding of the information. While certain methods are acceptable to one group or culture, they might be less acceptable to others. Therefore, it is important to match the methods to the content and audience needs. In addition, if time permits, health education specialists could pilot strategies with small audiences to receive feedback and evaluation of the best methods of presentation.

SECTION VI

Key stakeholders. Key stakeholders are individuals who are interested in the health information. They may be community, business, religious, health agency, or other leaders. Health education specialists should communicate with stakeholders regularly to increase the utilization of the health-related information. The presentation methods could include: an oral presentation, a one or two page executive summary, a short report, graphs or tables of data, or an oral presentation with a PowerPoint.

Health education specialists should consider whether the presentation will be formal (i.e., at an organized function), semiformal, or informal. Some steps for conducting effective presentations are:
1. Prepare for the presentation
2. Understand the presentation setting
3. Open the presentation
4. Use effective skills in delivering the presentation
5. End the presentation
6. Respond to the audience's questions

(Wagenschutz & Rivas, 2009)

Competency 6.2: Train Others to Use Health Education/PromotionSkills

Health education specialists should have the skills and abilities to analyze, prioritize, deliver, and evaluate training provided to interested groups. In this capacity, health education specialists will utilize their skills to develop a variety of training experiences that can address issues ranging from improving self-efficacy regarding diabetes management, conflict resolution skills among youth, car seat safety for children, or teambuilding to strategic planning in the workplace. Regardless of the area around which training is intended, health education specialists play an important role in delivering such training and should have the necessary skills to lead training sessions. Please refer to Competency 3.2 for more information on training personnel to deliver health promotion programs. The Council on Linkage between Academia and Public Health Practice (2012) has a short resource for training, called *Guide to Improving and Measuring the Impact of Training*.

❖6.2.1 Assess training needs of potential participants

Trainings are delivered to individuals or groups to increase the knowledge, skills, or proficiency in a topic area in order to improve job performance. Health education specialists may get requests for training from a variety of different organizations or for in-service training. Requests for training should be collected and assessed to determine if they fit the needs of the organization and produce positive outcomes for participants.

A training needs assessment is conducted to identify the gap between the actual and desired performance in organizations (Lawson, 2008). Health education specialists should involve key staff from the organization, planning committee, and other stakeholders to inform the assessment process. The five recommended steps in conducting a training needs assessment are to:
1. Identify the need or problem
2. Determine the needs assessment design

KEY: no symbol - entry level; ❖ advanced 1; ■ advanced 2

3. Collect data
4. Analyze data
5. Provide feedback

(Lawson, 2008)

In the identification of needs, health education specialists can learn about the organizational context, perform a gap analysis, and set objectives for the assessment. Next, health education specialists can establish criteria for the needs assessment design and evaluate the advantages and disadvantages of methods. The criteria for choosing data collection methods may be dependent on time, staffing, preference of the leaders of the organization, number of stakeholders, workplace disruptions, complexity of training issues, the validity and reliability of methods, and the training audience themselves. Data are then collected through a variety of methods, including interviews, surveys, document reviews (e.g., individual development plan, procedures, organizational plans, reports, or audits), proficiency tests, performance appraisals, training evaluations, job descriptions, or observations (Lawson, 2008). An individual development plan is a tool to create and track progress toward goals related to job performance. The individual development plan can be used for annual performance reviews or for training purposes. It is important to conduct the assessment at least three to four weeks before the training to allow for adequate time to review the data and plan for training content. Some examples of training assessment questions are:

- Topics for training:
    - What training have you received to prepare you for your job?
    - What additional training topics and skills would help you do your job better?
    - What are the most difficult aspects of your job that could be improved with more training?
    - What skills, knowledge, or behaviors do you think your participants/employees need to receive or improve upon in order to do their jobs better?

- Previous training:
    - What trainings have been offered in the past?
    - What types of training topics have you received?
    - What kinds of training do you personally deliver?

- Training logistics:
    - How would you like to receive training (e.g., in person, webinar, conference)?
    - What are barriers to the training efforts?
    - What helps you get to trainings? What types of incentives would encourage you to attend?

In the data analysis step, health education specialists conduct qualitative and/or quantitative analyses and determine some potential solutions or recommendations for training. Finally, they can disseminate needs assessment findings by writing a report or making oral presentations. The data and implications can be shared with the organization and other stakeholders to determine the next steps (Lawson, 2008).

Information collected through past training efforts, training needs assessments with the intended audience, training records, performance evaluations, and other organizational data will provide the basis for developing training goals and objectives.

❖ 6.2.2 Develop a plan for conducting training

Once it has been determined that trainings need to be conducted, health education specialists may have to prioritize the multiple requests for training. Different criteria may assist in making decisions on which trainings should occur first. Then, health education specialists can schedule and plan for high priority requests. Some considerations in prioritizing requests include the following:

- Urgency of the need for education
- Objectives of the training
- Potential impact on the organization or community
- Projected return on investment
- Training design needs
- Size of the audience and/or training
- Costs of the training
- Importance of the requester
- Projected workload associated with the training

(Lawson, 2008)

Identify priority populations. Health education specialists should select priority populations for the training. Some considerations for identifying these populations include: which individuals will benefit most from the training or has unmet needs for knowledge and skills, which individuals are the primary stakeholders, and which groups may have the greatest impact on the organization after receiving the training (Lawson, 2008). Past and current training needs assessment data and discussions with the stakeholders for the training can inform the selection of priority training populations. In addition, administrative factors may be taken into consideration as well, including time, budget, and staff capacity.

Use learning theory to develop or adapt training programs. Learning theories are incorporated into the development or adaptation of training programs to make learning more effective. Refer to Competency 3.2 for more information about learning theories. These theories may provide a foundation for how learning occurs or offer strategies to employ in training sessions. Training based on theoretical principles or concepts may have increased effectiveness. The following are examples of some considerations used in training.

Develop training plan. Trainings can enhance the knowledge and skills of professionals and communities. Effective training programs should follow these major steps:
1. Determine training needs
2. Set objectives
3. Determine subject content to accomplish the objectives
4. Select participants
5. Determine the best schedule

KEY: no symbol - entry level; ❖ advanced 1; ■ advanced 2

6. Select appropriate facilities
7. Select appropriate instructors
8. Select and prepare audiovisual aids
9. Coordinate the program
10. Evaluate the program

(Kirkpatrick & Kirkpatrick, 2009)

The training needs assessment or other formative research can help with steps one to six. Health education specialists can determine if it is appropriate to deliver training or if other content experts need to be recruited to best present the training content. Then, health education specialists should prepare the training curriculum based on training objectives and using appropriate strategies from learning theories to make learning successful. Please refer to Sub-competency 6.2.9 for a description of strategies.

The trainer should take into consideration:

- Priority audience
- Where training will be held
- Goals and objectives of the initiative/intervention
- Planned activities for the program
- Materials needed

❖ 6.2.3. Identify resources needed to conduct training

Health education specialists may also receive requests for information about skills related training or professional development in health promotion. They can start by evaluating if current training resources meet the needs of the organization. Training resources are often provided for professional development through workshops or conferences from local, regional, or national professional associations. Professional organizations may also offer annual meetings, workshops, distance learning, and Webinars (i.e., presentations delivered through the Internet) about health promotion issues. Health education specialists can locate training resources that fulfill continuing education requirements for CHES/MCHES credentialed individuals through the NCHEC Web site located at http://www.nchec.org/.

Health education or public health-related training may be offered by local health departments, colleges or universities, local or regional professional associations, extension services, area health education centers (AHECs), or through national professional associations. Some of these organizations or governmental agencies may also offer online training courses.

- The Community Tool Box also has practical information and skills for health education. It is created and maintained by the Work Group on Health Promotion and Community Development at the University of Kansas (http://ctb.ku.edu/en/).

- The Public Health Foundation has a learning resource center that has high quality training and health promotion materials (http://www.phf.org/). It also offers TrainingFinder Real-time Affiliate

SECTION VI

Integrated Network (TRAIN), a Web-based learning management clearinghouse of distance and on-site training for local, state, or national arenas. It is located at https://www.train.org/DesktopShell.aspx. Materials are in a variety of formats, including print, computer-based, and video.

- SOPHE has the Center for Online Resources & Education (CORE) that offers print materials and elearning on multiple topics. It is located at http://sophe.bizvision.com/.

- The National Associations of County & City Health Officials (NACCHO) has a Workforce Resource Center that offers some training resources. It is located at http://www.naccho.org/topics/workforce/workforce-resource-center.cfm.

- The Health Resources and Services Administration funds a Public Health Training Centers Network with regional centers that provide online and in-person training content to build workforce capacity for students and professionals. It is located at http://bhpr.hrsa.gov/grants/publichealth/trainingcenters/.

❖ 6.2.4 Implement planned training

Once finalized, the training plan needs to be implemented. The implementation plan should involve the following:
- Administrative details
- Promotion of the training
- Recruitment of the audience
- Schedules and venue selection
- Training objectives, curriculum and supporting materials
- Assignment of the trainers
- Evaluation procedures and instruments
- Budget

(Council on Linkages, 2012; Piskurich, Beckschi, & Hall, 2000)

Although one individual or group may take the lead in a training event, several individuals or groups could be involved in the marketing and arrangements related to the training event (McKenzie et al., 2013).

Use a variety of resources and strategies. Training may involve a variety of strategies based on its goals and audience. Some common strategies such as teaching and peer education strategies are presented below (McKenzie et al., 2013). Audiovisual materials, multimedia, and printed educational materials often support the instruction (See Table 6.3).

KEY: no symbol - entry level;   ❖ advanced 1;   ■ advanced 2

Table 6.3

Examples of Teaching Strategies

Teaching strategies	Lecture Brainstorming Case studies Coaching Group or cooperative learning Debates Demonstrations Discussion Drills Guest speakers Panel Peer teaching Simulations and games Role playing Problem solving
Audio visual materials	Audiotapes Charts, pictures, posters Computer Film/Video Television Projector
Printed educational materials	Handouts and worksheets Pamphlets Study guides Text and reference books Workbooks
Computer-based	Internet Distance learning Social media Video conferencing
Training simulations	Training on equipment Training simulators Computer simulation Gaming

Note. Adapted from McKenzie et al., 2013

❖ 6.2.5 Conduct formative and summative evaluation of trainings

Conducting an evaluation will help prove the worth of the training programs. Formative and summative evaluations may be helpful to describe the impact of training. Formative evaluation involves evaluation activities to generate information that will guide improvements for a program or health promotion efforts. Summative evaluation includes activities taken to create a judgment on program's performance and whether specific goals and objectives were met (McKenzie et al., 2013). In terms of training, formative evaluation could help get rapid reactions or input to make midcourse corrections or changes while training is being delivered, while summative evaluation will focus on assessing if the training goals and specific objectives were obtained. See Competency 4.1 for more information about formative and summative evaluation.

Kirkpatrick and Kirkpatrick (2009) recommend three primary reasons that training programs must be evaluated: (a) to justify the existence of the training and its contribution to the organization or participants, (b) to determine whether to continue the training program, and (c) to collect information on how to improve the training. Four levels of training and what they measure are proposed in Table 6.4. Evaluation should start at level one and move sequentially through the other levels

Table 6.4

Levels of Training

Level	Description	Tools
Level 1 – Reaction	Participants' feelings about the training	Surveys Feedback forms
Level 2 – Learning	Extent to which participants change attitudes, improve knowledge or competencies, and/or increase skills because of the training	Survey before and after the intervention
Level 3 – Behavior	Extent to which participants are employing the skills on the job	Interviews and observations over time
Level 4 – Results	Effects on the organization because of the training	Archival review of documents for the indicators of success

Note. Adapted from Kirkpatrick and Kirkpatrick, 2009

KEY: no symbol - entry level;   ❖ advanced 1;   ■ advanced 2

Quantitative and qualitative methods can be employed to evaluate training at all levels. Common quantitative methods for training evaluation may be surveys or self-assessments; qualitative methods may be interviews, focus groups or observations of training participants. For Level 1, the trainer could have ratings on a Likert scale or open-ended questions about the training in terms of meeting its objective, presentation content, presenter(s), and the training logistics. For Level 2, the trainer could have participants' rate changes in their attitudes, complete knowledge, or Competency items, or rate knowledge or skills changed as a result of the training. For Level 3 and 4, the trainer could follow up at times after the training to have the participant describe or rate their use of the acquired knowledge or skills, or the trainer could review organization documents for changes in the performance of the staff in attendance or the organization as a result of the training.

❖ 6.2.6 Use evaluative feedback to create future trainings

It is important to review the results of training evaluation to inform the development of future trainings. Sharing the results with key stakeholders and having discussions about the interpretation of the data and the actions to be taken as a result of the evaluations promotes the use of evaluation data. Training evaluation results could be summarized into the following formats:

- A short report with narrative and tables
- An executive summary of key findings (less than five pages)
- Graphs in an evaluation document, short summary in print or via social media (e.g., Facebook), or PowerPoint file
- A short newsletter article

Sharing can help inform discussions about keeping presenters and logistics the same or making changes based on the comments or ratings (e.g., reactions, satisfaction). Ideas or suggestions for how to improve acquisition of knowledge and skills could also be implemented in future training. Making refinements ensures that future trainings use the feedback given in evaluations.

Competency 6.3: Provide Advice and Consultation on Health Education/Promotion Issues

Sometimes health education specialists are asked by outside organizations and agencies to assist with a particular health or health education issue. Consultants might be asked to facilitate organizations in planning, implementing, or evaluating programs. Consultants might also be asked to give educational seminars on a health topic or to deliver a program, such as a smoking cessation program, to employees of a company that does not have a health education specialist on staff.

❖ 6.3.1 Assess and prioritize requests for advice/consultation

An effective consultative relationship requires knowledge about the health issue/problem, as well as resources, a helping attitude, and skills to provide advice and direction to meet the programmatic goals and objectives of an organization. Consultation or advice needs are similar to training needs. See Sub-competency 6.2.1 for more information about how to assess consultation needs. The need for consultation should be established by meeting with key stakeholders of the organization, discussing of the reasons for consultation, and reviewing organizational documents supporting the need. Once this information is gathered, health education specialists can better assess the need for assistance and begin the consultative relationship.

Prioritize requests for assistance. Sometimes the demand for consulting services may exceed resources; therefore, a number of considerations are taken into account in prioritizing these requests. These considerations may include:

- If the request matches the skills of the health education specialist
- If it falls into the major category of services offered
- What the scope and nature are of the request for assistance
- The level of commitment of the clients or organizations involved
- The presence of other consultants who may also provide the same services

❖ 6.3.2 Establish advisory/consultative relationships

Health education specialists act as liaisons between individuals, groups, and health care provider organizations. Often, when health education specialists serve as liaisons, they address group fears and experiences regarding a health issue. Health education specialists may also consider how the involved parties listen, reflect, and summarize ideas and questions.

Health education consultants that serve as liaisons between groups and organizations may need the following skills: facilitation, presentation, data collection, meeting management, resource material evaluation, networking, and report writing. Consultants may be asked to liaise among different groups and coordinate communication among and linkages with other public health agencies in the area. Consultants analyze and synthesize information about the problem or concern and interpret it for the client. They meet regularly with the client or other stakeholders, and assess the quality and appropriateness of resource materials. They must be able to write detailed reports covering problem diagnosis, actions, and recommendations, while keeping in mind barriers and the political climate of the client's organization (Dickert & Sugarman, 2005).

Define parameters of effective consultative relationships. Health education specialists often work as liaisons between individuals in systems, such as the local or state health department, voluntary health agencies, or health care facilities. They may collaborate with staff within their place of employment or with individuals in differing agencies and organizations. Health education specialist shares their knowledge and expertise with individual clients, groups, organizations, and community leaders when acting as consultants.

The expertise shared with the client includes:

- Health education and health promotion information
- Program assessment, planning, and evaluation skills
- Health education resources and materials
- Professional guidance on health-related procedures

KEY: no symbol - entry level; ❖ advanced 1; ■ advanced 2

Serve as a Health Education/Promotion Resource Person

Through this interpersonal process of consultation, health education specialists can provide technical assistance and special information to those clients or organizations in need of help. Health education specialists can act as either internal consultants (informally advising colleagues within an agency) or external consultants (outside of the agency, more formal). As internal consultants, health education specialists act as resource persons and respond to information requests, as well as organize materials (Dickert & Sugarman, 2005).

On the other hand, external consulting usually requires a contract between consultant and client. The services provided are more technical assistance- or process-oriented. As a direct health education service, formal consulting with outside groups requires health education specialists to provide technical expertise, current theory, and specialized knowledge.

The steps in formal consulting include:
1. Issue recognition (client awareness of problem and decision to use the consultant)
2. Consultant selection (meetings, proposals developed and evaluated, selection)
3. Engagement (identification of barriers/concerns; developing strategies for change)
4. Issue definition (data gathering)
5. Resolution pathways (developing alternatives)
6. Pathway implementation
7. Termination and evaluation (report writing and follow-up)

(Stryker, 2011)

Consultants generally assist in defining the health issue and developing a plan of action based on the current appraisal of all available information. Once the information is gathered, consultants help the client understand the concerns surrounding the health problem, analyze the implications of the problem, and develop an appropriate plan of action to effectively deal with the problem. After the consultation is completed, health education specialists can review the accomplishments, evaluate the consultative process, and make recommendations in the final report.

Requests for information and materials often come from outside organizations. Health education specialists must be able to answer specific questions, distribute educational resources, or make appropriate referrals to other agencies. Effective health education consultants in the role of liaisons will ensure that the learning environment is comfortable and positive, that they are available as a facilitator or teacher, and that the clients are open to learning (Dickert & Sugarman, 2005).

When working among staff or outside groups, health education specialists focus on:
- Trusting and respecting other leaders and groups
- Engaging individuals and groups
- Empathizing with individuals and groups
- Supporting individuals and groups

Health education specialists should also exhibit cultural competence or the ability to interact and provide effective care to people of different cultures. Cultural competence is important in the delivery of consultative services for health promotion. They should have knowledge of different cultures and how those cultures affect health status (e.g., cultural competence training), suggest that materials be in the language of the intended audience, and advocate for services that reflect awareness of cultural beliefs and practices or a diverse staff and linguistic services, if needed, when working with outside groups (Diaz-Cuellar & Evans, 2013).

❖ 6.3.3 Provide expert assistance and guidance

After the consultative relationship has been established, health education specialists will provide the assistance needed and outlined in the consultation agreement. Often, the tasks will involve the common skills of health education specialists, including assessing individual and community needs; planning, implementing and evaluating effective health education programs; coordinating the provision of health education services; acting as a resource person; or communicating health and health education needs and resources. Health education specialists should keep in communication with the client or organization frequently as defined in the consultation agreement. Monitoring progress and keeping open communications with the client will make the relationship more effective.

Technical assistance (TA) is the provision of direct, hands-on aid that builds capacity to complete with quality and prevention tasks (Chinman et al, 2005). The focus of TA is to: (a) develop individual skills and the conditions to use the skills effectively, (b) build effective organizations, (c) strengthen interrelationships between organizations, and (d) create enabling environments for addressing health issues across social sectors (Blasé, 2009). The provision of basic TA is to provide information and support (e.g., materials, overview workshops, tools) in an episodic or short-term timeframe. Intensive TA is required when new knowledge, skills, and abilities are called for and changes will need to occur at multiple levels to support and sustain the change (e.g., organization change, policy change) (Blasé, 2009).

TA methods can vary based on relationship and needs. Some formats of TA include:
- One-on-one consultation(s) (e.g., in person, telephone, e-mail, chat, etc.)
- Coaching (e.g., observation, feedback, data reviews)
- Group-based capacity building (e.g., group intensives, service learning)
- Informal (e.g., unplanned conversations at conferences) and formal networking among colleagues of similar interest (e.g., communities of practices)

Facilitate collaborative efforts to achieve program goals. Often, health education specialists may be asked to serve as partners, individuals, or groups who work with or convene other organizations to accomplish a shared goal to promote the health of the community. These may be called partnerships, collaboratives, or coalitions. Some benefits of partnering are:
- Increasing credibility beyond individual organizations
- Leveraging or maximizing resources

KEY: no symbol - entry level;   ❖ advanced 1;   ■ advanced 2

- Improving the reach to the community
- Increasing broad support for an effort
- Minimizing the duplication of efforts

(Olson, 2014)

Skillful networking can provide health education specialists with an extensive contact list of other professionals working in a variety of settings who can be called upon for guidance, such as opinions, answers, and referrals, when appropriate. Many agencies, organizations, hospitals, and businesses (especially those that cannot afford full-time, in-house technical experts) hire consultants to create interventions, conduct evaluations, or make program recommendations. Health education specialists often use the expertise of health education consultants when planning or modifying their programs.

❖ 6.3.4 Evaluate the effectiveness of the expert assistance provided

Evaluation should be ongoing in the consultative relationship. Generally, it is divided into three steps:

1. Identification of the evaluation questions or criteria
2. Assessment of the achievement of the questions or criteria
3. Dissemination of findings

In the evaluation, data can be gathered from the clients, consultants, and other stakeholders. Different methods may be employed to evaluate the consultation, including qualitative methods, such as observation, organizational documents, checklists, and/or quantitative methods including surveys or databases. Using multiple methods allows for triangulation of results from different sources.

Some examples of evaluation questions of consultation include:

- To what extent have the goals of the contract been met?
- To what degree has the timeline for the consultation plan been achieved?
- In what ways has the organization changed as a result of the consultation?
- How does the organization feel about the consultant's behavior throughout the consultative relationship?
- What is the level of satisfaction with the consultant and their reports?

Formative evaluation allows for continual assessment of the relationship throughout. It allows for monitoring progress, troubleshooting, and corrective actions. Some specific items that can be evaluated are:

- Number and length of contacts between consultant and client
- Progress made to date
- Degree client is satisfied with what has happened
- Clients' impression of consultant
- Any changes needed in the manner that the consultation is being conducted

Summative evaluation focuses on the outcomes or products of the consultation. Once evaluation questions are defined, collected, and analyzed, the results can be shared with all parties to discuss their implications and make recommendations for improvements in the relationship or next steps

(Dougherty, 2013).

SECTION VI

❖ 6.3.5 Apply ethical principles in consultative relationships

Consultants must have a set of principles that define ethical behavior and guide their actions toward those behaviors. Ethical practice may be based on deciding what is right and wrong, then performing the right behavior. Therefore, health education specialists must practice integrity in the conduct of health education. Please see Appendix A for the Code of Ethics for the Health Education Profession.

Some other important issues in ethical practice are informed consent and privacy of information. Health education specialists may also have to submit a proposal to an agency or university's IRB for review and approval of their procedures, data collection instruments, and informed consent documents. Furthermore, once individuals participate in health education services, health education specialists have a duty to protect the information provided by any participants, or privacy of information. The enactment of the HIPPA stressed the importance of standards and use of participant or patient information (Cottrell et al., 2014).

Some important ethical guidelines to consider when working with organizations are listed below.

- Do no harm to your client. Health education specialists should, in their actions and work with other organizations, protect clients and other stakeholders from harm.
- Keep client information private or confidential unless the client or law requests otherwise.
- Avoid conflicts of interest. For example, health education specialists should not represent two opposing interests at one time.
- Do not act in the official capacity as an advocate for the client.
- Do not go beyond your own expertise or qualifications. Health education specialists should know their level of competence with various health education skills and perform actions that match their own education, training, or professional experiences (i.e., not exceeding those boundaries of competence).
- Respect others. Consultants should respect the opinions, values, and beliefs of others different from their own.
- Ensure that all participation in research and data collection is voluntary and has informed consent.
- Represent accurately potential services and outcomes to their employers.
- Maintain competence in their field of practice.

(American Psychological Association, 2010; Authenticity Consulting, 2005)

KEY: no symbol - entry level;   ❖ advanced 1;   ■ advanced 2

CHAPTER VII

Area of Responsibility VII
Communicate, Promote, and Advocate for Health, Health Education/Promotion, and the Profession

7.1 Identify, develop, and deliver messages using a variety of communication strategies, methods, and techniques

  7.1.1   Create messages using communication theories and/or models
  7.1.2   Identify level of literacy of intended audience
  7.1.3   Tailor messages for intended audience
  7.1.4 ❖ Pilot test messages and delivery methods
  7.1.5 ❖ Revise messages based on pilot feedback
  7.1.6   Assess and select methods and technologies used to deliver messages
  7.1.7   Deliver messages using media and communication strategies
  7.1.8   Evaluate the impact of the delivered messages

7.2 Engage in advocacy for health and health education/promotion

  7.2.1   Identify current and emerging issues requiring advocacy
  7.2.2   Engage stakeholders in advocacy initiatives
  7.2.3   Access resources (for example, financial, personnel, information, data) related to identified advocacy needs
  7.2.4   Develop advocacy plans in compliance with local, state, and/or federal policies and procedures
  7.2.5   Use strategies that advance advocacy goals
  7.2.6   Implement advocacy plans
  7.2.7   Evaluate advocacy efforts
  7.2.8   Comply with organizational policies related to participating in advocacy
  7.2.9   Lead advocacy initiatives related to health

7.3 Influence policy and/or systems change to promote health and health education

  7.3.1   Assess the impact of existing and proposed policies on health
  7.3.2   Assess the impact of existing and proposed policies on health education
  7.3.3   Assess the impact of existing systems on health
  7.3.4   Project the impact of proposed systems changes on health education
  7.3.5   Use evidence-based findings in policy analysis
  7.3.6 ❖ Develop policies to promote health using evidence-based findings
  7.3.7 ❖ Identify factors that influence decision-makers
  7.3.8 ❖ Use policy advocacy techniques to influence decision-makers
  7.3.9   Use media advocacy techniques to influence decision-makers
  7.3.10 Engage in legislative advocacy

7.4 Promote the health education profession

7.4.1   Explain the major responsibilities of the health education specialist

7.4.2   Explain the role of professional organizations in advancing the profession

7.4.3   Explain the benefits of participating in professional organizations

7.4.4   Advocate for professional development of health education specialists

7.4.5   Advocate for the profession

7.4.6   Explain the history of the profession and its current and future implications for professional practice

7.4.7   Explain the role of credentialing (for example, individual, program) in the promotion of the profession

7.4.8   Develop and implement a professional development plan

7.4.9 ■   Serve as a mentor to others in the profession

7.4.10 ■   Develop materials that contribute to the professional literature

7.4.11 ■   Engage in service to advance the profession

The Role. Health education specialists are charged with the responsibility of providing information to diverse audiences. Whether through individual, small group, or mass communication strategies and techniques, health education specialists use their professional background to create, tailor, pilot test, deliver, and evaluate the impact of their communication. Their ability to communicate effectively provides health education specialists with the foundation to advocate for health and health education/promotion. As advocates, they create, implement, and evaluate plans that influence both policy and systems. Health education specialists' advocacy efforts also promote the profession of health education/promotion by explaining the history of the profession, the major responsibilities of health education specialists, and the role of professional organizations and credentialing in advancing the profession.

Settings. The following text is used to describe how communication and advocacy are used in different health education practice settings.

Community Setting. In a community setting, health education specialists develop communication messages to be delivered through a variety of channels and program materials in the language of the priority population and at appropriate reading levels. Health education specialists also act as advocates for community health needs. Such advocates may lobby the local government to use funds in ways that help promote the community's health or create policy that promotes community health. Additionally, health education specialists promote the health education/promotion profession through service and mentorship.

School (K-12) Setting. When employed in a school setting, health education specialists may promote the Whole School, Whole Community, Whole Child (WSCC) model by presenting curriculum information and student health information needs and/or concerns to groups of parents. In the event of parental concerns, health education specialists must consider the multiple value systems represented by the group and

KEY: no symbol - entry level; ❖ advanced 1; ■ advanced 2

employ appropriate strategies to communicate the material and respond to parents' questions. Depending on the topic, health education specialists may use illustrations from classroom instruction, student presentations, videos, or Web technology to enhance the presentation. Health education specialists also can advocate for students' and/or faculty members' health in a school setting by creating school health councils or teaching advocacy skills in the curriculum.

Health Care Setting. In this setting, health education specialists are often responsible for creating and updating all patient education materials. These materials include brochures, posters, flyers, public service announcements, and the health care facility's Web site. Health education specialists often serve as the voice for patient education and must advocate for its inclusion in the health care setting. Health education specialists also work with others in the health care system to ensure that the patient education materials are consistent throughout the system. Like health education specialists in other settings, health education specialists in this setting promote the health education/promotion profession through service and participation in professional health education organizations.

Business/Industry Setting. Health education specialists in the workplace might become aware of previously unrecognized health needs among employees. Health education specialists must communicate those needs (e.g., insufficient opportunity for physical activity) to management. Using their background in behavioral and biological sciences, health education specialists interpret the problem for management and articulate the possible ways of addressing the problem, such as offering a program or screening or changing organizational policy. Health education specialists must

acknowledge concerns specific to management to communicate ways in which a specific health education program or policy might benefit management and employees.

College/University Setting. Health education specialists in a college/university setting may face the challenge of ensuring health education's place in the college/university curricula. Communication supporting the program might be handled through reports to curricula committees, presentations to administrators, electronic communications, or small group discussions with members and students. University health education specialists may develop advocacy plans for improving the health of current and future students. They also teach their students how to communicate, promote, and advocate for health and health education. Beyond the university, health education specialists need to advocate for various community, state, and national health issues, as well as for the health education profession as a whole. Advocating may involve population-based strategies and the use of various media and social media outlets.

College/University Health Services Setting. In this setting, heath education specialists utilize a variety of communication techniques and technology platforms to develop, evaluate, and deliver messages to the campus community. These messages may be advocating for resources, policy, and system changes to improve health or promote the profession. Health education specialists must explain their role on campus relative to other areas, the benefits of participating in professional organizations, and how to become credentialed. Communication, promotion, and advocacy intersect in the college/university setting. For example, health education specialists may be responsible for implementing a social norm campaign to improve students' decisions concerning the use of alcohol and other drugs. They must communicate the need for the campaign to stakeholders. These needs may include the educational purpose, relevant social norms data, and an interpretation of the program's value relative to the established needs and concerns of the community. This communication may be distributed via electronic or print channels (e.g., posters placed around campus, social media postings), as well as face-to-face (i.e., presentations to stakeholder groups). Health education specialists also work with select student organizations to encourage policy development regarding alcohol consumption on campus and alternatives to alcohol. They also may advocate for local laws or ordinances that strengthen alcohol or drug related offenses for businesses.

Key Terms

Advocacy is "the process of influencing outcomes such as policy decisions in organizations by taking into consideration how the political, economic, social systems impact people's lives" (World Health Organization [WHO], 2010).

Cultural Sensitivity is understanding, valuing, and respecting the similarities and differences between culturally-based attitudes, beliefs, and behaviors (Diaz-Cuellar & Evans, 2013).

Health communication informs and influences practices, behaviors, or policies in an effort to improve individual or community health (Schiavo, 2013).

Health literacy is the degree to which an individual has the capacity to obtain, communicate, process, and understand basic health information and services to make appropriate health decisions (CDC, 2014d).

Health marketing is the creation and delivery of health promotion programs using multidisciplinary, evidence-based strategies to motivate the public toward positive health practices (CDC, 2011).

Lobbying is any attempt to influence specific legislation according to federal law (IRS, 2014).

A **lobbyist** is a person who tries to influence legislation on behalf of a special interest (Doyle et al., 2010).

Persuasive communication involves tailored health-related messages to meet audience needs and persuade them to adopt healthy attitudes and behaviors (Doyle et al., 2010).

KEY: no symbol - entry level;   ❖ advanced 1;   ■ advanced 2

Policies are sets of rules and objectives to guide activities (Doyle et al., 2010).

Social Marketing is using marketing principles in planning, implementation, and evaluation of health education programs designed to bring about social change. The ultimate objective of marketing is to influence action (Resnick & Siegel, 2013).

Social Media is online interaction or communication that allows users to share information, ideas, personal messages, and other content (Merriam Webster, 2014). For example, blogs, videos, image sharing, and social networking sites like Facebook, Twitter, and LinkedIn are all examples of social media.

Competency 7.1: Identify, develop, and deliver messages using a variety of communication strategies, methods, and techniques

In order to engage stakeholders in health and health education, it is often necessary for health education specialists to employ a variety of communication strategies, methods, and techniques. Health education specialists are often required to use behavioral theories to design communication-based interventions and determine the best channel through which to disseminate messages. Please refer to Sub-competency 3.3.2 for a description of common behavior change theories and models. The following section discusses the role of a health education specialist in developing, testing, and delivering health messages.

7.1.1 Create messages using communication theories and/or models

Consumers are increasingly seeking health information not only about disease treatment but also about disease prevention and health promotion (ODPHP, 2014.). Consumer-focused health education specialists learn as much as possible about the target audience and influence behavior change by crafting messages that address consumer needs. Public perceptions about health-related messages are influenced by the following characteristics: ease of solution and immediate results, perceived susceptibility, and personal beliefs (National Cancer Institute (NCI), 2008).

Several behavior change theories and models (see Sub-competency 3.3.2) can be applied to communication. Health communications should represent an ecological perspective and foster multilevel strategies, such as tailored messages at the individual level, targeted messages at the group level, social marketing at the community level, media advocacy at the policy level, and mass media campaigns at the population level (NCI, 2005).

Communications alone are likely not enough to sustain behavior change. Health education specialists can ask the question: "How do communication processes and messages contribute to behavior change?" For example, communications can increase knowledge and awareness of an issue, influence perceptions and attitudes, debunk misconceptions, and potentially prompt action (NCI, 2005).

SECTION VII

According to the Elaboration Likelihood Model, finding out how much the audience cares about an issue will help health education specialists craft effective messages. A person who feels directly impacted by a topic will be more likely to pay attention to a message and want the details (Petty, Barton, & Wheeler, 2009). On the other hand, a person who is not engaged in a topic will need peripheral stimuli (e.g., images) to grab their attention.

No matter how much a person may care about a topic, everyone is limited in the amount of information we can retain. Information Processing Theory suggests that a health education specialist:
- Keep communications simple
- Include no more than 2-3 main messages
- Break information into small chunks

In the **social marketing** model (CDC, 2007), health education specialists listen to the needs and wants of the consumer by looking at the marketing mix, traditionally consisting of the 4 "P's":
- Product: health behavior, program, or idea
- Price: financial, physical, psychological, time
- Place: How and where learning will take place
- Promotion: approach used to reach the audience

Resnick & Siegel (2013) add a fifth "P," Partners. This "P" refers to the importance of mobilizing resources by working with other organizations.

7.1.2 Identify level of literacy of intended audience

Health education specialists should assess the literacy and health literacy levels of their audience before developing materials and messages. Literacy and health literacy are not the same thing, but they are related. About half of adults have limited literacy skills; this means they struggle with basic reading and writing tasks. Approximately nine out of ten adults have limited health literacy skills; this means they struggle with complex health information, including navigating the United States healthcare system. Many factors contribute to a person's health literacy status, including age, education, income, health status, and stress (USDHHS, 2010).

Health literacy is defined as the extent to which individuals have the ability to obtain, process, and understand basic health information and health care services to make appropriate health decisions (USDHHS, 2009). Some consequences of poor health literacy are inappropriate or no usage of health care services, improper use of medicines, poor health outcomes, or poor self-management of chronic conditions (Zarcadoolas, Pleasant, & Greer, 2006).

Because so many people struggle with health information, health education specialists should use plain, everyday language when communicating health information to consumers. For example, health education specialists can pick resources that use simple language and have short sentences, define medical or technical terms, and supplement the education with other materials such as videos and

KEY: no symbol - entry level; ❖ advanced 1; ■ advanced 2

pictures (Plain Language Action and Information Network, 2014). Health education specialists can use readability formulas like SMOG, Fry Readability formula, or Flesch-Kincaid readability tests to evaluate the reading grade level of a text. However, it is important to remember that readability formulas are often inaccurate, and they cannot predict how well your intended audience will understand the material.

In verbal communication, health education specialists should:
- Speak slowly
- Focus on and repeat key messages
- Explain things in plain language (i.e., avoid jargon)
- Avoid using statistics
- Allow time for questions
- Use the "teach back" technique in which individuals have a chance to show that they are understanding the messages
- Use other communication materials or strategies to compliment the interaction

In addition to literacy, **numeracy**, or the ability to understand numbers, can also affect individuals' health care decisions and behaviors (Peters et al., 2007). Some strategies to assist people in their numeracy processing is to:
- Present fewer health statistics
- Reduce the need for inferences and calculations
- Use visual cues or displays to show numbers

Other strategies include focusing on one numeric idea at a time (e.g., one per sentence), using analogies or physical items to represent quantity (e.g., fist as a serving size for fruits), or teaching with stories. For example, in teaching about walking two times a day for 30 minutes, health education specialists might talk about a man who takes a long walk around his neighborhood after breakfast and dinner.

7.1.3 Tailor messages for intended audience

When it comes to health communication and promotion, one size does not fit all. Health education specialists must identify and understand the characteristics of the intended audience in order to communicate effectively. Some characteristics include ethnicity, socioeconomic status, sex, age, geographical location, health status, health-related knowledge, and literacy skills. It is also important to consider the trusted sources of information for your intended audience. Tailoring is creating communication individualized for the receiver to increase the relevance of the information presented. Information about the individual is used to determine the type of context and channels of the communication. Conversely, targeting is creating communications to shared characteristics of populations such as seniors at a senior center or college students (Kreuter et al., 2000).

Many factors, including culture, influence the perception of health messages. It is important to be aware of the advantages of segmenting the population into the priority audience according to behavioral, cultural, demographic, physical, and psychographic characteristics. Psychographics refer to more complex variables that describe individuals such as personalities, lifestyles, attitudes, and interests. Health education specialists should respect the diversity between cultures, understand attitudes and values related to cultures, and involve the priority audience in material and message development and testing (NCI, 2008).

Effective campaigns are audience centered and developed by professionals with specific knowledge of the psychographics and demographics of the intended audience. Specific communication is intended to reach a subgroup of a population with shared characteristics (e.g., black women); tailored information is intended to reach one specific individual (Kreuter et al., 2003). Both targeting and tailoring take into consideration the cultural practices and needs of the priority audience and can improve the effectiveness of a message or campaign (ODPHP, 2009). Every culture has a value system in which health practices are reflected. When serving multicultural and diverse populations, health education specialists train providers to work toward **cultural competency**. For example, they may seek to overcome language barriers by involving bilingual community members and create partnerships with community resources and coalitions (Doyle et al., 2010).

Whenever possible, the health education specialist should choose words, examples, and images that reflect the intended audience.

❖ 7.1.4 Pilot test messages and delivery methods

It is important to pilot test (using focus groups, interviews, questionnaires, readability tests) draft materials to make sure they are understandable and relevant (Plomer & Bensley, 2009). The pilot testing methods should fit the program's budget and timeline. Include individuals who share similar characteristics as the intended audience such as gatekeepers, opinion leaders, and community influences as test segments where appropriate.

Pilot testing can be used to assess comprehension and recall, determine personal relevance, and evaluate controversial elements, but health education specialists need to consider the time it takes to revise the communication message based on the findings of the pilot test (NCI, 2008).

The CDCynergy Social Marketing Edition outlines steps for piloting and revising materials:
1. Test creative concepts with intended audiences to see if the ideas resonate
2. Pretest specific messages with intended audiences to ensure that they hear what you want them to hear
3. Pretest products and materials with intended audiences to ensure that your products and materials elicit the intended response and produce the desired actions
4. Choose pretest settings – the places where you hope to provide your service(s) or expose your audience to messages
5. Pretest product distribution plans (CDC, 2007)

In addition to pilot testing messages, health education specialists can pilot test their delivery methods (e.g., Web, e-mail, social media, or print).

KEY: no symbol - entry level;   ❖ advanced 1;   ■ advanced 2

❖ 7.1.5 Revise messages based on pilot feedback

Health education specialists can think of message creation and testing as an iterative process; after piloting test messages, health education specialists can revise them to incorporate audience feedback. This participatory process can enhance the effectiveness and reach of health education messages. After modifications, the communication message should be tested again.

Pilot testing and modification should be integrated into the overall timeline to ensure that products, services, and communication materials will be ready for program launch. The creation of materials, including the pretesting process, can be time-consuming (Plomer & Bensley, 2009). However, feedback received is necessary to improve message efficacy.

Health education specialists responsible for revising health education communication materials based on the feedback acquired from the pilot must take into consideration the following:

- The nature of the message (e.g., style, sensitivity, complexity)
- The function of the message (e.g., calling attention to an issue or teaching a new skill)
- Goals and objectives of the message
- Activities and channels to reach (e.g., senior centers, schools, universities, churches, health clinics)
- Additional effort and implications by modifying the message
- Costs and accountability
- Budget and/or in-kind resources from other sources

(CDC, 2007; NCI, 2008)

Depending on the extent of revisions, costs may range from minimal to extensive. In order to minimize cost, program planners should share revised messages with the priority population to ensure changes are appropriate. Also, results from pilot testing will help program planners to identify new, old, or a combination of new and old channels through which revised messages will be disseminated.

Regardless of the channel utilized to disseminate revised messages, they must be scientifically accurate, consistent, clear, credible, and relevant to the intended audience (NCI, 2008; Kreps, Barnes, Neiger, & Thackeray, 2009). Revised messages should take into account key primary cultural factors that include: race, ethnicity, language, nationality, and religion (Schiavo, 2013). In addition, other secondary cultural factors should be taken into consideration, such as age, gender, educational level, occupation, and income level (NCI, 2008). Program planners must stay in touch with the norms, perceptions, and views of their priority populations. Therefore, through the use of a participatory approach, it is necessary to periodically revise messages in order to enhance their effectiveness and reach to priority populations.

SECTION VII

7.1.6 Assess and select methods and technologies used to deliver messages

Health education specialists should take into consideration the advantages and disadvantages of different methods of disseminating educational materials (NCI, 2008) as described in Table 7.1. Health education specialists should make sure the intended audience, message, and channel align. For example, mass media (e.g., radio or television) can be good for raising awareness among a general audience; social media is good for delivering targeted messages that can be easily acted on and shared; and one-on-one counseling can be good for teaching.

When choosing a delivery method, consider your message:
- Is it a sensitive or embarrassing topic?
- Is the message complex?
- Is it time sensitive?

Also consider your audience:
- Are they online (and if so, on a smart phone or computer)?
- Where do they go for health information?

Table 7.1

Communication Channels and Activities: Pros and Cons

Type of Channel	Activities	Pros	Cons
Interpersonal channels	Hotline counseling • Patient counseling • Instruction • Informal discussion • Fact sheet with a list of questions for patients to ask health care providers • How-to booklets and points for discussions in private homes or within the family • Videos for discussion	• Can be credible • Permit two-way discussion • Can be motivational, influential, supportive • Most effective for teaching and helping/caring • Can supply messages in culturally sensitive format	• Can be expensive • Can be time consuming • Can have limited intended audience reach • Can be difficult to link into interpersonal channels
Organizational channels	• Organizational meetings and conferences • Workplace campaigns • Newsletters • Educational programs (in-person, audiovisual, computerized, print)	• May be familiar, trusted, and influential • May provide more motivation/support than media alone • Can offer shared experiences	• Can be time consuming to establish • May not provide personalized attention • Organizational constraints may require message approval

KEY: no symbol - entry level; ❖ advanced 1; ■ advanced 2

Organizational channels	• In-house radio or video broadcasts • Add-ons to regular communication (e.g., messages handed out with paychecks or organization notices)	• Can reach larger intended audience in one place	• May lose control of message if adapted to fit organizational needs
Community channels	• Town hall meetings and other events • School campaigns • Faith-based organization campaigns • Educational programs • Speeches • Kiosks or displays in shopping malls, post offices, or other public venues	• May be familiar, trusted, and influential • Can reach larger intended audience in one place • Requires collaborative approach • Can evaluate knowledge change in some cases	• Can be time consuming to establish • Difficulties with establishing lead agency in collaborations can arise • Evaluating behavior change is difficult • No or limited one-on-one time with intended audience
Mass media channels *Newspaper*	• Advertisements • Inserted sections on a health topic (paid) • Letters to the editor • Op-Ed pieces • Cartoons/comics • Newspaper inserts • Media kits	• Can reach broad intended audiences rapidly • Can convey health news more thoroughly than TV or radio and faster than magazines • Intended audience has opportunity to clip, reread, contemplate, and pass along material • Small circulation papers may take Public Service Announcements (PSA)	• Coverage demands a newsworthy item • Larger circulation papers may take only paid ads and inserts • Exposure usually limited to one day • Article placement requires contacts and may be time-consuming • Stories can be difficult to "pitch"
Mass media channels *Radio*	• Ads (paid or public service placement) • Radio • News	• Range of formats available to intended audiences with known listening preferences	• Reaches smaller audiences than TV • Public service ads run infrequently and at low listening times

KEY: no symbol - entry level; ❖ advanced 1; ■ advanced 2

Mass media channels *Radio*	• Public affairs/talk shows • Dramatic programming (entertainment education) • Audio news releases • Media kits • Music news releases/music videos	• Opportunity for direct intended audience involvement • Can distribute ad scripts that are flexible and inexpensive • Ads or programming can reach intended audience when they are most receptive • Paid ads can be relatively inexpensive	• Many stations have limited formats that may not be conducive to health messages • Difficult for intended audiences to retain or pass on material
Mass media channels *Television*	• Ads (paid or public service placement) • News • Public affairs/talk shows • Dramatic programming (entertainment education) • Audio or video news releases • Media kits • Music news releases/music videos	• Largest audience reach • Visual combined with audio good for emotional appeals and demonstrating behaviors • Can reach low income intended audiences • Ads or programming can reach intended audience when most receptive • Ads allow message and its execution to be controlled	• Ads can be expensive • PSAs run infrequently and at low viewing times • Message might be difficult for audience to retain • Promotion can result in overwhelming demand
Mass media channels *Internet*	• Web sites • E-mail lists • Chat rooms • Newsgroups • Ads (paid or public service placement) • Social networking sites	• Large reach • Can instantaneously update and disseminate information • Can control and tailor information • Can be interactive and visually appealing • Can use banner ads to direct intended audience to your program's Web site	• Can be expensive to design and maintain • Intended audiences may not have access to the Internet • Newsgroups and chat rooms may require monitoring • Can require maintenance over time

KEY: no symbol - entry level;   ❖ advanced 1;   ■ advanced 2

SECTION VII

| Mass media channels
Social media | • Facebook
• Twitter
• Blogs
• LinkedIn
• Podcasts | • Can have large reach
• Can be interactive and visually appealing
• Takes advantage of those comfortable with technology | • Requires training on how to use these tools
• Can require larger commitment with timing to implement and evaluate |

Note. Adapted from NCI, 2008.

Health communication informs and influences health-related decisions (NCI, 2008). A health communication campaign can support a multicomponent approach to solving public health problems. Prior to campaign material distribution and promotion, health education specialists should remember to carefully define the market, segment the market, analyze the segments, and choose a target market with shared consumer preferences (CDC, 2007). Health education specialists are in a unique position to determine the format/type of materials to be developed by evaluating the nature and function of the message, as well as how it best fits with the channels selected.

7.1.7 Deliver messages using media and communication strategies

After identifying and developing appropriate communication strategies, methods, and techniques, and selecting the appropriate channel(s), health education specialists must deliver messages to the intended audience. Message delivery requires continual monitoring. Health education specialists should fine tune their delivery to ensure intended audiences are being reached and use process evaluation to keep track of message and material delivery (e.g., quantities of materials distributed, number of special events held, number of Web site visits, or phone inquiries).

7.1.8 Evaluate the impact of the delivered messages

Evaluating the impact of the delivered messages will provide evidence of success that health education specialists need to demonstrate and improve effectiveness. Three common measures for health communication include change in (a) knowledge, (b) attitude, and (c) behavior. Health education specialists should start by asking, "What do we want people to think or do as a result of the communication intervention?" (e.g., get a flu shot or wear a bike helmet).

First, health education specialists should define the data they want to collect. Next, they need to decide on the data collection methods (e.g., survey). Finally, they need to collect and analyze the data. Health education specialists should plan to disseminate the evaluation report to others in the field who can learn from the findings.

Common metrics to evaluate the impact of delivered messages include:
- Reach (i.e., number of people exposed to the message)
- Recall (i.e., how well people remember seeing or hearing the message)

- Traffic driven to a Web site (i.e., number of unique visitors or hits)
- User interactions and engagement with social media (e.g., number of "likes" or "retweets")• Impressions or mentions in the media
- Changes in behavior (e.g., number of people getting the flu shot)
- Changes in attitudes or beliefs (e.g., number of people who believe the flu shot will help protect them from the flu)

The simplest evaluation design is a pre (before) and post (after) measurement. However, this evaluation design does not account for the influence of external factors. Health education specialists' goal in evaluating a communication effort is to get the most reliable and accurate information possible, given:

- The specific evaluation questions
- Nature of the communication initiative
- Availability and willingness of participants
- Time and resource constraints

(University of Kansas, 2014b)

Evaluation can and needs to occur on many different levels, including evaluation of communication strategies, methods, or techniques. This can include several surveillance and evaluation efforts. For example, since 2002, evaluation of the statewide Strategic Tobacco Retail Effort Campaign (STORE, n.d.), a campaign designed to look strategically at tobacco retail licensing to minors, has consisted of several surveillance and evaluation efforts. These efforts include: tobacco purchase surveys, point of marketing surveys, law enforcement surveys, surveillance studies, media tracking, opinion polls, and ordinance tracking, among others.

Competency 7.2: Engage in advocacy for health and health education/promotion

The word advocate comes from the Latin word for "voice." **Advocacy** has been defined as a way to systematically alter policy and infrastructure (Caira et al., 2003). Advocacy skills are essential for health education specialists because advocacy embraces the concept of influencing organizational decision-makers, as well as public officials or the legislative body. It is essential for health education specialists to build advocacy skills and become active participants in the process. Individuals can take small steps in supporting advocacy efforts. Health education specialists must find and use their "voice" in important issues within their community, state, or nation (Lachenmayr, 2009). Advocacy can take several forms and can be for social change, policy development and implementation, awareness, and even to strengthen the profession of health education.

7.2.1 Identify current and emerging issues requiring advocacy

To be an effective advocate, it is essential to be aware of new developments that require action. Most health education professional associations have Web sites and electronic mailing lists that can help disseminate information to professionals regarding current advocacy initiatives and needs. Topics for advocacy can be centered on determinants of health or social justice issues. Social justice is the equal opportunity of individuals or groups to have basic human needs met (Levy & Sidel, 2013).

KEY: no symbol - entry level;   ❖ advanced 1;   ■ advanced 2

When considering issues to advocate for, health educational professionals may want to consider the scope of the problem to be addressed, the possible solutions and their outcomes, the acceptability of the advocacy efforts to the community or population affected, and the resources or financial costs associated with advocating or choosing to not advocate for the issue. The following list includes potential sources of advocacy related information:

- SOPHE has an entire section of their Web site devoted to advocacy priorities. This can be found at http://www.sophe.org/advocacy.cfm.
- The American Public Health Association also has a Web site that identifies legislative priorities and even provides advocacy tools such as form letters and talking points. This can be found at http://apha.org/policies-and-advocacy.
- To track the current status of federal legislation the Web site (https://www.congress.gov/) provides the latest information and also provides congressional voting records.

7.2.2 Engage stakeholders in advocacy initiatives

In order for advocacy efforts to be effective, health education specialists must engage stakeholders in the community who often are also gatekeepers to grass roots mobilization. By conducting key informant interviews, holding focus groups, reviewing case studies, and conducting surveys of settings that are specific to political context, health education specialists begin the process of building a stakeholder base for their advocacy efforts. Once an advocacy issue is identified, health education specialists can ask the following questions when engaging stakeholders:

- What community resources are available?
- Who are the allies and adversaries on this issue?
- Who else shares the problem?
- What would those groups who share the problem gain or lose by joining the campaign?
- Would you be willing to help with advocacy efforts?

(Adapted from Lachenmayer, 2009, p. 337)

7.2.3 Access resources (for example, financial, personnel, information, data) related to identified advocacy needs

When determining advocacy resources to be used, it is important to select sources on the characteristics of data needed and also to select sources that are credible with the advocate's partners and policymakers the advocate wishes to influence. Sources might include:

- Peer-reviewed publications which provide the background and science behind issues and planned action. However, there can be a time gap between the research and publication that causes the information to be seen as dated.

- Health education professional organizations (see list in Sub-competency 7.6.4 in Table 7.4) provide position papers, resolutions, model policies, and tool kits addressing multiple health education issues.

SECTION VII

- Federal Web sites can be used, such as the National Institutes of Health, which has 27 institutes and centers (http://www.nih.gov/icd/index.html). The CDC's 11 centers and other offices provide reports, evidence-based tools, and best practice resources. From either of these Web sites, health education specialists can subscribe to RSS feeds. These Web sites provide health topic information, data sources, model policies, and news. Federal Web sites provide timely and credible information often updated in nearly real time.

- National nongovernmental organization Web sites including The American Heart Association, American Lung Association, and American Cancer Society offer a broad range of content and policy tools and advice. Research!America and Trust for America's Health are examples of credible national Web sites focused on environmental change and policy.

- Nationally recognized health philanthropies such as the Robert Wood Johnson Foundation and Kellogg Foundation maintain Web sites with white papers and model programs, policies, and practices that are highly credible.

- Professional organizations of policymakers are information sources valued as credible and practical by policymakers. The National Governors Association and National Conference of State Legislatures monitor policy initiatives across the country and provide resources. National health policy resources include the Association of State and Territorial Health Officials and the National Association of County and City Health Officials, the national organization representing local health departments.

- State health agency Web sites and state health and human services agencies provide background and policy tools relevant to each state.

7.2.4 Develop advocacy plans in compliance with local, state, and/or federal policies and procedures

In developing an advocacy plan, health education specialists are tasked with collecting and analyzing quantitative and qualitative data, selecting effective tools, and evaluating the impact of policy decisions (Brownson et al., 2009).

Health education specialists should be aware of advocacy policies and procedures for the setting in which they work. For example, nonprofit agencies can perform lobbying as long as that lobbying meets the federal guidelines and does not exceed a certain percentage of the nonprofit's activities. Lobbying is any attempt to influence specific legislation according to federal law (IRS, 2014). Lobbying can be direct via communications with a member or employee of the legislature, while grants roots lobbying attempts to influence public opinion with respect to the legislation or issue and encouraging them to take action (IRS, 2014). **Lobbying** is different from advocacy in that it involves asking policy makers to pass or dismiss a certain policy or piece of legislation. Advocacy tends to take a more general form of creating awareness or mobilizing the communities. It should be noted that health education specialists working for some state and federal agencies are not allowed to conduct lobbying activities. Health education specialists should know polices that govern them in their workplace to avoid any potential violations.

KEY: no symbol - entry level; ❖ advanced 1; ■ advanced 2

SECTION VII

7.2.5 Use strategies that advance advocacy goals

Advocacy initiatives are designed to influence policy and law, and often include activities such as education, lobbying, and mobilization, among others (Dorfman & Krasnow, 2014). Advocacy strategies can also be categorized into several areas:

1. Voting behavior (i.e., register to vote and encourage others to do the same)
2. Electioneering (i.e., contributing to the campaign of a candidate supportive of public health and health education)
3. Direct lobbying (i.e., contacting a policy maker)
4. Grassroots lobbying (e.g, town hall meetings, starting a petition drive to advocate for a specific policy)
5. Use of the Internet to access information on health issues
6. Media advocacy (e.g., responding to members of the media for health-related information)
7. Social media (e.g., use of Facebook, Twitter, Blogs)

(Centola, 2013)

7.2.6 Implement advocacy plans

An advocacy plan includes five elements:

1. Goals
2. Organizational considerations
3. Constituents, allies and opponents
4. Targets
5. Tactics

In the first two steps, health education specialists should identify the goals of the advocacy effort and identify organizational issues that can facilitate or impede efforts. Health education specialists should then begin to identify their allies, constituents, and opponents. Allies are a critical part of any campaign and, therefore, play an essential part in the implementation of advocacy efforts. Allies are the way that health education specialists have connections to and influence over their targets.

Once health education specialists know their campaign goals, organizational issues, and have developed a list of allies and opponents, a list of the targets for their campaign needs to be developed. Health education specialists must also identify which individuals can make the final decision and should keep good records of whether these individuals are considered a target, supporter, opponent, or undecided on the issue. As a final step to the development of an advocacy campaign, health education specialists need to begin to strategically think about the tactics that they can use with their allies to influence their targets and help them to achieve their campaign goal. A good resource to utilize in the development and implementation of advocacy plans is the Community Health Toolbox available at http://ctb.ku.edu/en.

As health education specialists plan their action steps, it is useful to ask these questions:
- What will be the scope of this action?
- Who will carry it out?
- When will the action take place, and for how long?
- Do we have the resources to make it happen?
- What resources are available?
- Which allies and constituents should be involved?
- Which individuals and organizations might oppose or resist?

7.2.7 Evaluate advocacy efforts

Since advocacy has become a more common activity for health education specialists, it is becoming increasingly important to evaluate those efforts (Jackson, 2014). Because successful implementation of advocacy strategies is determined in real time and, by nature, must be responsive to continuously shifting social and political environments, advocacy evaluation is most likely to be proactive than retrospective in approach and emphasize assessment of continuous progress over time toward the policy goal (Jackson, 2014).

Common advocacy evaluation questions include:
- How are advocates building their professional capacities by learning skills such as communications, media relations, strategy development, and campaign planning?
- Based on influential factors in the political, social, and economic environments, what advocacy strategies are likely to be most effective for policy change efforts?
- How can multiple agencies work together effectively to advocate for mutually desirable policy changes?
- How can advocacy strategies be changed during a campaign to more effectively influence desired policy changes?

(Fagen et al., 2009, p. 483)

Table 7.2 below describes resources to assist health education specialists in developing competency in advocacy evaluation.

Table 7.2

Advocacy Evaluation Resources

Innovation Network http://www.innonet.org	Free clearinghouse of more than 100 advocacy evaluation resources; free newsletter Advocacy Evaluation Update; free report Speaking for Themselves: Advocates' Perspectives on Evaluation
The California Endowment http://www.calendow.org	Sections of Web site on advocacy and evaluation; free down-loadable materials including The Challenges of Assessing Advocacy: Parts I and II
The Evaluation Exchange http://www.hfrp.org/evaluation/the-evaluation-exchange	Freely downloadable publication from the Harvard Family Research Project, Evaluation Exchange Spring 2007 issue focused on advocacy evaluation

Note. Adapted from Fagen et al., 2009, pp. 483-484.

KEY: no symbol - entry level; ❖ advanced 1; ■ advanced 2

In addition to the above evaluation suggestions, it is essential to plan for evaluation from the beginning through the advocacy plan. Specific questions you may want to consider are:

- How will you assess process, impact, and outcome?
- How will you disseminate these results?
- How will you loop back and use these to improve your advocacy initiatives?

7.2.8 Comply with organizational policies related to participating in advocacy

Federal, state, and organizational laws and policies affect health education specialists' ability to participate in certain types of advocacy efforts while "on" organizational time. It is the responsibility of health education specialists to comply with state and federal law, as well as the organizational policy regarding such activities. Formal organizational policy, as well as departmental or individual management policy, may apply.

The Code of Ethics for the Health Education Profession (CNHEO, 2011) states that health education specialists have a responsibility to promote, maintain, and improve individual, family, and community health. The Health Education Code of Ethics encourages actions and social policies that support and facilitate the best balance of benefits over harm for all affected parties.

Outside of their daily role, health education specialists can strengthen advocacy efforts as members of a professional organization that advocates and may lobby for issues of interest. Health education specialists can also use the organization's name in support of an issue, if that organization has an established position on the issue and approves such use.

An individual acting as a private citizen can participate in any level of advocacy or lobbying. Care must be taken not to use any resources (e.g. time, computers, phones, letterhead, etc.) that belong to an employer when acting as a private citizen. It may also be necessary to declare views belonging to the individual and not the organization from which they are employed.

7.2.9 Lead advocacy initiatives related to health

Making public policy and leading advocacy initiatives is a continuous process that relies heavily upon proven approaches and other factors that include resources, personal experiences, ideology, interest groups, and advocacy organizations. Health education specialists must become and remain committed to staying current on effective approaches to mobilize their stakeholders, disseminate success with other health education specialists, and participate in training opportunities to sharpen skills and abilities to lead advocacy initiatives. Leading advocacy initiatives requires health education specialists to demonstrate leadership in prioritizing key issues in public health and education, identifying appropriate social networks, mobilizing other health education organizations, and engaging in fundraising, strategic planning, and evaluating advocacy efforts.

Competency 7.3: Influence policy and/or systems change to promote health and health education

Ecological models of health recommend interventions at various levels from individuals to institutions to policies (Bartholomew et al., 2011). The following forces affect the organization, financing, and delivery of health-related policy: congress, federal health agencies, states, health care providers, businesses, and local communities (Barr, 2002). Because health policy and systems changes are constantly evolving endeavors, it is essential for health education specialists to stay abreast of developments for advocacy work and policy/systems change.

The role of health education specialists to influence health policy to promote health is very important. It is important to focus on health promotion interventions at this level because personal choices are often made in the context of a larger environment, and health problems may be related to factors outside of a person's control (Bartholomew et al., 2011). Health policies are actions and decisions that are implemented to achieve specific health care goals (WHO, 2014). Public policy can significantly influence community health and also can impact all other factors that influence overall health. Public policy can affect income, housing, education, access to food and resources, the availability and quality of health care, and the environment in which people live. Systems change is modification in how a collective unit makes decisions about policies, program services, and the allocation of resources.

Longest (2010) describes four forms of policies:
1. Laws enacted at any level of government (i.e., 1965 federal public law P.L. 89-97 creating Medicare and Medicaid)
2. Rules and regulations from agencies responsible for implementing laws (e.g., FDA regulation to restrict sales of cigarettes to minor)
3. Operational decisions that may be authoritative procedures or protocols
4. Judicial decisions

Public policies can also be further divided into allocative and regulatory categories. Allocative policies offer benefits to some distinct class of individuals. Funding to support medical education or groups who are impoverished is an example of these polices. Regulatory policies influence the actions and decisions of others. They can be divided into: (a) economic regulations such as those that limit market restrictions (e.g., licensing of health providers or organizations), price set (e.g., rates of reimbursement for Medicare), provide for quality control of provisions for health services (e.g., safety standards, medical device regulations), or (b) social regulations (e.g., safe worksites, non-discrimination in health care delivery) (Longest 2010).

Some newer public health initiatives have centered on the focus of "health in all policies." The rationale for these initiatives is to develop a collaborative approach to addressing health through the partnership of multiple sectors in the community (Rundolph et al., 2013). This approach improves health by including health impacts into decision-making in all sectors and policy areas. Usually, health education specialists can participate in these efforts by being part of partnership discussions of how their organization's or sector's work can influence or improve the health and well-being of the community and develop a collective policy or policies to bring sustained change.

KEY: no symbol - entry level; ❖ advanced 1; ■ advanced 2

7.3.1 Assess the impact of existing and proposed policies on health

Policies play a major role in delivering and financing health care and public health efforts in the United States; they influence or structure health care, communities, and society. Commonly recognized steps in the policy making process are: (1) formulation, (2) enactment, (3) implementation, and (4) maintenance/modification. Formulation activities involve program identification, agenda setting, selecting a policy solution, and drafting the policy or legislation. The policy is then enacted. During implementation, activities include policy makers or actors guiding the implementation of policies and making it operational (e.g., setting up protocols, communications, and enforcement). During maintenance, the policy becomes institutionalized. Sometimes, policies have to be changed due to new evidence, unintended consequences, consumer sentiment, or evaluation findings (Longest, 2010).

Recently there has been greater emphasis on policy change for health. Frieden's Health Impact Pyramid (2010) recommends interventions that change the context for individual behavior (Tier 2) as more effective public health actions than one-on-one, clinical interventions. These interventions can impact more people and environments than individual programs. Tier 2 can include laws (e.g., restrictions in sale of alcohol to minors, helmet laws) and systems changes (e.g., smoke-free public buildings). For example, the provision of funding for such programs as the Women and Infant Children program (WIC) can provide needed infant formula and preventative care for at-risk families and improve health outcomes.

National health policies guide the establishment of health program priorities. Resources exist for monitoring the passing and impact of health policies. THOMAS tracks federal legislation (http://thomas.loc.gov/home/thomas.php) and the United States Health Policy Gateway (http://ushealthpolicygateway.com/) offers detailed resources related to different health topics. The Health Policy Gateway provides a profile of health issues at the federal, state, and city levels and presents information key health issues. Important considerations in health policy development include community needs assessment and a scientific assessment of the results, impacts of current programming, and available resources to support and maintain the policy (Doyle et al., 2010). Health education specialists' role often includes preparing data for quick and practical dissemination. For success in the process, health education specialists often need to proactively analyze and assemble data in order to ensure evidence is ready when a policy window or opportunity emerges (Greenlick, Goldberg, Lopes, & Tallon, 2005).

Health policies affect health and its determinants through behavior, social factors, physical environment, and health services (Longest, 2010). These health determinants offer some potential areas to evaluate to determine the effects of policies. The following table presents the health impacts and examples of measures.

Table 7.3

Impact of Selected Health Policies

Impacts	Measures
Behaviors	Cigarette consumptions of teens impacted by minor sales laws or seat belt use through national/regional/local surveillance surveys Women screened by the CDC's National Breast and Cervical Cancer Early Detection Program (Breast and Cervical Cancer Mortality Prevention Act of 1990 (Public Law 101-354) each year through data systems % of children vaccinated for mandated childhood vaccines for school entries through surveys or medical claims data
Physical environments (e.g., exposure to harmful agents, conducive to health)	Enactment of policies such as Clean Air Act or smoke-free ordinances in legislation registries Mitigation of homes affected by asbestos or lead in state lead program databases Cities who have adopted complete street policy initiatives for safe usage of streets by all users and all ages in registries
Social factors (e.g., poverty, unemployment)	Children covered by the State Children's Health Insurance Program (SCHIP) (P.L. 111-3) in reports Adults covered by Affordable Care Act (ACA) health plans through healthcare.gov
Health services availability and access (e.g., expenditures, workforce regulations)	Dollars spent on chronic disease programs in a state in state budget expenditures Loan repayment recipients (providers) in program databases Number of diabetes prevention or self-management programs in an area through an inventory

KEY: no symbol - entry level; ❖ advanced 1; ■ advanced 2

Policy evaluation documents the impact of policies. It can be defined as a systematic collection and analysis of data to make judgments about contexts, activities, or effects of the policy process (CDC, 2014f). It often requires a combination of quantitative and qualitative data. Quantitative policy tracking can include surveys, media tracking, measurement from direct observation (e.g., seat use), or tracking of policy through registries. Conversely, qualitative data may involve content analysis of policy language or modifications, key informant interviews, focus groups, case studies of states/organizations enacting or implementing polices, observations, and media tracking (CDC, 2014f). There are several types of health policy evaluations or studies that could be undertaken: (a) policy making studies to identify factors that polices would be adopted and the process), (b) implementation studies to analyze policy implementation and enforcement, (c) intervention studies to assess policy effects on health outcomes or its mediators, or (d) mechanism studies to ascertain methods which policies impact behaviors, environments, or health outcomes (Dodson, Brownson, & Weiss, 2012). The RE-AIM evaluation framework also can be employed for policy evaluation. It has five dimensions: (a) reach (i.e., who will be affected by the policy), (b) effectiveness (e.g., short or longer term impacts, unintended consequences), (c) adoption (e.g., organizations adopting, policy diffusion, participation level), (d) implementation (e.g., support, steps taken, costs, enforcement, compliance), and (e) maintenance (institutionalizing the policy over time) (Brownson et al., 2009).

Health education specialists can work with other health agencies to track or collect evaluation data after the implementation of policy. These impacts could span the typical health promotion outcomes of change in behavior, health status, morbidity or mortality, or quality of life or policy process. Table 7.4 offers some purposes of evaluation and potential evaluation questions for each stage of the policy process (CDC, 2014c).

Table 7.4

Evaluation of Policy

Policy Process	Purpose of evaluation	Evaluation questions
Problem identification	Describe the content and case of the issues	• To what extent was the problem defined to be amendable to a policy solution? • Were the right stakeholders engaged in the problem identification?
Policy analysis	Describe how the policy options were analyzed in terms of support, health impacts, and budget impacts	• How were the policy options identified and assessed? • What is the public health impact of a solution? • What is the economic impact of a policy solution?

Policy Process	Purpose of evaluation	Evaluation questions
Policy development	Assess the development process	• What were the sources of the policy content? • Who were the policy actors involved? • What resources were used in policy enactment?
Policy enactment	Assess adoption or enactment of the policy	• Who enacted the policy? • What steps were taken to enact the policy? • What were the barriers and facilitators to the enactment of the policy?
Policy implementation	Describe how the policy was translated into practice	• What were the barriers and facilitators to implementation? • To what extent was the policy implementation consistent with the policy language/content? • What are the benefits of the policy? • How is the policy enforced? • Is the policy achieving its intended outcomes?

7.3.2 Assess the impact of existing and proposed policies on health education

It is a responsibility of health education specialists to effectively assess and communicate important health education information and policy impacts to key decision-makers. Health education specialists must communicate the role of health education in generating policy changes that lead to creating optimal conditions that promote health. Across multiple determinants of health at the individual (e.g., behaviors, attitudes), family (e.g., structure, support), neighborhood or community (e.g., toxins, crime, poverty), cultural groups (e.g., shared beliefs, values), and organizational (e.g., educational system, health care, polices) levels, health education specialists play an important role in identifying strategies around which to improve the conditions that promote health—all of which should be communicated at local, state, and national levels (Schulz & Northridge, 2004).

As professionals, health education specialists interact with a variety of individuals ranging from legislative correspondents, health care providers, and patients. Health education specialists have to be skilled in written and verbal communication, as well as able to understand and interpret mass media and convey any potential challenges or benefits in implementing health education policy. To facilitate the use of this information, health education specialists may develop tools, such as guidelines, educational materials, practice recommendations, talking points, and translation of reports into activities (Atkins, Fink, & Slutsky, 2005).

KEY: no symbol - entry level;   ❖ advanced 1;   ■ advanced 2

SECTION VII

7.3.3 Assess the impact of existing systems on health

Systems strategies are changes that impact all elements of an organization, institution, or system. A system is an organized collection of integrated elements that work as a whole to accomplish an overall goal. Systems can be simple (e.g., clinical reminder system) or complex (e.g., more coordination between elements, engagement of actors, and organization) (Holmes et al., 2012). A systems change is modification in how a collective unit decides upon policies, program services, decision-making, and the allocation of resources (United States Department of Justice, 2014a). Systems thinking and change requires action at multiple levels. Meadows has identified these places to intervene in systems to address public health problems (Holmes et al., 2012). These provide areas of leverage points for systems change. Table 7.5 provides a description of these levels.

Table 7.5

Levels for Systems Change

Level	Description
Paradigm	The mindset or beliefs of how the systems works and refer to goals, policies and structure Change: shift or reinforcement of the paradigm
Goals	Aims of the system Change: Focus or change the aims of the system
System structure	Parts of the systems, actors (e.g., leadership, staff, partners), and interconnections between the parts Change: modifying linkages within the system or incorporating new elements
Feedback and delays	Providing information about the results of different actions by system elements to the source/administration of the actions. Change: create or change feedback loop, adding feedback loops or changing feedback delays
System elements	Actors and physical elements of the system connection through activities and information flow (communication) Change: changes to subsystems, actors or elements

Note. Adapted from Holmes et al., 2012

SECTION VII

Examples of systems are neighborhoods, schools, communities, health systems, worksites, or health insurers. The benefit of system change is that is impacts more than a single entity (e.g., school, worksite, clinic) and maximizes the reach of its effects. For example, the ACA has a policy that all health plans under it must provide free preventive services to all enrollees; therefore, individuals enrolled in the various plans will have access and no costs for vaccines, cancer screening, blood pressure, cholesterol, etc. Other examples of system changes may include a state school board that has adopted healthy nutrition standards for procurement of meals for students across their school, a community health initiative that involves multiple sectors in addressing active living (e.g., faith, schools, urban planning), or a health system that employs a comprehensive patient electronic care portal from electronic medical records, telemedicine, and integrated online support disease management for all of their locations.

Systems change can take a long period of time, so impacts may be years away. It is important to consider interim milestones. Evaluations of systems change can have the same methods and impacts of those for policies, including process, context, and short-term and longer terms outcomes. See Sub-competency 7.3.1 for a description of those health impacts. Evaluation methods could include organizational interviews with leaders and staff, observations of events or structure, surveys of key informants, and patient/population oriented outcomes for more process-oriented questions. System thinking examines systems components not as separate pieces, but in terms of how they interact. Some evaluation questions could be asked about the system parts, including shifts in systems interdependence, communications or interactions, and system choices (e.g., attitudes about change, change fit alignment with mission). Evaluation of systems change is often more complex and involves data collection at multiple stakeholder levels (e.g., leadership, staff, partners, consumers/clients).

7.3.4 Project the impact of proposed systems changes on health education

Understanding the implementation and impacts of systems changes in communities, community sectors, or health systems is critical to future strategic actions for health organizations or systems. Health education specialists can be actively involved in systems change to plan for future improvements in systems change, assist in evaluation of these changes, and communicate the updates about the implementation and outcome of these changes. They can also be instrumental in the dissemination of their effectiveness and disseminate their results to different audiences and actors. If a system change is shown to be effective, then methods should be taken to share the evaluation results and sustain it. In addition, health education specialists can help disseminate the effective system change to other systems to increase the impact of this strategy. Dissemination is defined as actively spreading evidence-based interventions to different audiences through predetermined channels with a communication plan with outlined strategies (Rabin & Brownson, 2012). Using planned active dissemination strategies with multiple methods for diffusing evidence-based systems change will be more effective (Rabin et al., 2010).

KEY: no symbol - entry level; ❖ advanced 1; ■ advanced 2

7.3.5 Use evidence-based findings in policy analysis

Health education specialists should use evaluation and research findings in policy analysis to inform health policy debates and to help address decision-makers' information needs regarding longstanding critical issues, such as people who lack health insurance, efficient operation of government health insurance programs, effective care delivery, chronic disease and long-term care, health care financing, and public health. Further, the utilization of evaluation and research findings can help health education specialists assess needs of their stakeholders that remain unmet. Use of evaluation and research findings in policy analysis will serve as a key resource to help health education specialists remain current with reported policy implications, identify of solutions, and translate effective policy and media advocacy techniques to influence decision-makers into practice.

As professionals, health education specialists interact with a variety of individuals ranging from legislative correspondents, health care providers, and patients. Health education specialists have to be skilled in written and verbal communication, as well as in understanding and interpreting mass media.

Conceptually, health policy includes factors and forces that affect the health of the public. Policies play a major role in delivering and financing health care and public health efforts in the United States; they influence or structure health care, communities, and society.

The following forces affect the organizing, financing, and delivery of health-related policy: congress, federal health agencies, states, health care providers, businesses, and local communities (Barr, 2011). Because health policy is an ever-changing endeavor, it is essential for health education specialists to stay abreast of developments for advocacy work and policy change.

❖ 7.3.6 Develop policies to promote health using evidence-based findings

Hartsfield , Moulton, & McKie (2007) reviewed public health laws, identifying over 100 covering a variety of topics, most commonly tobacco control, injury prevention, and school health (Brownson et al., 2009). However, only 6.5% of the reviewed laws provided research evidence supporting such legislation (Brownson, et. al, 2009).

Policy change to impact health status should include evidence that can be in two forms: quantitative (e.g., epidemiological or economic data, evaluation findings) or qualitative (e.g., health expert testimonies, expert opinions, narrative accounts). Studies have shown that the combination of both of these types of evidence has a stronger persuasive impact than one alone. Quantitative evidence may be derived from peer-reviewed journal articles, data from surveillance systems, and evaluation of programs or policies. Evidence-based resources have often used as evidence for policymaking such as the Guide to Community Preventive Services or Cochrane Reviews (Brownson et al., 2009).

The Guide to Community Preventive Services is a free resource to help practitioners choose programs and policies to improve health and prevent disease at the community level. Systematic reviews are used to answer these questions:

- Which program and policy interventions have been proven effective?
- Are there effective interventions that are right for my community?
- What might effective interventions cost?
- What is the likely return on investment?

Laws and policies can affect population health and reduce long-term medical and other costs. Examples include:

- Broad-based policies, such as smoking bans and laws
- Targeted laws, such as child safety seat laws
- Educational requirements, such as vaccinations for child care and school attendance
- Community-wide interventions, such as water fluoridation

(CDC, 2014a)

The Community Guide (http://www.thecommunityguide.org/uses/policy_development.html) provides information on public health interventions and policies that have been shown to be effective. As a result, legislators, policy makers, community leaders, and community members interested in specific issues can use it to:

- Identify what laws and policies promote public health and at what cost
- Draft evidence-based policies and legislation
- Justify funding decisions and proposals
- Support policies and legislation that promote the health of their communities and change policies and legislation that do not

Cochrane reviews provide systematic reviews of health care and policy. Each review begins with a research question and interventions, matching search criteria are found. The reviews aim to determine if there is or is not conclusive evidence for a recommended policy or intervention. The library is found at http://www.cochrane.org/cochrane-reviews.

❖ 7.3.7 Identify factors that influence decision-makers

Legislative advocacy, media advocacy, and grassroots activities are ways to influence decision-makers (Doyle et al., 2010). The following presents definition of these strategies. **Legislative advocacy** is contacting a policy maker to discuss a public health problem. Health education specialists can provide well-documented data and empirical evidence to help decision-makers create laws and regulations to support health (Lachenmayr, 2009).

Media Advocacy attempts to change the normative behavior of the media to alter public policy/practice and create environmental change. The first step is to set the agenda to garner media attention in order to alter the public's perception of the importance of a public health issue. The next step is to frame the issue by selecting specific content to present as important (Doyle et al., 2010). Media advocacy is a

KEY: no symbol - entry level; ❖ advanced 1; ■ advanced 2

powerful tool for health education specialists and their advocacy efforts. Media advocacy is an effective way to gain support for health education efforts and initiatives. When health education specialists are developing the strategies for the media advocacy efforts, they should ask the following questions:

- What is the problem they are trying to solve?
- What is the possible solution to the problem?
- Who will support the effort?
- What needs to be said and how can attention be gained?

(Dorfman, 2009)

Methods such as news, press, video, or radio releases, as well as interviews, letters to the editor, and media alerts, are all strategies to build support and communicate the need for health programs or health policy change and implementation (Schiavo, 2013).

Grassroots activities are efforts that originate from individuals within a community, rather than originating with health agencies. Health education specialists can help individuals and communities organize efforts to reach health-related goals (Doyle and Ward, 2010).

Although television and radio reach a broad population, these methods tend to offer insufficient details for the target audience. Online resources and social media, such as Facebook, Twitter, LinkedIn, and others, can spread the message about an issue quickly as individual users pass on content. Additionally, information can instantaneously be updated and can be tailored for intended audiences (NCI, 2008).

❖ 7.3.8 Use policy advocacy techniques to influence decision-makers

The developers of policy vary across levels. At the national level, congress and federal health agencies have prominent roles in developing health policy. Federal laws such as the Affordable Care Act, Medicare, and Medicaid impact the financing and delivery of care for Americans. At the state level, states can enact legislation and set guidance for professional licensure for health care providers and professionals. At the community level, business and their health plans, hospital systems, medical centers, and health departments all can implement policies to affect the local community (Barr, 2011).

There are many techniques that can be used to help influence policy makers. Policy makers are held accountable to their constituents and as civil servants. Many people do not exercise their right to influence policy makers, so those professionals who do choose to advocate or lobby can be extremely effective. The following is a list of potential techniques that can be used either by themselves or in combination to influence decision-makers:

- Voting
- Legislative meetings with staffer or policy maker
- Develop policy tool kits or resolutions that can be disseminated to others to advocate with
- Use policy makers to help influence other policy makers
- Hold town hall meetings with policy makers present

SECTION VII

- Write an opinion piece for the local newspaper
- Send a tailored advocacy letter with a clear "ask" to the policy maker

Longest (2010) also suggests that there are certain ways to influence policymaking depending on the stage of the process. During policy formulation, health education specialists could help set the agenda by defining the problem and evaluating policy solutions, as well as recommending content and evidence to draft the policy or legislation. During policy implementation, they can offer public comment on draft rules or policies and serve on advisory bodies. After enactment, they can recommend changes based on operational experience, evaluations, or new health evidence.

7.3.9 Use media advocacy techniques to influence decision-makers

Capwiz and other Internet action networks are vital resources for health education specialists to utilize when working on advocacy issues (http://action.apha.org/site/PageNavigator/Advocacy). For example, there are e-advocacy tools to help mobilize their members to send letters to members of congress electronically.

Often these action network sites have various components that can be utilized, for example the APHA Advocacy link offers:
- *Legislation Updates* contains information about health-related legislation.
- *Media Guide* allows members to send electronic letters to local media.
- *Legislative Action Center* posts regular updates on legislation, and allows members to email local political representatives.

In addition to Internet action networks, mobile technologies can also be used as tools for advocacy efforts. These involve "any device and application that uses cellular (or wireless) technology to send information or communication across distances to other devices or people" (Lefebvre, 2009, p. 491).

7.3.10 Engage in legislative advocacy

Before contacting an elected official, it is important to have an understanding of the issue being discussed. Bills, resolutions and other legislation can be found at THOMAS. THOMAS is a Web site of federal legislative information maintained by the Library of Congress (http://thomas.loc.gov/home/thomas.php). Prepare brief and clear "talking points" that state the problem, proof of the problem, and the solution being advocated. Many individuals contact their elected officials by phone, e-mail, fax, letter, or in-person. E-mailed or faxed letters are a preferred written method, because unlike mailed letters they do not have to go through a bioterrorism screening process. Because of the changing dynamics of the mail screening processes, individuals should check for the best way to contact an elected official.

Prior to a first meeting with a legislator, it is vital for health education specialists to conduct research on the legislator. This will help identify personal and professional information about the legislator, as well as endorsers, committees, sponsors, and influencers of the legislator.

After contacting a legislator, advocacy efforts are not over. It is important to take the time to show appreciation with a "thank you" and to follow-up with the representative or an appropriate staff person.

KEY: no symbol - entry level; ❖ advanced 1; ■ advanced 2

Find others who support the issue and encourage them to make a phone call, write a letter, sign a petition, or schedule a meeting. By using a variety of strategies to advocate for health issues, health education specialists have the potential to shape and change policy to impact the health of many people (Galer-Unti et al., 2004).

Health education specialists conducting media advocacy can follow some basic steps to improve effectiveness: develop a strategy, understand the media, develop messages, and attract journalists' attention and trust (Dorfman, 2009).

Individuals involved in advocacy work and policy change often question their impact on the system. Evaluating the progress of policy change created by advocacy efforts can be challenging. The California Endowment (Guthrie, Louie & Foster, 2006) recommends the following steps in a policy evaluation approach:
1. Adopting a conceptual model for understanding the process of policy change
2. Developing a theory about how and why planned activities lead to desired outcomes
3. Selecting benchmarks to monitor progress
4. Measuring progress toward benchmarks and collecting data

The California Endowment also advocates creating benchmarks to represent key milestones in creating change. Table 7.6 represents an example of a benchmark framework:

Table 7.6

Example of Benchmark Development from Framework

Benchmark Category	Project-Specific Interim Benchmarks of Progress
Changing definitions/ reframing	Change official purpose of vending machines to include providing nutritious food for students.
Community or individual behavior	Recruit 100 students to submit requests for healthy snack choices into the school suggestion box.
Shifts in critical mass	Have four of seven school board members to make a motion to hold a hearing on the issue of vending machines in schools.
Institutional policy	School board passes a resolution banning sodas from being sold in school vending machines.
Holding the line	Stop vending machine lobby from introducing resolution to allow vending machines in junior high and high schools.

Note. Adapted from Guthrie et al., 2006

SECTION VII

Research regarding health care policy provides evidence-based information that affects health care outcomes. In addition, research influences quality, cost, use, and access to public health and health care. The research background helps public health stakeholders to make informed decisions and improve the quality of health education and public health efforts.

Competency 7.4: Promote the health education profession

One responsibility of health education specialists is to promote the health education profession. This includes explaining the responsibilities of health education specialists, the history of the profession, and the role of professional organizations and credentialing in advancing professional practice. Health education specialists may also engage in service to advance the health education profession such as serving as a mentor or contributing to professional literature.

7.4.1 Explain the major responsibilities of the health education specialist

The Seven Areas of Responsibility of health education specialists include:

I. Assess needs, resources, and capacity for health education/promotion
II. Plan health education/promotion
III. Implement health education/promotion
IV. Conduct evaluation and research related to health education/promotion
V. Administer and manage health education/promotion
VI. Serve as a health education/promotion resource person
VII. Communicate, promote, and advocate for health, health education/promotion, and the profession

(NCHEC et al., 2014)

The United States Department of Labor Bureau of Labor Statistics (BLS) (2009) defines health education specialists (SOC 21-1091.00) as those who promote, maintain, and improve individual and community health. The BLS recognizes that health education specialists are responsible for a range of responsibilities that include:

- Assisting individuals and communities to adopt healthy behaviors
- Collecting and analyzing data to identify community needs prior
- Planning, implementing, monitoring, and evaluating programs

They may also serve as a resource to assist individuals, other professionals, or the community and may administer fiscal resources for health education programs (BLS, 2009).

7.4.2 Explain the role of professional organizations in advancing the profession

Professional associations in health education carry out many of the functions necessary for continuing education in the profession. Their purposes include, but are not limited to, conducting continuing education programs, disseminating research findings, legislative advocacy, and establishing ethics and standards for the profession (Cottrell et al., 2009).

KEY: no symbol - entry level;   ❖ advanced 1;   ■ advanced 2

The CNHEO is a collaboration of membership organizations. Members of the CNHEO are listed in Table 7.7. The primary mission of the CNHEO is to "mobilize resources of the health education profession in order to expand and improve health education, regardless of the setting" (CNHEO, 2014). CNHEO:

- Facilitates national-level communication, collaboration, and coordination among the member organizations
- Provides a forum for the identification and discussion of health education issues
- Formulates recommendations and takes appropriate action on issues affecting member interests
- Serves as a communication and advisory resource for agencies, organizations, and persons in the public and private sectors on health education issues
- Serves as a focus for the exploration and resolution of issues pertinent to professional health education specialists

(CNHEO, 2014)

Table 7.7

Members of the Coalition of National Health Education Organizations

Member	Mission	Publication
American College Health Association (ACHA)	ACHA is the principal advocate and leadership organization for college and university health.	*Journal of American College Health*
http://www.acha.org		
American Public Health Association (APHA)	To be a strong advocate for health education, disease prevention and health promotion directed to individuals, groups and communities in all activities of the association. To set, maintain and exemplify the highest ethical principles and standards of practice on the part of all professionals whose primary purpose is health education and disease prevention.	*American Journal of Public Health* *The Nation's Health*
http://www.apha.org		

SECTION VII

Member	Mission	Publication
American School Health Association (ASHA)	To protect and promote the health of children and youth by supporting coordinated school health programs as a foundation for school success.	*Journal of School Health* *Health in Action*
http://www.ashaweb.org		
Directors of Health Promotion and Education (DHPE)	To strengthen, promote and enhance the professional practice of health promotion and public health education nationally and within State health departments.	*The Voice*
http://www.dhpe.org		
Eta Sigma Gamma (ESG)	To foster professional competence and dedication of members in the health education profession.	*The Health Educator* *Eta Sigma Gamma Student Monograph*
http://www.etasigmagamma.org		
Society for Public Health Education (SOPHE)	To provide leadership in facilitating and promoting initiatives to achieve national health and education goals and objectives. The society promotes effective school programs and practices that involve collaboration with parents and community groups to positively impact healthy and active lifestyles.	*Health Promotion Practice* *Health Education and Behavior* *Pedagogy in Health Promotion*
http://www.sophe.org		

7.4.3 Explain the benefits of participating in professional organizations

A **professional association** is an organization formed to unite and inform people who work in the same occupation (Santiago, 2014). The establishment of professional standards and a credentialing process raises the level of practice in the profession. Membership in one or more of the professional organizations in Table 7.7 allows health education specialists to update skills and knowledge, network with peers and mentors, and identify collaborators for research and publication opportunities. In addition, many associations provide job banks, which assist members, both in locating a new position and in recruiting professional talent. Joining state and local professional organizations can increase networking that supports health education specialists' ability to influence local and state policy, as well as grow and maintain supportive partnerships.

KEY: no symbol - entry level; ❖ advanced 1; ■ advanced 2

7.4.4 Advocate for professional development of health education specialists

For both academics and practitioners, professional growth opportunities include providing and participating in continuing education opportunities via professional organizations at the state and national level. With so many changes in health education and health-related policy on a daily basis, it is essential that health education specialists participate in and advocate for professional development. This is particularly important for those desiring to maintain their CHES and MCHES certifications. The following are some potential opportunities for advocating for professional development:

- Identify opportunities and apply for funding for professional development workshops such as a health education advocacy summit
- Publish articles in peer-reviewed journal on the importance of professional development
- Create shadowing or volunteering opportunities for health education professionals
- Help to provide continuing education units contact hours (CECH) for various programs that are health education related in their community.

7.4.5 Advocate for the profession

Advocacy for the profession can take on many forms. Attending conferences, educating others about the profession, mentoring young professionals, and advocating for policies to advance the profession are all examples. Although relatively speaking, health education is a newer discipline, and many people may not understand the professional role and responsibilities our profession requires. By advocating for the profession, health education specialists help to distinguish the profession from others, secure potential jobs, and help improve collaboration between health education specialists and other allied and public health professionals.

7.4.6 Explain the history of the profession and its current and future implications for professional practice

The history of health education in the United States dates back to the late 19th century with the establishment of the first academic programs preparing school health educators (Allegrante et al., 2004). Interest in quality assurance and the development of standards for professional preparation of health educators emerged in the 1940s. Over the next several decades, professional associations produced guidelines for preparing health educators, and accreditation efforts were introduced. Yet, it was not until the 1970s that health education began evolving as a true profession in terms of a sociological perspective (Livingood & Auld, 2001). In addition to defining a body of literature, efforts were initiated to promulgate a Health Education Code of Ethics, a skill-based set of Competencies, rigorous systems for quality assurance, and a health education credentialing system (NCHEC et al., 2010).

Beginning in the mid-1970s, the health education profession began the process of developing the steps necessary to establish the credentialing of health educators. This process is outlined in more detail in the publication, *A Competency-Based Framework for Health Education Specialists – 2010* (NCHEC et al., 2010a). The landmark Role Delineation Project (United States Department of Health, Education and

Welfare, 1978) was officially funded in 1978. Through a series of conferences, workshops, and a national survey of health educators, the responsibilities, functions, skills, and knowledge expected of entry-level health educators were delineated. In the 1985 document, *A Framework for the Development of Competency-Based Curricula for Entry-level Health Educators,* the Areas of Responsibility, Competencies, and Sub-Competencies were delineated for the preparation and practice of health educators. The concept of a "generic role" common to all health educators, regardless of work setting, emerged and formed the basis for the credentialing process for health education specialists (NCHEC et al., 2010a).

The planning committee for the First Bethesda Conference in 1978 became the National Task Force on the Preparation and Practice of Health Educators (NTFPPHE). NTFPPHE formally became incorporated as the National Commission for Health Education Credentialing, Inc. (NCHEC) in 1988. In 1989, experienced health education professionals had the opportunity to become Certified Health Education Specialists via a charter certification phase that included meeting eligibility requirements, submitting an application, and a review of documented education and experience. The first CHES exam was administered in 1990 and is now offered twice a year at more than 120 testing locations nationwide.

The role of the health educator was further defined in a six-year (1998-2004) study known as the National Health Educator Competencies Update Project (CUP), which outlined the roles of entry- and advanced-level health educators (Gilmore et al., 2005). Results from the CUP study led to the release of a new Framework (NCHEC, SOPHE, & AAHE, 2006), a new study guide (NCHEC, 2007), and revisions to the CHES examination in October 2007 to reflect the updated Responsibilities, Competencies, and Sub-competencies of the entry-level health educator. Very significantly, the CUP model introduced a hierarchical model in which advanced-levels built on the entry-level (Gilmore et al. 2005).

In June of 2008, the CHES certification program was granted accreditation by the National Commission for Certifying Agencies (NCCA), a government-recognized accrediting body for professional certification organizations. This accreditation signifies that the CHES exam complies with stringent testing and measurement standards among certification organizations. The NCCA standards require that a certification program conduct a periodic job analysis to verify the Competencies that are the basis of an exam.

The subsequent job analysis was held in 2008-2009 to again validate the contemporary practice of entry- and advanced-level health educators. This 18-month research project, known as the Health Educator Job Analysis-2010 (HEJA 2010) and confirmed a hierarchical model of entry- and advanced-level Competencies. As with the previous study, the results were used to update the framework publications, *A Competency-Based Framework for Health Education Specialists-2010,* and to revise the study material, *The Health Education Specialist: A Companion Guide for Professional Excellence, 6th Edition.*

KEY: no symbol - entry level; ❖ advanced 1; ■ advanced 2

The presence of a hierarchical model of the advanced-level which builds upon the entry-level Competencies confirmed the concept first introduced in the CUP study and led to the creation of a second level of certification. The advanced-level Competencies were first used in the Experience Documentation Opportunity (2010-2011) of current CHES to obtain the MCHES first awarded in April 2011 (NCHEC, 2010a). The first MCHES exam was released in October 2011.

The next research study was held in 2013-2014 and known as the Health Education Specialist Practice Analysis- 2015 (HESPA 2015). The name was changed to reflect the change in the recognized name from health educator to health education specialist. The purpose of this study was to validate the current practice of entry- and advanced-level health education specialists to determine any changes in health education practice since the last major job analysis study, HEJA 2010, and to inform certification, professional preparation, and continuing education initiatives. More details are available in *A Competency-based Framework for Health Education Specialists – 2015* (NCHEC & SOPHE, 2015). The HESPA 2015 results are also the basis of this publication, *The Health Education Specialist: A Companion Guide for Professional Excellence, 7th Edition* (NCHEC, 2015).

The health education profession has a proud history of scientifically validating the Competencies that have become the basis of the professional credential(s), professional preparation, and professional development. The verified Responsibilities, Competencies and Sub-competencies (currently 7, 26, and 258, respectively) define the profession and distinguish individuals from those trained in other disciplines.

Health Education Certification History Timeline
- 1978 – National Task Force on the Preparation & Practice of Health Educators established
- 1978 – 1981 Role Delineation Project conducted
- 1985 – A Framework for the Development of Competency-Based Curricula for Entry Level Health Educators published
- 1988 – NCHEC incorporated as a nonprofit organization
- 1989 – Charter CHES certification phase
- 1990 – First CHES exam given
- 1997 – CHES exam offered twice a year
- 2000 – Code of Ethics for Health Education Profession adopted
- 2005 – National Health Educator Competencies Update Project (CUP) results released (1998 – 2004 study)
- 2006 – Revised framework, A Competency- Based framework for Health Educators -2006, published
- 2007 – Revised study guide, The Health Education Specialist: A Companion Guide for Profession Excellence, 6th Edition, published
- 2007 – CHES exam revised based on CUP results.

- 2008 – CHES certification program accredited by National Commission on Certifying Agencies (NCCA)
- 2010 – Health Educator Job Analysis (HEJA) Results Released (2008-2009 study)
- 2010 – Revised framework, A Competency-Based Framework for Health Education Specialists-2010, published
- 2010 – Revised study material, The Health Education Specialist: A Companion Guide for Professional Excellence 6th Edition, published
- 2011 – CHES exam revised based on HEJA results
- 2011 – MCHES certification first conferred via Experience Documentation Opportunity (EDO) for existing CHES
- 2011 – MCHES first examination offered. EDO closed
- 2013 – The CHES certification program is re-accredited and the MCHES certification program received accreditation by NCCA
- 2015 – Health Education Practice Analysis (HESPA) results released (2013-2014 study)

7.4.7 Explain the role of credentialing (for example, individual, program) in the promotion of the profession

Credentialing is an umbrella term that refers to several processes put in place to ensure that persons who deliver a given service have obtained a minimum level of competency (skills, ability, and knowledge). These processes include the accreditation of institutions and licensure or certification/registration of individuals (National Task Force on the Preparation and Practice of Health Education Specialists, 1985; Taub, Birch, Auld, Lysoby, & Rasar King, 2009; Cottrell, Auld, Birch, Taub, Rasar King, & Allegrante, 2012). Certification is the method of individual credentialing for the profession.

The CHES certification was developed by and for the health education profession to demonstrate the mastery of a set of fundamental skills across all practice settings. It is a voluntary certification. The CHES credential has three components: academic preparation specifically in health education, successfully passing a written exam, and continued professional development (continuing education) of a minimum of 75 continuing education contact hours over a five year period. In order to obtain and maintain the CHES credential, all three components must be met.

As a result of the CUP and the HEJA 2010 research findings, an advanced-level certification, MCHES, was introduced in 2010. The MCHES credential has four components: academic preparation in health education, experience in the field, successfully passing a written exam, and continued professional development (continuing education) of a minimum of 75 contact hours over a five year period. "CHES" or "MCHES" after a health education specialist's name is one indication of professional competence and a commitment to continued professional development.

NCHEC has committed to maintaining accreditation for the CHES and MCHES certification programs through NCCA. Among the NCCA *Standards for the Accreditation of Certification Programs is the requirement that a professional role* delineation or job analysis be conducted and periodically validated. NCHEC has therefore committed to ongoing re-verification of the Responsibilities,

KEY: no symbol - entry level;   ❖ advanced 1;   ■ advanced 2

Competencies, and Sub-competencies of health education specialists, which has implications beyond certification, including the areas of professional development and professional preparation in the field of health education.

In addition to individual certification, the health education profession has mechanisms for accreditation of institutions/programs preparing health education specialists. Efforts have been made to coordinate the system of quality assurance of health education programs under the guidance of three task forces starting with the National Task Force on Accreditation in Health Education (Allegrante, 2004; Taub et al., 2009). The Council on Education for Public Health (CEPH) accredits schools of public health, graduate programs in public/community health, and undergraduate programs affiliated with graduate program. The SOPHE/AAHE Baccalaureate Program Approval Committee (SABPAC), which previously approved undergraduate programs, ended in 2014 as CEPH began to also accredit standalone undergraduate programs in public health. The National Council for Accreditation of Teacher Education (NCATE) and Teacher Accreditation Council (TEAC) accredited teacher preparation programs recently unified under the Council for the Accreditation of Educator Preparation (CAEP) (Taub et al., 2014).

7.4.8 Develop and implement a professional development plan

A professional development plan documents the goals, required knowledge and skills, and objectives which individuals will need to attain in order to support their career development. Sources of professional growth for health education specialists can come through job experience and training, other professional experiences, formal academic preparation, and obtaining individual certification. Professional development opportunities include:

- Reading professional journals
- Attending professional meetings
- Taking courses or in service workshops
- Authoring journal articles, chapters, or books
- Presenting at professional meetings
- Participating in other professional development activities

At some point, health education specialists who do not already have an advanced degree may consider obtaining a master or doctoral degree. Typical graduate degrees include:

- Master of Education (MEd)
- Master of Science (MS)
- Master of Arts (MA)
- Master of Public Health (MPH)
- Master of Science in Public Health (MSPH)
- Doctor of Philosophy (PhD)
- Doctor of Public Health (Dr.PH)

The individual's personal plan for growth should help inform the choice of degree, as well as college or university. In pursuing continuing education opportunities, health education specialists should be cognizant of how the activities may further develop their knowledge and skills in the Seven Areas of Responsibility. Many health education specialists choose to gain the nationally recognized CHES and/or MCHES certification to promote, demonstrate, and continue their professional development. Please refer to Sub-competency 7.4.7 for more information on credentialing. Once employed, health education specialists can revisit a professional development plan annually with their supervisor to continually support their career goals.

■ 7.4.9 Serve as a mentor to others in the profession

Mentoring is assisting another person either with short-term or long-term development through a learning relationship. The mentor is a trusted, faithful guide to the mentee for their personal, professional, or career development. The mentee learns by gaining new awareness, knowledge, ideas, and skills (Connor & Pokora, 2012). A mentor is someone who teaches or gives help and advice to a less experienced and often younger person (Merriam-Webster, 2014). In order to grow the profession and elevate its importance in society, it is important for health education specialists to reach out to new and emerging health education specialists to help them develop and build their professional growth. Therefore, health education specialists are encouraged to become an official mentor or coach to someone in the profession and help them succeed by finding ways to use their strengths while developing new skills and knowledge. Both parties can benefit from mentoring; it offers the opportunity to exchange skills. Many more seasoned health education specialists can upgrade their technology skills by working with and learning from younger colleagues. Previous research has shown that robust mentorship helps people with their career development and career satisfaction, supports faculty retention, and contributes to academic productivity (Straus et al., 2013).

■ 7.4.10 Develop materials that contribute to the professional literature

From any practice setting, health education specialists can participate in research/practice collaboration, including participating on writing teams for publication in peer-reviewed journals, or electronic or print books. Participation as a member of a cross disciplinary team in research or practice initiatives can enrich both health education literature and the other participating disciplines. Health education specialists staying current in reading one or more professional journals regularly can respond to articles in peer-reviewed journals in letters to the editor or commentaries.

Practitioners can publish lessons learned and evaluation findings in "notes for the field" opportunities in research journals or by contributing to more practice-oriented journals (such as *Health Promotion Practice*). Practitioners and researchers can serve on dissertation or master's thesis committees, co-author articles with masters or doctoral candidates, and mentor them to continue as contributors to the field. Research and practice collaborations can also lead to submission of theory driven practice tested model programs, policies, or practices to listings such as the Substance Abuse and Mental Health Services Administration's (SAMHSA) National Registry of Evidence-based Programs and Practices (NREPP) (SAMHSA, 2014).

KEY: no symbol - entry level; ❖ advanced 1; ■ advanced 2

All health education specialists can submit abstracts or presentations to local, state, and national meetings that can lead to them being included as a part of meeting proceedings. Volunteering to be a reviewer for such abstracts or for health education, health communication, health promotion, or related journals not only contributes to the professional literature of the field but can also improve health education specialists' research and writing skills.

■ 7.4.11 Engage in service to advance the profession

Previous sections have discussed service opportunities such as joining local, state, and national professional organizations, serving on committees or as an elected officer, and volunteering as a reviewer for conference abstracts or professional publications. Health education specialists can also contribute their skills and experience by serving on boards of local, state, or national health and human service nonprofit organizations or on community health coalitions. They can lead their expertise on health assessment or planning to these efforts. In addition, they can also serve on grant review panels for organizations. Recruiting the best and brightest of our students and colleagues to the profession of health education, engaging them in professional organizations and mentoring them in our various roles and settings is a service that will continue to elevate all aspects of our profession.

Advocating for health education resources and making legislative visits to promote the inclusion of health education in state or federally funded health education, health communication, and health promotion activities are other ways to serve. Running for public office at the local, state, or federal level represents a long-term way to engage in service, thus working to reach the "best in advocacy" (Galer-Unti et al., 2004). Health education specialists should seek positions of authority with responsibilities for making policy and apply many of the health education skills discussed in this study guide to improve organizational effectiveness.

The value of professional involvement and service is unquestionable. It is through service that health education specialists can derive the greatest satisfaction. The struggles, accomplishments, and networking that emerge from working with peers who share a similar interest will help health education specialists develop an appreciation for how much can be accomplished by working collectively to achieve a common goal. More importantly than building resumes, service helps health education specialists to make connections, develop skills, and gain confidence in their abilities. All of these attributes yield rich rewards.

SECTION VII

This page was
intentionally left blank

Adams, S.A. (2012). Revisiting the online health information reliability debate in the wake of "web 2.0": An inter-disciplinary literature and website review. *International Journal of Medical Informatics, 79*(6), 391- 400.

Aday, L.A., & Cornelius, L.J. (2006). *Designing and conducting health surveys: A comprehensive guide* (3rd ed.). San Francisco, CA: Jossey-Bass.

Ajzen, I. (1988). *Attitudes, personality, and behavior.* Chicago, IL: Dorsey Press.

Allegrante, J.P., Airhihenbuwa, C.O., Auld, M.E., Birch, D.A., Roe, K.M., Smith, B.J., & National Task Force on Accreditation in Health Education. (2004). Toward a unified system of accreditation for professional preparation in health education: Final report of the National Task Force on Accreditation in Health Education. *Health Education and Behavior, 31*(6), 668-83.

American Joint Committee on Standards for Educational Evaluation. (2008). *Program evaluation standards: Summary of the standards.* Retrieved from http://www.eval.org.

American Psychological Association. (2010). Ethical principles of psychologists and code of conduct. Retrieved from http://psycnet.apa.org/index.cfm?fa=buy.optionToBuy&id=2010-14198-011

American School Health Association. (2009). *What is school health?* Retrieved from http://www.ashaweb.org/about/what-is-school-health/

American Society for Training and Development [ASTD]. (2014). *5 best practices of training and development professionals.* Retrieved from https://www.td.org/Offers/2013/08/5-Best-Practices-of-Training-and-Development-Professionals

Ammary-Risch, N.J., Zambon, A., & Brown, K.M. (2010). Communicating health information effectively. In C.I. Fertman & D.D. Allensworth (Eds.), *Health promotion programs: From theory to practice* (pp. 203-231). San Francisco, CA: Jossey-Bass.

Anspaugh, D.J., Dignan, M.B., & Anspaugh, S.L. (2000). *Developing health promotion programs.* Boston, MA: McGraw-Hill.

Armstrong, S. (2010). *The essential performance review handbook.* Franklin Lakes, NJ: Career Press.

Authenticity Consulting. (2005). *Field guide to consulting and organizational development with nonprofits: A collaborative and systems approach to performance, change and learning.* Minneapolis, MN: Authenticity Consulting, LLC.

Babbie, E.R. (2012). *The practice of social research* (13th ed.). Belmont, CA: Cengage Learning.

Bandura, A. (1986). *Social foundations of thought & action: A social cognitive theory.* Englewood Cliffs, NJ: Prentice Hall.

Barr, D.A. (2011). *Introduction to U.S. health policy: The organization, financing, and delivery of health care in America* (3rd ed.). Baltimore, MD: Johns Hopkins University Press.

Bartholomew, L.K., Parcel, G.S., Kok, G., Gottlieb, N.H., & Fernandez, M.E. (2011). *Planning health promotion programs: An intervention mapping approach* (3rd ed.). San Francisco, CA: Jossey-Bass.

Bastida, E., Tseng, T., McKeever, C., & Jack, L., Jr. (2010). Ethics and community-based participatory research: Perspectives from the field. *Health Promotion Practice, 11*(16), 16-20.

Baumgartner, T.A., & Hensley, L.D. (2012). *Conducting and reading research in kinesiology* (5th ed.). Boston, MA: McGraw-Hill.

Bensley, L.B., Jr. (2009). Using theory and ethics to guide method selection and application. In R.J. Bensley & J. Brookins-Fisher (Eds.), *Community health education methods: A practical guide* (3rd ed.) (pp. 3-30). Sudbury, MA: Jones and Bartlett Publishers.

Beaulieu, L.J. (2002). *Mapping the assets of your community: A key component for building local capacity* [PDF Document]. Retrieved from http://www.nebhands.nebraska.edu/files/227_asset_mapping.pdf

REFERENCES

Blase, K. (2009). *Technical assistance to promote service and system change: Roadmap to effective intervention practices #4.* Tampa, Florida: University of South Florida, Technical Assistance Center on Social Emotional Intervention for Young Children.

Brownson, R.C., Baker, E.A., Left, T.L., Gillespie K.N., & True, W.R. (2010). *Evidence-based public health* (2nd ed.). New York, NY: Oxford University Press.

Brownson, R.C., Chriqui, J.F., & Stamatakis, K.A. (2009). Understanding evidence-based public health policy. *American Journal of Public Health, 99*(9), 1576-1583.

Brownson, R., Fielding, J., & Maylahn, C. (2009). Evidence-based public health: A fundamental concept for public health practice. *Annual Review of Public Health, 30,* 175–201.

Bryan, R.L., Kreuter, M.W., & Brownson, R.C. (2008). Integrating adult learning principles into training for public health practice. *Health Promotion Practice, 10*(4), 557-563.

Burke, R.E., & Friedman, L.H. (2010). *Essentials of management and leadership in public health.* Sudbury, MA: Jones and Bartlett.

Butterfoss, F.D. (2007). *Coalitions and partnerships in community health.* San Francisco, CA: Jossey-Bass.

Butterfoss, F.D. (2009). Building and sustaining coalitions. In R.J. Bensley & J. Brookins Fisher (Eds.), *Community health education methods: A practical guide* (3rd ed.) (pp. 299-332). Sudbury, MA: Jones and Bartlett.

Butterfoss, F.D. (2013). *Ignite! Getting your community coalition "fired up" for change.* Bloomington, IN: Author.

Caira, N.M., Lachenmayr, S., Sheinfeld, J., Goodhart, F.W., Cancialosi, L., & Lewis, C. (2003). The health educator's role in advocacy and policy: Principles, processes, programs, and partnerships. *Health Promotion Practice, 4*(3), 303-313.

Capurro, D., Cole, K., Echavarría, M.I., Joe, J., Neogi, T., & Turner, A.M. (2014). The use of social networking sites for public health practice and research: A systematic review. *Journal of Medical and Internet Research, 16*(3), e79.

Castro, F. G., Barrera, Jr, M., & Holleran Steiker, L. K. (2010). Issues and challenges in the design of culturally adapted evidence-based interventions. *Annual Review of Clinical Psychology, 6,* 213-239.

Centers for Disease Control and Prevention. (1999). Framework for program evaluation in public health. *Morbidity and Mortality Weekly Report, 48,* 11.

Centers for Disease Control and Prevention. (2003). *CDCynergy 3.0: Your guide to effective health communication* (Version 3). [CD ROM]. Atlanta, GA: Author.

Centers for Disease Control and Prevention. (2007). *CDCynergy social marketing edition* (Version 2). Retrieved from http://www.orau.gov/cdcynergy/soc2web/

Centers for Disease Control and Prevention. (2010). *Introduction to program evaluation for public health programs.* Retrieved from http://www.cdc.gov/getsmart/program-planner/Step3.html

Centers for Disease Control and Prevention. (2011). *Health marketing basics.* Retrieved from http://www.cdc.gov/healthcommunication/ToolsTemplates/Basics.html

Centers for Disease Control and Prevention, Division of Community Health. (2013). *A practitioner's guide for advancing health equity: Community strategies for preventing chronic disease.* Atlanta, GA: US Department of Health and Human Services.

Centers for Disease Control and Prevention. (2014a). *Community guide: Public policy.* Retrieved from http://www.thecommunityguide.org/uses/policy_development.html

Centers for Disease Control and Prevention. (2014b). *A sustainability planning guide for healthy communities* [PDF Document]. Atlanta, GA: U.S. Department of Health and Human Services, Centers for Disease Control and Prevention, National Center for Chronic Disease Prevention and Health Promotion, Division of Adult and Community Health. Retrieved from http://www.cdc.gov/nccdphp/dch/programs/healthycommunitiesprogram/pdf/sustainability_guide.pdf

Centers for Disease Control and Prevention. (2014c). *Best practices for comprehensive tobacco control programs—2014* [PDF Document]. Atlanta, GA: U.S. Department of Health and Human Services, Centers for Disease Control and Prevention, National Center for Chronic Disease Prevention, & Health Promotion, Office on Smoking and Health. Retrieved from http://www.cdc.gov/tobacco/stateandcommunity/best_practices

Centers for Disease Control and Prevention. (2014d). *Health literacy.* Retrieved from http://www.cdc.gov/healthliteracy

Centers for Disease Control and Prevention. (2014e). *Social determinants of health.* Retrieved from http://www.cdc.gov/socialdeterminants/FAQ.html

Centers for Disease Control and Prevention. (2014f). *Using evaluation to inform CDC's policy process.* Atlanta, GA: Centers for Disease Control and Prevention, US Department of Health and Human Services.

Centola, D. (2013). Social media and the science of health behavior. *Circulation, 127*(21), 2135-2144.

Cheadle, A., Schwartz, P. M., Rauzon, S., Beery, W. L., Gee, S., & Solomon, L. (2010). The Kaiser Permanente community health initiative: Overview and evaluation design. *American Journal of Public Health, 100*(11), 2111-2113.

Chen, W.W., Sheu, J.J., & Chen, H.S. (2010). Making decisions to create and support a program. In C.I. Fertman & D.D. Allensworth (Eds.), *Health promotion programs: From theory to practice* (pp.121-150). San Francisco, CA: Jossey-Bass.

Chenoweth, D.H. (2011). *Worksite health promotion* (3rd ed.). Champaign, IL: Human Kinetics.

Chinman, M., Hannah, G., Wandersman, A., Ebener, P., Hunter, S. B., Imm, P., & Sheldon, J. (2005). Developing a community science research agenda for building community capacity for effective preventive interventions. *American Journal of Community Psychology, 35*(3-4), 143-157.

Cleary, M.J., & Neiger, B.L. (1998). *The certified health education specialist: A self-study guide for professional competency* (3rd ed.). Allentown, PA: National Commission for Health Education Credentialing, Inc.

Coalition of National Health Education Organizations. (2011). *Code of ethics for the health education profession* [PDF Document]. Retrieved from http://www.cnheo.org/files/coe_full_2011.pdf

Coalition of National Health Education Organizations. (2014). *What does the Coalition do?* Retrieved http://www.cnheo.org/aboutus.html

Connor, M., & Pokora, J. (2012). *Coaching and mentoring at work: Developing effective practice.* (2nd ed.). New York: Open University Press.

Cottrell, R.R., Girvan, J.T., & McKenzie, J.F. (2014). *Principles and foundations of health promotion and education* (6th ed.). San Francisco, CA: Pearson/Benjamin Cummings.

Cottrell, R. R., & McKenzie, J. F. (2010). *Health promotion and education research methods: Using the five chapter thesis/dissertation model.* Burlington, MA: Jones & Bartlett Learning.

Council on Linkages. (2012). *Improving and measuring the impact of trainings: Strategies & methods.* Washington, DC: Council on Linkages.

Crosby, R. A., DiClemente, R. J., & Salazar, L. F. (2006). *Research methods in health promotion.* San Francisco, CA: Jossey-Bass.

REFERENCES

DeCenzo, D.A., & Robbins, S.P. (2012). *Human resource management* (11th ed.). Danvers, MA: John Wiley and Sons.

Deeds, S.G. (1992). *The health education specialist: Self-study for professional.* Los Alamitos, CA: Loose Cannon.

Diaz-Cuellar, A.L., & Evans, S.F. (2013). Diversity and health education. In M.A Perez & R.R. Luquis (Eds.), *Cultural competence in health education and health promotion* (2nd ed.) (pp. 43-65). San Francisco, CA: Jossey-Bass.

Dickert, N., & Sugarman, J. (2005). Ethical goals of community consultation in research. *American Journal of Public Health, 95*(7), 1123-1127.

DiClemente, R.J., Crosby, R.A., & Kegler, M.C. (2009). *Emerging theories in health promotion practice and research.* San Francisco, CA: Jossey-Bass.

Doak, C.C., Doak, L.G., Gordon, L., & Lorig, K. (2001). Selecting, preparing, and using materials. In K. Lorig (Ed.), *Patient education: A practical approach* (3rd ed.) (pp. 183-197). Thousand Oaks, CA: Sage Publications, Inc.

Doak, C.C., Doak, L.G., & Root, J.H. (1996). *Teaching patients with low literacy skills* (2nd ed.). Philadelphia, PA: JB Lippincott.

Doak, C.C., Doak, L.G., & Root, J.H. (Eds.). (2002). *Pfizer health literacy principles: A handbook for creating patient education materials that enhance understanding and promote health outcomes.* New York, NY: Pfizer.

Dodson, E.A., Brownson, R.C., & Weiss, S.M. (2012). Policy dissemination research. In R.C. Brownson, G.A., Colditz, & E.K. Proctor (Eds.), *Dissemination and implementation research in health: Translating science to practice* (pp. 437-459). New York: Oxford.

Dorfman, L. (2009). Using media advocacy to influence policy. In R.J. Bensley & J. Brookins-Fisher (Eds.). *Community health education methods: A practical guide* (3rd ed.) (pp. 361-389). Sudbury, MA: Jones and Bartlett.

Dorfman, L., & Krasnow, I. D. (2014). Public health and media advocacy. *Annual Review of Public Health, 35,* 293-306.

Dougherty, A.M. (2013). *Psychological consultation and collaboration in school and community settings* (6th ed.). Belmont, CA: Cengage Learning.

Doyle, E., Ward, S., & Oomen-Early, J. (2010). *The process of community health education and promotion.* Mountain View, CA: Mayfield Publishing Company.

Dreier, M., Borutta, B., Seidel, G., Kreusel, I., Töppich, J., Bitzer, E.M., Dierks, M., & Walter, U. (2013). Development of a comprehensive list of criteria for evaluating consumer education materials on colorectal cancer screening. *BMC Public Health, 13*(1), 1-12.

Edberg, M. (2007). *Social and behavioral theory in public health.* Sudbury, MA: Jones and Bartlett.

Eysenbach, G., Powell, J., Kuss, O., & Sa, E. (2002). Empirical studies assessing the quality of health information for consumers on the World Wide Web: A systematic review. *JAMA, 287*(20), 2691-2700.

Fagen, M., Reed, E., Kaye, J., & Jack, L. (2009). Advocacy evaluation: What is it and where to find out more about it. *Health Promotion Practice, 10*(4), 482-484.

Fallon, L. F., & Zgodzinski. (2011). *Essentials of public health management* (3rd ed.). Sudbury, MA: Jones and Bartlett.

Fertman, C.I., Spiller, K.A., & Mickalide, A.D. (2010). Developing and increasing program funding. In C.I. Fertman & D.D. Allensworth (Eds.), *Health promotion programs: From theory to practice* (pp.233-225). San Francisco, CA: Jossey-Bass.

Fink, A. (2013). *Conducting research literature reviews: From the internet to paper* (4th ed.). Thousand Oaks, CA: Sage Publications, Inc.

Fitzpatrick, J.L., Sanders, J.R., & Worthen, B.R. (2010). *Program evaluation: Alternative approaches and practical guidelines* (4th ed.). Boston, MA: Pearson, Allyn, & Bacon.

Fjeldsoe, B.S., Marshall, A.L., & Miller, Y.D. (2009). Behavior change interventions delivered by mobile telephone short-message service. *American Journal of Preventive Medicine, 36*(2), 165-173.

Fodor, J.T., Dalis, G.T., & Giarratano, S.R. (2010). *Health instruction in schools.* Bradenton, FL: BookLocker.

Freitas, F. A., & Leonard, L. J. (2011). Maslow's hierarchy of needs and student academic success. *Teaching and Learning in Nursing, 6*(1), 9-13.

Frieden, T.R. (2010). A framework for public health action: the health impact pyramid. *American Journal of Public Health, 100*(4), 590-595.

Frieden, T.R. (2014). Six components necessary for effective public health program implementation. *American Journal of Public Health, 104*(1), 17-22.

Freudenberg, N., Bradley, S.P., & Serrano, M. (2009). Public health campaigns to change industry practices that damage health: An analysis of 12 case studies. *Health Education and Behavior, 36*(2), 230-249.

Friere, P. (2000). *Pedagogy of the oppressed.* New York, NY: Continuum.

Friis, R.H., & Sellers, T.A. (2013). *Epidemiology for public health practice* (5th ed.). Sudbury, MA: Jones and Bartlett.

Fixsen, D.L., Blase, K.A., Naoom, S.F., & Wallace, F. (2009). Core implementation components. *Research on Social Work Practice, 19*(5), 531–540.

Gagne, R.M., Wager, W.W., Golas, K,. & Keller, J.M. (2005). *Principles of instructional design* (5th ed.). Independence, KY: Cengage Learning.

Galer-Unti, R., Tappe, M.K., & Lachenmayr, S. (2004). Advocacy 101: Getting started in health education advocacy. *Health Promotion Practice, 5*(3), 280-288.

Gardner, H. (2011). *Frames of mind: The theory of multiple intelligences.* NY: Basic Books.

Georgia Health Policy Center. (2011). *Sustainability framework* [PDF Document]. Atlanta, GA: Georgia Health Policy Center. Retrieved from http://www.raconline.org/sustainability/pdf/georgia-health-policy-center-sustainability-framework.pdf

Gilbert, G.G., Sawyer, R.G., & McNeill, E.B. (2011). *Health education: Creating strategies for school and health* (3rd ed.). Sudbury, MA: Jones and Bartlett.

Gilmore, G.D. (2012). *Needs and capacity assessment strategies for health education and health promotion (4th ed.).* Sudbury, MA: Jones and Barlett.

Gilmore, G.D., Olsen, L.K., Taub, A., & Connell, D. (2005). Overview of the national health educator competencies update project 1998-2004. *Health Education & Behavior, 32*(6), 725-737.

Ginter, P.M. (2013). *Strategic management of health care organization* (7th ed.). San Francisco, CA: Jossey-Bass.

Glanz, K., Rimer, B.K., & Viswanath, K. (Eds.). (2008a). *Health behavior and health education: Theory research and practice* (4th ed.). San Francisco, CA: Jossey-Bass.

Glanz, K., Rimer, B.K., & Viswanath, K. (2008b). Theory, research and practice in health behavior and health education. In Glanz, K., Rimer, B.K., & Viswanath, K (Eds.) *Health behavior and health education: Theory research and practice* (4th ed.) (pp. 23-40). San Francisco, CA: Jossey-Bass.

REFERENCES

Goldman, K.D. (2009). Social marketing concepts. In R.J. Bensley & J. Brookins-Fisher (Eds.), *Community health education methods: A practical guide* (3rd ed.) (pp. 103-128). Sudbury, MA: Jones and Bartlett Publishers.

Goldman, K.D., & Schmaltz, K.J. (2005). How great groups do it: Improving group effectiveness. In K.D. Goldman & K.J. Schmaltz (Eds.), *Health education tools of the trade: Tools for tasks that didn't come with the job description* (pp.77-80). Washington, D.C: Society for Public Health Education.

Goodson, P. (2010). *Theory in health promotion research and practice: Thinking outside the box.* Sudbury, MA: Jones and Bartlett.

Gorman-Smith, D. (2006). *How to successfully implement evidence-based social programs: A brief overview for policymakers and program providers.* Washington, DC: Coalition for Evidence-Based Policy working paper. Retrieved from http://coalition4evidence.org/wp-content/uploads/2012/12/PublicationHowToSuccessfullyImplement06.pdf

Green, L.W., & Kreuter, M.W. (2005). *Health program planning: An educational and ecological approach* (4th ed.). Boston, MA: McGraw-Hill.

Greenlick, M.R., Goldberg, B., Lopes, P., & Tallon, J. (2005). Health policy roundtable—view from the state legislature: translating research into policy. *Health Services Research, 40*(2), 337-346.

Gronlund, N.E. (1995). *How to write and use instructional objectives* (5th ed.). Englewood Cliffs, NJ: Prentice Hall.

Gronlund, N.D., & Brookhart (2008). *Gronlund's writing instructional objectives* (8th ed.). Upper Saddle River, NJ: Pearson.

Guthrie, K., Louie, J. & Foster, C.C. (2006). *The challenge of assessing policy and advocacy activities: PART II—Moving from theory to practice.* San Francisco, CA: California Endowment.

Harkness, J. A. (2008). Comparative survey research: Goals and challenges. In E. D. de Leeuw, J. J. Hox & D. A. Dillman (Eds.), International handbook of survey methodology (pp. 56-77). New York, NY/London: Lawrence Erlbaum Associates.

Harris, M.J. (2010). *Evaluating public and community health programs.* San Francisco, CA: Jossey-Bass.

Hartsfield, D., Moulton, A.D., & McKie, K.L. (2007). A review of model public health laws. *American Journal of Public Health, 97*(supl1), S56-S61.

Hayden, J. (2014). *Introduction to health behavior theory* (2nd ed.). Sudbury, MA: Jones and Bartlett.

Healey, B.J., & Zimmerman, R.S. (2010). *The new world of health promotion: New program development, implementation, and evaluation.* Boston, MA: Jones and Bartlett.

Heldman, A. B., & Schindelar, J. (2013). Social media engagement and public health communication: Implications for public health organizations being truly "social". *Public Health Reviews, 35*(1), 1-18.

Hellriegel, D., & Slocum, J.W. (2013). *Organizational behavior* (13th ed.). Mason, OH: Cengage Learning.

Hernandez, S.R., & O'Connor, S.J. (2009). *Strategic management of human resources in health services organizations* (3rd ed.). Albany, NY: Cengage Learning.

Hochbaum, G.M. (1958). *Public participation in medical screening programs: A socio-psychological study* [PHS Publication No. 572]. Washington, DC: US Public Health Service.

Hodges, B.C., & Videtto, D.M. (2011). *Assessment and planning in health programs.* Sudbury, MA: Jones & Bartlett Learning.

Hrastinski, S. (2008). Asynchronous and synchronous e- learning. *Educause Quarterly, 31*(4), 51-55.

Institute of Medicine. (2002). *Speaking of health: Assessing health communication strategies for diverse populations.* Committee on Communication for Behavior Change in the 21st Century: Improving the Health of Diverse Populations. Washington, DC: National Academy Press.

REFERENCES

Institute of Medicine. (2004). *Health literacy: A prescription to end confusion.* Washington, DC: National Academy Press.

Internal Revenue Service. (2014). *"Direct" and "grass roots" lobbying defined.* Washington, DC: International Revenue Service. Retrieved from http://www.irs.gov/Charities-&-Non-Profits/Direct—and—Grass-Roots—Lobbying-Defined

Issel, L. M. (2014). *Health program planning and evaluation: A practical, systematic approach for community health* (3rd ed.). Sudbury, MA: Jones and Bartlett.

Jack, L., Jr., Hayes, S., Scharalda, J.G., Stetson, B., Jones-Jack, N., Valliere, M., Kirchain, W.R., LeBlanc, C. (2010). Appraising quantitative research in health education: Guidelines for public health educators. *Health Promotion Practice, 11*(2), 161-165.

Jackson, A. (2014). Evaluation of public policy advocacy: Challenges, principles and best-ac case study. *International Journal of Public Sector Management, 27*(4), 2-2.

Jeanfreau G., & Jack, L., Jr. (2010). Appraising qualitative research in health education: guidelines for public health educators. *Health Promotion Practice, 11*(2), 161-65.

Johnson, B., & Turner, L.A. (2010). Data collection strategies in mixed methods research. In A. Tashakkori & Teddlie (Eds.), *Handbook of mixed methods in social and behavioral research* (pp. 297-320). Thousand Oaks, CA: Sage Publications, Inc.

Johnson, D.W., & Johnson, F.P. (2012). *Joining together: Group theory and group skills* (11th ed.). Boston, MA: Pearson.

Johnson, J., & Breckon, D. (2007). *Managing health education and promotion programs: Leadership skills for the 21st century.* Boston, MA: Jones and Bartlett.

Joint Center for Political and Economic Studies. (2012). Place matters for health in Orleans parish: Ensuring opportunities for good health for all. Washington DC: Author.

Joint Committee on Health Education Terminology. (2002). Report of the 2000 joint committee on health education and promotion terminology. *Journal of School Health, 72*(1), 3-7.

Journal of the National AHEC Organization. (2010). *Health literacy toolkit* [PDF Document]. Retrieved from http://www.nationalahec.org/documents/MarchApril2010CenterfoldHealthLiteracy.pdf

Kaplan, A.M., & Haenlein, M. (2010). Users of the world, unite! The challenges and opportunities of social media. *Business Horizons, 53*(1), 59-68

Kaplan, R.M., Riley, W.T., & Mabry, P.L. (2014). News from the NIH: Leveraging big data in the behavioral sciences. *Translational Behavioral Medicine, 4*(3), 229-231.

Karlsson, J., & Beaufils, P. (2013). Legitimate division of large data sets, salami slicing and dual publication, where does a fraud begin? *Knee Surgery, Sports Traumatology, Arthroscopy, 21*(4), 751-752.

Kemm, J., Parry, J., & Palmer, S. (2004). Health impact assessment: Concepts, theory, techniques and applications. New York, NY: Oxford University Press.

Kimberlin, C. L., & Winterstein, A. G. (2008). Validity and reliability of measurement instruments used in research. *American Journal of Health-System Pharmacy, 65*(23), 2276-2284.

Kingdon, J.W. (2010). *Agendas, alternatives, and public policies* (2nd ed.). San Francisco, CA: Pearson.

Kirkpatrick, D.L., & Kirkpatrick. J.D. (2009). *Evaluating training programs: The four levels* (3rd ed.). San Francisco, CA: Berrett-Koehler.

Klasnjal, P., & Pratt, W. (2012). Healthcare in the pocket: Mapping the space of mobile-phone health interventions. *Journal of Biomedical Informatics, 45*(1), 184-198.

REFERENCES

Knowles, M.S., Holton III, E.F., & Swanson, R.A. (2005). *The adult learner: The definitive classic in adult education and human resource development* (6th ed.). Burlington, MA: Butterworth-Heinemann.

Kreps, G., Barnes, M., Neiger, B. & Thackeray. (2009). Health communication. In R.J. Bensley & J. Brookins-Fisher (Eds.), *Community health education methods: A practical guide* (3rd ed.) (pp. 87). Sudbury, MA: Jones and Bartlett.

Kreuter, M.W., Farrell, D., Olevitch, L., & Brennan, L. (2000). *Tailoring health messages: Customizing communications with computer technology.* Mahwah, NJ: Lawrence Erlbaum and Associates.

Kreuter, M.W., Lezin, N.A., Kreuter, M.W., & Green, L.W. (2003). *Community health promotion ideas that work* (2nd ed.). Sudbury, MA: Jones and Bartlett.

Lachenmayr, S. (2009). Using advocacy to affect policy. In R.J. Bensley & J. Brookins-Fisher (Eds.), *Community health education methods: A practical guide* (3rd ed.) (pp. 333-360). Sudbury, MA: Jones and Bartlett.

Lawson, K. (2008). *The trainer's handbook: Updated edition* (3rd ed.). San Francisco, CA: Pfieffer.

Levy, B. & Sidel, V.W. (2013). *The nature of social injustice and its impact on public health.* New York: Oxford.

Livingood,W.C., & Auld, M.E. (2001).The credentialing of a population-based profession: Lessons learned from health education certification. *Journal of Public Health Management & Practice, 7*(4), 38-45.

Livet, M., Courser, M., & Wandersman, A. (2008). The prevention delivery system: Organizational context and use of comprehensive programming frameworks. *American Journal of Community Psychology, 41*(3-4), 361-378.

Longest, B.B., Jr. (2010). *Health policy-making in the United States* (5th ed.). Chicago, IL: Health Administration Press.

Longest, B.B., Jr. (2011). *Managing health programs and projects.* San Francisco, CA: Jossey-Bass.

Mager, R. F. (1997). *Preparing instructional objectives: A critical tool in the development of effective instruction.* Atlanta, GA: Center for Effective Performance.

Mas, F.S., Allensworth, D.D., & Jones, F.S. (2010). Health promotion programs designed to eliminate health disparities. In C.I. Fertman & D.D. Allensworth (Eds.), *Health promotion programs: From theory to practice* (pp.29-55). San Francisco, CA: Jossey-Bass.

McKenzie, J.F., Neiger, B.L., & Thackeray, J. L. (2013). *Planning, implementing, & evaluating health promotion programs: A primer* (6th ed.). San Francisco, CA: Pearson/Benjamin Cummings.

McKenzie, J.F., Pinger, R.R., & Kotecki, J.E. (2011). *An introduction to community health* (7th ed.). Sudbury, MA: Jones and Bartlett.

Merriam, S.B., Caffarella, R.S., Baumgartner, L.M. (2007). *Learning in adulthood: A comprehensive guide* (3rd ed.). San Francisco: Jossey-Bass.

Merriam-Webster. (2014). *Mentor.* Retrieved from http://www.merriam-webster.com/dictionary/mentor

Miles, M. B., Huberman, A. M., & Saldaña, J. (2013). *Qualitative data analysis: A methods sourcebook* (3rd e.d). Thousand Oaks, CA: Sage Publications, Inc.

Miner, K.R., Childers, W.K., Alperin, M., Cioffi, J., & Hunt. N. (2005). The MACH model: From competencies to instruction and performance of public health professionals. *Public Health Reports, 120,* 9-15.

Miner, J.T., & Miner, L.E. (2013). *Proposal planning & writing* (5th ed.). Santa Barbara, CA: Greenwood.

Minelli, M.J., & Breckon, D.J. (2009). *Community health education: Settings, roles, and skills for the 21st century* (5th ed.). Sudbury, MA: Jones and Barlett.

REFERENCES

Minkler, M., & Wallertein, N. (2008). *Community-based participatory research for health from process to outcomes* (2nd ed.). San Francisco, CA: Jossey-Bass.

Montano, D.E., & Kasprzyk, D. (2008). Theory of reasoned action, theory of planned behavior, and the integrated behavioral model. In K. Glanz, B.K. Rimer, & K. Viswanath (Eds.), *Health behavior and health education: Theory research and practice* (4th ed.) (pp. 67-96). San Francisco, CA: Jossey-Bass.

Moore, J. E., Bumbarger, B. K., & Cooper, B. R. (2013). Examining adaptations of evidence-based programs in natural contexts. *The Journal of Primary Prevention, 34*(3), 147-161.

Malterud, K. (2012). Systematic text condensation: a strategy for qualitative analysis. *Scandinavian Journal of Public Health, 40*(8), 795-805.

National Association of County and City Health Officials. (2010). *Mobilizing for action through Planning and Partnerships (MAPP).* Retrieved from http://www.naccho.org/topics/infrastructure/MAPP/index.cfm

National Association of City and County Health Officers. (2013). *Mobilizing for action through planning and partnerships – achieving healthier communities through MAPP - A users handbook.* Washington DC: Author.

National Cancer Institute [NCI]. (2005). *Theory at a glance* (2nd ed.). Washington, DC: Author.

National Cancer Institute. (2006). *Using what works: Adapting evidence-based programs to fit your needs.* Retrieved from http://cancercontrol.cancer.gov/use_what_works/start.htm

National Cancer Institute. (2008). *Making health communications work* [PDF Document]. Retrieved from http://www.cancer.gov/pinkbook

National Cancer Institute. (2015). *Using trusted resources.* Retrieved from http://www.cancer.gov/cancertopics/managing-care/using-trusted-resources.

National Cancer Institute. (2014). *Evaluating online sources of health education.* Retrieved from http://www.cancer.gov/cancertopics/cancerlibrary/health-info-online

National Center on Quality Teaching and Learning (2014). *Creating a learning environment for children.* Retrieved from http://eclkc.ohs.acf.hhs.gov/hslc/tta-system/teaching/eecd/learning%20environments/planning%20and%20arranging%20spaces/edudev_art_00400_060906.html

National Commission for Health Education Credentialing, Inc., & Society for Public Health Education. (2015). *A competency-based framework for health educators - 2015.* Whitehall, PA: Author.

National Commission for Health Education Credentialing, Inc., Society for Public Health Education, & American Association for Health Education. (2010a). *A competency-based framework for health educators - 2010.* Whitehall, PA: Author.

National Commission for Health Education Credentialing, Inc., Society for Public Health Education, & American Association for Health Education [AAHE]. (2010b). *Health education specialist job analysis -2010: Executive summary and recommendations.* Retrieved from http://www.nchec.org/credentialing/competency/

National Implementation Research Network. (2014). *Implementation defined.* Retrieved from http://nirn.fpg.unc.edu/learn-implementation/implementation-defined

National Institutes of Health. (2011). *Principles of community engagement* (2nd ed.). Washington, DC: Author.

National Library of Medicine. (2009). *Resources: A user's guide to finding and evaluating health information on the web.* Retrieved from http://www.mlanet.org/resources/userguide.html

REFERENCES

National Task Force on the Preparation & Practice of Health Education Specialists. (1985). *A framework for the development of competency-based curricula for entry-level health education specialists.* New York, NY: National Commission for Health Education Credentialing, Inc.

Newman, S.D., Andrews, J.O., Magwood, G.S., Jenkins, C., Cox, M.J., & Williamson, D.C. (2011). Community advisory boards in community-based participatory research: A synthesis of best processes. *Preventing Chronic Disease, 8*(3), A70.

Neutens, J.J., & Rubinson, L. (2010). *Research techniques for the health sciences* (4th ed.). San Francisco, CA: Pearson/Benjamin Cummings.

Northwest Center for Public Health Practice (2012). *Effective adult learning: A toolkit for teaching adults* [PDF Document]. Retrieved from http://www.nwcphp.org/documents/training/Adult_Education_Toolkit.pdf

Occupational Health and Safety Administration. (2010). *Best practices for development, delivery, and evaluation of Susan Harwood training grants* [PDF Document]. Washington, DC: U.S. Department of Labor, Occupational Safety & Health Administration. Retrieved from https://www.osha.gov/dte/sharwood/best-practices-booklet.pdf

Olson, S.J. (2014). Partnerships and collaboration: Critical components to promoting health. In B.J. Healey & R.S. Zimmerman (Eds.). *The new world of health promotion: New program development, implementation and evaluation.* (pp. 283-213). Sudbury, MA: Jones and Bartlett.

Orfaly, R.A., Francis, J.C., Campbell, P., Whittemor, B., Joly, B., & Koh, H. (2005). Train-the-trainer as an educational model in public health preparedness. *Journal of Public Health Management and Practice (Supplement S)*, 123-127.

Parvanta, C. (2011). Public health communication: a planning framework. In C.F. Parvanta, D.E. Nelson, S.A. Parvanta, & R.N. Harner (Eds.), *Essentials of Public Health Communication* (pp. 19-38). Sudbury, MA: Jones and Bartlett Learning.

Patton, M.Q. (2008). *Utilization-focused evaluation* (4th ed.). Thousand Oaks, CA: Sage Publications, Inc.

Patton, M.Q. (2014). *Qualitative research & evaluation methods: Integrating theory and practice* (4th ed.). Thousand Oaks, CA: Sage Publications, Inc.

Perrin, K. M. (2014). *Essentials of planning and evaluation for public health.* Burlington, MA: Jones & Bartlett Learning.

Peters, E., Hibbard, J., Slovic, P., & Dieckmann, N. (2007). Numeracy skill and the communication, comprehension, and use of risk-benefit information. *Health Affairs, 26*(3), 741-748.

Piskurich, G.M., Beckschi, P., & Hall, B. (2000). *The ASTD handbook for training and delivery.* New York: McGraw-Hill.

Plain Language Action and Information Network. (2014). *Plain language.gov: Improving communication from the federal government to the public.* Retrieved from http://www.plainlanguage.gov

Plain Language Action and Information Network. (2014). *Plain Language Websites.* Retrieved from http://www.plainlanguage.gov/webPL/index.cfm

Plomer, K.D. & Bensley, R.J. (2009). Developing and selecting print materials. In R.J. Bensley & J. Brookins Fisher (Eds.), *Community health education methods: A practical guide* (3rd ed.) (pp. 209-236). Sudbury, MA: Jones and Bartlett.

Poland, B. (2009). Settings for health promotion: An analytic framework to guide intervention design and implementation. *Health Promotion Practice, 10*(4), 505-516.

Prevention Institute. (2014). *Improving environments for health & health equity.* Retrieved from http://www.preventioninstitute.org/index.php?option=com_content&view=article&id=81&Itemid=180

Project Management Institute. (2014). *What is project management?* Retrieved from http://www.pmi.org/About-Us/About-Us-What-is-Project-Management.aspx.

Prochaska, J. (2005). Stages of change, readiness, and motivation. In J. Kerr, R. Weitkunat, & M. Moretti (Eds.). *ABC of behavior change: A guide to successful disease prevention and health promotion* (pp. 111-123). Edinburgh: Elsevier.

Prochaska, J., Redding, C., & Evers, K. (2008). The transtheoretical model and stages of change. In K. Glanz, B.K. Rimer, & K. Viswanath (Eds.), *Health behavior and health education: Theory, research, and practice* (4th ed.) (pp. 170-222). San Francisco, CA: Jossey-Bass.

Rabin, B. A., & Glasgow, R. E. (2012). Dissemination of interactive health communication programs. *Interactive Health Communication Technologies: Promising Strategies for Health Behavior Change.* New York, NY: Routledge.

Rabin, B.A., Glasgow, R.E., Kerner, F.J., Klump, M.P., & Brownson, R.C. (2010). Dissemination and implementation research on community-based cancer prevention: A systematic review. *American Journal of Preventive Medicine, 38*(4), 443-456.

Rees, K.S., & Goldsmith, M. (2009). Selecting presentation methods. In R.J. Bensley & J. Brookins-Fisher (Eds.), *Community health education methods: A practical guide* (3rd ed.) (pp. 265-298). Sudbury, MA: Jones and Bartlett.

Resnick, E., & Siegel, M. (2013). *Marketing public health: Strategies to promote social change* (3rd ed.). Sudbury, MA: Jones and Bartlett.

Robbins, S. & Judge, T. (2015). *Essentials of organizational behavior* (13th ed.) Upper Saddle River, NJ: Prentice Hall.

Roe, K.M., Roe, K., & Strona, F.V. (2009). Facilitating groups. In R.J. Bensley & J. Brookins-Fisher (Eds.), *Community health education methods: A practical guide* (3rd ed.) (pp. 293-323). Sudbury, MA: Jones and Bartlett.

Rogers, E.M. (2003). *Diffusion of innovation* (5th ed.). New York, NY: Free Press.

Rosenstock, I.M., Strecher, V.J., & Becker, M.H. (1988). Social learning theory and the health belief model. *Health Education Quarterly, 15*(2), 175-183.

Rossi, P. H., Lipsey, M.W., & Freeman, H.E. (2003). Evaluation: A systematic approach (7th ed.). Thousand Oaks, CA: Sage.

Rowitz, L. (2013). *Public health leadership: putting principles into practice* (3rd ed.). Sudbury, MA: Jones and Bartlett.

Rudolph, L., Caplan, J., Ben-Moshe, K. & Dillon L. (2013). *Heath in all policies: a guide for state and local governments.* Washington, DC: American Public Health Association and Public Health Institute.

Saks, A. M., Haccoun, R. R., & Belcourt, M. (2010). *Managing performance through training and development.* Boston, MA: Cengage Learning.

Sallis, J.F., Owen, N., & Fisher, E.B. (2008). Ecological models of health behavior. In K. Glanz, B.K. Rimer & K. Viswanath (Eds), *Health behavior and health education: Theory, research, and practice* (4th ed.) (pp. 465-486). San Francisco, CA: Jossey-Bass.

Schell, S.F., Luke, D.A., Schooley, M.W., Elliott, M.B., Herbers, S.H., Mueller, N.B., & Bunger, A.C. (2013). Public health program capacity for sustainability: A new framework. *Implementation Science, 8*(15).

Schiavo, R. (2013). *Health communication: From theory to practice* (2nd ed.). San Francisco, CA: Jossey-Bass.

Schulz, A., & Northridge, M. E. (2004). Social determinants of health: implications for environmental health promotion. *Health Education & Behavior, 31*(4), 455-471.

REFERENCES

REFERENCES

Sharma, M., & Petosa, R., L. (2012). *Measurement and evaluation for health educators.* Burlington, MA: Jones & Bartlett Learning.

Sharma, M. & Romas, J.A. (2010). *Theoretical foundations of health education and health promotion.* Sudbury, MA: Jones and Bartlett.

Sherow, S., Weinberg, J., Sloan, J., & Morin, E. (2002). *Planning for change: A coalition building technical assistance system.* Philadelphia, PA: Author.

Shi, L., & Johnson, J. A. (2013). *Novick & Morrow's public health administration: Principles for population-based management.* Sudbury, MA: Jones and Bartlett.

Simons-Morton, B.G., Greene, W.H., & Gottlieb, N.H. (1995). *Introduction to health education and health promotion* (2nd ed.). Prospect Heights, IL: Waveland Press.

Sleet, D.A., & Cole, S.L. (2010). Leadership and change for sustainability. In C.I. Fertman & D.D. Allensworth (Eds.), *Health Promotion Programs: From Theory to Practice* (pp.291-310). San Francisco, CA: Jossey-Bass.

Strategic Tobacco Retail Effort. *STORE: Strategic Tobacco Retail Effort.* (2014). Retrieved from http://www.tcsstore.org/stages/index.html

Straus, S. E., Johnson, M. O. , Marquez, C., & Feldman, M. (2013). Characteristics of successful and failed mentoring relationships: A qualitative study across two academic health centers. *Academic Medicine, 88*(1), 82-89.

Stryker, S.C. (2011). *Principles and practices of professional consulting.* Lanham, MD: Government Institutes.

Substance Abuse and Mental Health Services Administration. (2012). *The non-researcher's guide to evidence-based program evaluation.* Retrieved from http://www.nrepp.samhsa.gov/Courses/ProgramEvaluation/NREPP_0406_0090.html

Substance Abuse and Mental Health Services Administration. (2014). *National registry of evidence-based programs and practice.* Retrieved from http://www.nrepp.samhsa.gov/

Taub, A., Birch, D. A., Auld, M. E., Lysoby, L., & Rasar King, L. (2009). Strengthening quality assurance in health education: Recent milestones and future directions. *Health Promotion Practice, 10*(2), 192-200.

Taub, A., Kreuter, M., Parcel, G., & Vitello, E. (1987). Report from the AAHE/SOPHE Joint Committee on Ethics. *Health Education Quarterly, 14*(1), 79-90.

Teddlie, C., & Tashakkori, A. (2009). *Foundations of mixed methods research: Integrating quantitative and qualitative approaches in the social and behavioral sciences.* Thousand Oaks, CA: Sage Publications, Inc.

Trochim, W.M., & Donnelly, J. (2006). *Research methods knowledge base* (3rd ed.) (pp. 6-8). Mason, OH: Atomic Dog.

Turnock, B.J. (2004). *Public health: What it is and how it works* (3rd ed.). Sudbury, MA: Jones and Bartlett.

U.S. General Services Administration. (2014). *Section 508: Opening doors to IT.* Retrieved from http://www.section508.gov/

United States Department of Health and Human Services, Office of Minority Health. (2014). *National standards for culturally and linguistically appropriate services in health care (The National CLAS Standard).* Retrieved from http://minorityhealth.hhs.gov/omh/browse.aspx?lvl=2&lvlid=53

United States Department of Health and Human Services. Office of Disease Prevention and Health Promotion. (2014). *Healthy people 2020.* Washington, DC. Retrieved from http://www.healthypeople.gov/.

United States Department of Health and Human Services, Office of Disease Prevention and Health Promotion. (2009). *Quick guide to health literacy.* Retrieved from http://www.health.gov/communication/literacy/quickguide/.

United States Department of Health and Human Services, Office of Disease Prevention and Health Promotion. (2010). *National action plan to improve health literacy.* Washington, DC: United States Department of Health and Human Services.

United States Department of Health and Human Services, Office of Disease Prevention and Health Promotion. (2014). *Healthy People 2020.* Retrieved from http://www.healthypeople.gov/

United States Department of Health and Human Services, Office of Disease Prevention and Health Promotion. (2014). *Healthy people 2020: Health communication and health information technology.* Retrieved from http://www.healthypeople.gov/2020/topics-objectives/topic/health-communication-and-health-information-technology

United States Department of Health and Human Services. (2014a). *HealthIT.gov: Finding quality resources.* Retrieved from http://www.healthit.gov/patients-families/find-quality-resources

United States Department of Health and Human Services. (2014b). *Information Collection/Paperwork Reduction Act.* Retrieved from http://www.hhs.gov/ocio/policy/collection/

United States Department of Justice. (2014a). *A comprehensive tool for federal employees who work with comprehensive community initiatives.* Retrieved from http://www.ccitoolsforfeds.org/systems_change.asp

United States Department of Justice. (2014b). *Limited English proficiency: A federal interagency website.* Retrieved from http://www.justice.gov/crt/lep

United States Department of Labor, Bureau of Labor Statistics. (2014). *Occupational outlook handbook, 2014-15 edition: Health educators and community health workers.* Retrieved from http://www.bls.gov/ooh/community-and-social-service/health-educators.htm

United States General Services Administration. (n.d.). *Section 508 Laws.* Retrieved from http://www.section508.gov/section508-laws

University of Kansas. (2014a). Welcome to the community toolbox. *Community Toolbox.* Retrieved from http://ctb.ku.edu

University of Kansas. (2014b). Section 4. Selecting an appropriate design for the evaluation. *Community Toolbox.* Retrieved from http://ctb.ku.edu/en/table-of-contents/evaluate/evaluate-community-interventions/experimental-design/main

University of Kansas. (2014c). Section 1. An overview of strategic planning or "VMOSA" (vision, mission, objectives, and action plans). *Community Toolbox.* Retrieved from http://ctb.ku.edu/en/tablecontents/sub_section_main_1085.htm

University of Wisconsin, Cooperative Extension, Program Development and Evaluation. (2010). *Logic models.* Retrieved from http://www.uwex.edu/ces/pdande/evaluation/evallogicmodel.html

Van Korlaar, C. (2012). *Guide to creating mission and vision statements.* Retrieved from http://topnonprofits.com/vision-mission

Virginia Tech. (2015). *RE-AIM.org.* Retrieved from http://www.re-aim.hnfe.vt.edu/

Wagenschutz, H.M., & Rivas, J. (2009). Developing effective presentations. In R.J. Bensley, & J. Brookins-Fisher (Eds.), *Community health education methods: A practical guide* (3rd ed.) (pp. 183-208). Sudbury, MA: Jones and Barlett.

Wang, C., & Burris, M.A. (1997). Photovoice: Concept, methodology, and use for participatory needs assessment. *Health Education and Behavior, 24*(3), 369-387.

REFERENCES

REFERENCES

Weiner, B. J. (2009). A theory of organizational readiness for change. *Implement Science, 4*(1), 67.

West, G.R., Clapp, S.P., Averill, E.M., & Cates W. Jr. (2012). Defining and assessing evidence for the effectiveness of technical assistance in furthering global health. *Global Public Health, 7*(9), 915-930.

World Health Organization. (2014a). *Health policy.* Retrieved from http://www.who.int/topics/health_policy/en/

World Health Organization. (2014b). *Social determinants of health.* Retrieved from http://www.who.int/social_determinants/en/

Windsor, R., Clark, N., Boyd, N., & Goodman, R. M. (2004). *Evaluation of health promotion, health education, and disease prevention programs* (3rd ed.). Boston, MA: McGraw-Hill.

W.K. Kellogg Foundation. (2004). *Logic model development guide.* Retrieved from http://www.wkkf.org/resource-directory/resource/2006/02/wk-kellogg-foundation-logic-model-development-guide.

W.K. Kellogg Foundation. (2010). Evaluation handbook. Retrieved from https://www.wkkf.org/resource-directory/resource/2010/w-k-kellogg-foundation-evaluation-handbook

Wurzbach, M.E. (Ed.). (2004). *Community health education and promotion: A guide to program design and evaluation* (2nd ed.). Gaithersburg, MD: Aspen Reference.

Zarcadoolas, C., Pleasant, A., & Greer, D.S. (2006). *Advancing health literacy: A framework for understanding and action.* San Francisco, CA: Jossey-Bass.

Code of Ethics for the Health Education Profession

The Code of Ethics for the Health Education Profession was developed by the Coalition of National Health Education Organizations (CNHEO). As the health education profession progresses and meets new challenges, the Code of Ethics is revised to reflect new realities. The Code of ethics was last revised in 2011. NCHEC policies and procedures adhere to the Health Education Code of Ethics. Violation of the code of ethics can result in enforcement of the NCHEC disciplinary policy.

PREAMBLE

The Health Education profession is dedicated to excellence in the practice of promoting individual, family, group, organizational, and community health. Guided by common goals to improve the human condition, Health Educators are responsible for upholding the integrity and ethics of the profession as they face the daily challenges of making decisions. Health Educators value diversity in society and embrace a multiplicity of approaches in their work to support the worth, dignity, potential, and uniqueness of all people.

The Code of Ethics provides a framework of shared values within the professions in which Health Education is practiced. The Code of Ethics is grounded in fundamental ethical principles including: promoting justice, doing good, and the avoidance of harm. The responsibility of each Health Educator is to aspire to the highest possible standards of conduct and to encourage the ethical behavior of all those with whom they work.

Regardless of job title, professional affiliation, work setting, or population served, Health Educators should promote and abide by these guidelines when making professional decisions.

Article I: Responsibility to the Public

A Health Educator's responsibilities are to educate, promote, maintain, and improve the health of individuals, families, groups, and communities. When a conflict of issues arises among individuals, groups, organizations, agencies, or institutions, Health Educators must consider all issues and give priority to those that promote the health and well being of individuals and the public, while respecting the principles of individual autonomy, human rights, and equality.

Section 1: Health Educators support the right of individuals to make informed decisions regarding their health, as long as such decisions pose no risk to the health of others.

Section 2: Health Educators encourage actions and social policies that promote maximizing health benefits and eliminating or minimizing preventable risks and disparities for all affected parties.

Section 3: Health Educators accurately communicate the potential benefits, risks and/o r consequences associated with the services and programs that they provide.

APPENDIX A

Code of Ethics for the Health Education Profession

Section 4: Health Educators accept the responsibility to act on issues that can affect the health of individuals, families, groups, and communities.

Section 5: Health Educators are truthful about their qualifications and the limitations of their education, expertise, and experience in providing services consistent with their respective level of professional competence.

Section 6: Health Educators are ethically bound to respect, assure, and protect the privacy, confidentiality, and dignity of individuals.

Section 7: Health Educators actively involve individuals, groups, and communities in the entire educational process in an effort to maximize the understanding and personal responsibilities of those who may be affected.

Section 8: Health Educators respect and acknowledge the rights of others to hold diverse values, attitudes, and opinions.

Article II: Responsibility to the Profession

Health Educators are responsible for their professional behavior, for the reputation of their profession, and for promoting ethical conduct among their colleagues.

Section 1: Health Educators maintain, improve, and expand their professional competence through continued study and education; membership, participation, and leadership in professional organizations; and involvement in issues related to the health of the public.

Section 2: Health Educators model and encourage nondiscriminatory standards of behavior in their interactions with others.

Section 3: Health Educators encourage and accept responsible critical discourse to protect and enhance the profession.

Section 4: Health Educators contribute to the profession by refining existing and developing new practices, and by sharing the outcomes of their work.

Section 5: Health Educators are aware of real and perceived professional conflicts of interest, and promote transparency of conflicts.

Section 6: Health Educators give appropriate recognition to others for their professional contributions and achievements.

Section 7: Health educators openly communicate to colleagues, employers, and professional organizations when they suspect unethical practice that violates the profession's Code of Ethics.

Code of Ethics for the Health Education Profession

Article III: Responsibility to Employers

Health Educators recognize the boundaries of their professional competence and are accountable for their professional activities and actions.

Section 1: Health Educators accurately represent their qualifications and the qualifications of others whom they recommend.

Section 2: Health Educators use and apply current evidence-based standards, theories, and guidelines as criteria when carrying out their professional responsibilities.

Section 3: Health Educators accurately represent potential and actual service and program outcomes to employers.

Section 4: Health Educators anticipate and disclose competing commitments, conflicts of interest, and endorsement of products.

Section 5: Health Educators acknowledge and openly communicate to employers expectations of job related assignments that conflict with their professional ethics.

Section 6: Health Educators maintain competence in their areas of professional practice.

Section 7: Health Educators exercise fiduciary responsibility and transparency in allocating resources associated with their work.

Article IV: Responsibility in the Delivery of Health Education

Health Educators deliver health education with integrity. They respect the rights, dignity, confidentiality, and worth of all people by adapting strategies and methods to the needs of diverse populations and communities.

Section 1: Health Educators are sensitive to social and cultural diversity and are in accord with the law, when planning and implementing programs.

Section 2: Health Educators remain informed of the latest advances in health education theory, research, and practice.

Section 3: Health educators use strategies and methods that are grounded in and contribute to the development of professional standards, theories, guidelines, data, and experience.

Section 4: Health Educators are committed to rigorous evaluation of both program effectiveness and the methods used to achieve results.

Section 5: Health Educators promote the adoption of healthy lifestyles through informed choice rather than by coercion or intimidation.

Code of Ethics for the Health Education Profession

Section 6: Health Educators communicate the potential outcomes of proposed services, strategies, and pending decisions to all individuals who will be affected.

Section 7: Health educators actively collaborate and communicate with professionals of various educational backgrounds and acknowledge and respect the skills and contributions of such groups.

Article V: Responsibility in Research and Evaluation

Health Educators contribute to the health of the population and to the profession through research and evaluation activities. When planning and conducting research or evaluation, health educators do so in accordance with federal and state laws and regulations, organizational and institutional policies, and professional standards.

Section 1: Health Educators adhere to principles and practices of research and evaluation that do no harm to individuals, groups, society, or the environment.

Section 2: Health Educators ensure that participation in research is voluntary and is based upon the informed consent of the participants.

Section 3: Health Educators respect and protect the privacy, rights, and dignity of research participants, and honor commitments made to those participants.

Section 4: Health Educators treat all information obtained from participants as confidential unless otherwise required by law. Participants are fully informed of the disclosure procedures.

Section 5: Health Educators take credit, including authorship, only for work they have actually performed and give appropriate credit to the contributions of others.

Section 6: Health Educators who serve as research or evaluation consultants maintain confidentiality of results unless permission is granted or in order to protect the health and safety of others.

Section 7: Health Educators report the results of their research and evaluation objectively, accurately, and in a timely fashion to effectively foster the translation of research into practice.

Section 8: Health Educators openly share conflicts of interest in the research, evaluation, and dissemination process.

Article VI: Responsibility in Professional Preparation

Those involved in the preparation and training of Health Educators have an obligation to accord learners the same respect and treatment given other groups by providing quality education that benefits the profession and the public.

Code of Ethics for the Health Education Profession

Section 1: Health Educators select students for professional preparation programs based upon equal opportunity for all, and the individual's academic performance, abilities, and potential contribution to the profession and the public's health.

Section 2: Health Educators strive to make the educational environment and culture conducive to the health of all involved, and free from all forms of discrimination and harassment.

Section 3: Health Educators involved in professional preparation and development engage in careful planning; present material that is accurate, developmentally and culturally appropriate; provide reasonable and prompt feedback; state clear and reasonable expectations; and conduct fair assessments and prompt evaluations of learners.

Section 4: Health Educators provide objective, comprehensive, and accurate counseling to learners about career opportunities, development, and advancement, and assist learners in securing professional employment or further educational opportunities.

Section 5: Health Educators provide adequate supervision and meaningful opportunities for the professional development of learners.

Approved by the Coalition of National Health Education Organizations February 8, 2011

Task Force Members:
Michael Ballard
Brian Colwell
Suzanne Crouch
Stephen Gambescia
Mal Goldsmith, Chairperson
Marc Hiller
Adrian Lyde
Lori Phillips
Catherine Rasberry
Raymond Rodriquez
Terry Wessel

The Code of Ethics is reprinted by permission of the Coalition of National Health Education Organizations http://www.cnheo.org/.

This page was
intentionally left blank

The Certified Health Education Specialist (CHES) and Master Certified Health Education Specialist (MCHES) Examinations

To implement a certification program, it is necessary to develop examinations that accurately measure practice-related knowledge and skills. The National Commission for Health Education Credentialing, Inc. (NCHEC) utilizes the CHES and the MCHES examinations to assess the extent to which a candidate can possess, apply, and interpret knowledge relative to the Seven Areas of Responsibility, delineated from *A Competency-Based Framework for Health Education Specialists – 2015.*

Both the CHES and MCHES examinations are criterion-referenced examinations that consist of a total of 165 (150 scored plus 15 pilot test) multiple choice questions in paper and pencil format. The passing score for each exam is determined by a modified Angoff method and represents a fixed standard of knowledge, independent of candidate performance. Essentially, this method allows subject-matter experts to establish a level of knowledge that is expected of professionals who are minimally competent. This passing point is reviewed, and statistics are analyzed to ensure reliability and validity of both the CHES and MCHES examinations. By using this methodology, there is no curve, and candidates do not compete against one another. There is also no penalty for guessing.

In constructing the exams, NCHEC works with a national testing organization with more than 50 years' experience in developing credentialing examinations. Together, the organizations develop the examinations according to the process mentioned above. The percentage of questions in the exam pertaining to each Area of Responsibility is based on the results of the Health Education Specialist Practice Analysis 2015. The percent of questions coming from each Area of Responsibility for the current examinations are presented in the tables below. When preparing for either the CHES or MCHES exams, it is recommended that a candidate take into account these percentages.

Areas of Responsibility	CHES % of exam	MCHES % of exam
I. Assess Needs, Resources, and Capacity for Health Education/Promotion	15% (25)	10% (17)
II. Plan Health Education/Promotion	18% (29)	16% (26)
III. Implement Health Education/Promotion	25% (41)	15% (25)
IV. Conduct Evaluation and Research Related to Health Education/Promotion	9% (15)	20% (33)
V. Administer and Manage Health Education/Promotion	12% (20)	18% (29)
VI. Serve as a Health Education/Promotion Resource Person	9% (15)	12% (20)
VII. Communicate, Promote, and Advocate for Health, Health Education,/Promotion and the Profession	12% (20)	9% (15)
Total	**100% (165)**	**100% (165)**

This page was
intentionally left blank

Certified Health Education Specialist Practice Examination Questions

The following practice examination questions address Sub-competencies identified as Entry-level as defined by the Health Education Specialist Practice Analysis (refer to pages 6 and 235) and outlined and addressed within this study companion. The practice questions, written by health education specialists, may assist the user in preparing for the Certified Health Education Specialist (CHES) examination and/or to identify areas of concentration for professional development and training of practicing health education specialists. The questions are not on the current certification examination. Some of the questions have been altered from discarded certification examination questions. The practice questions in this publication have not been subjected to the same rigorous psychometric testing procedures as questions appearing on the CHES or MCHES examinations. Specifically, a passing score on the practice examination questions does not in any way predict or guarantee a passing score on the CHES/MCHES examinations. The practice questions should only be used to direct study efforts.

The practice questions are meant to be challenging. Initially, the user may find that more than one answer appears to be correct. In these instances, the user is encouraged to conduct careful analysis of the questions and possible answers to identify the correct responses. It might be helpful to use the practice examination questions under similar conditions in which the CHES examination is officially administered. For example, the user would be allowed no more than three hours to complete the examination. The user would not utilize or depend on resources such as the study guide, textbooks, publications, or calculators to complete the examination.

An answer key is provided at the end of the practice examination questions. In addition to providing the user with the correct answer, the user will find at least one Area of Responsibility that aligns with the question identified. A review of the number of incorrect answers from any particular Area of Responsibility may help the user to target areas of weakness where more study would be beneficial. ***It is strongly recommended that resources beyond the use of this study companion are used to adequately prepare for the certification examination.***

In closing, feedback from candidates who were successful in passing previous certification examinations and previous study guide users indicates that being part of a small group that allowed participants to "work through" the practice examination questions and discuss why answers are were correct or incorrect can be beneficial.

Certified Health Education Specialist Practice Examination Questions

Select the *best* answer.

1. According to which theory or model do people assess the threat of an emerging disease by assessing their perceived susceptibility against the severity of the disease?
   a. Diffusion of Innovations
   b. Social Cognitive Theory
   c. Health Belief Model
   d. Social Marketing

2. A health education specialist is considering how people might adopt a program in order to understand how best to tailor specific messages. If the health education specialist wants to get the first people to adopt the program using the Diffusion of Innovations, which strategy might be best?
   a. Show the audience how most people have been enjoying the program
   b. Focus on how new and different the program is from what exists
   c. Wait for the opinion leaders to adopt
   d. Focus on how the program adheres to social norms

3. In a priority population, the infant mortality rate and overall death rate for mothers with less than a high school education is almost twice as high as mothers with 13 or more years of education. These are examples of:
   a. health equity.
   b. health determinants.
   c. health capacity.
   d. health disparities.

4. Data storage is an example of which type of technology need?
   a. Infrastructure
   b. Program delivery
   c. Collaboration technology
   d. Knowledge

5. Newsletters, community meetings, public service announcements, and social networking sites are examples of:
   a. social norms.
   b. communication campaigns.
   c. social media.
   d. communication channels.

6. Smoking bans in restaurants are which type of strategy in a community-based smoking prevention program?
    a. Health communication
    b. Health engineering
    c. Health policy
    d. Health mobilization

7. Which section of an original research paper presents evidence tested against the stated hypotheses or research questions and presents the statistical findings?
    a. Methodology
    b. Results
    c. Discussion
    d. Conclusion

8. Which of the following statements about informed consent is correct?
    a. It only has to be completed when a health education specialist is working with children or adolescents
    b. It explains the benefits, risks, and participation is voluntary and may be terminated at any time
    c. It protects the health education specialist in cases of negligence from being sued by participants who were harmed
    d. It is necessary for medical research, but not behavior-focused health education programs

9. The health department administrator just returned from a meeting where someone used a focus group to gather data and now has a great idea. The administrator tasks the health education specialist with conducting a focus group of low income citizens from the south side of town to answer questions about which heart disease intervention the department should offer city wide. Knowing the limitations of this strategy, the health education specialist is rightfully concerned about:
    a. the reliability of the findings.
    b. the generalizability of the findings.
    c. the validity of the findings.
    d. the accuracy of the findings.

10. When developing advocacy plans, which questions would be considered last?
    a. What tactics should be used to influence people?
    b. What are the goals of the advocacy effort?
    c. Who are our allies and opponents?
    d. What organizational issues might facilitate the effort?

Certified Health Education Specialist Practice Examination Questions

Graph 1: *Rates of Traumatic Brain Injury (TBI)*

Use for questions 11 and 12.

Rates of TBI-related Emergency Department Visits, Hospitalizations, and Deaths — United States, 2001–2010

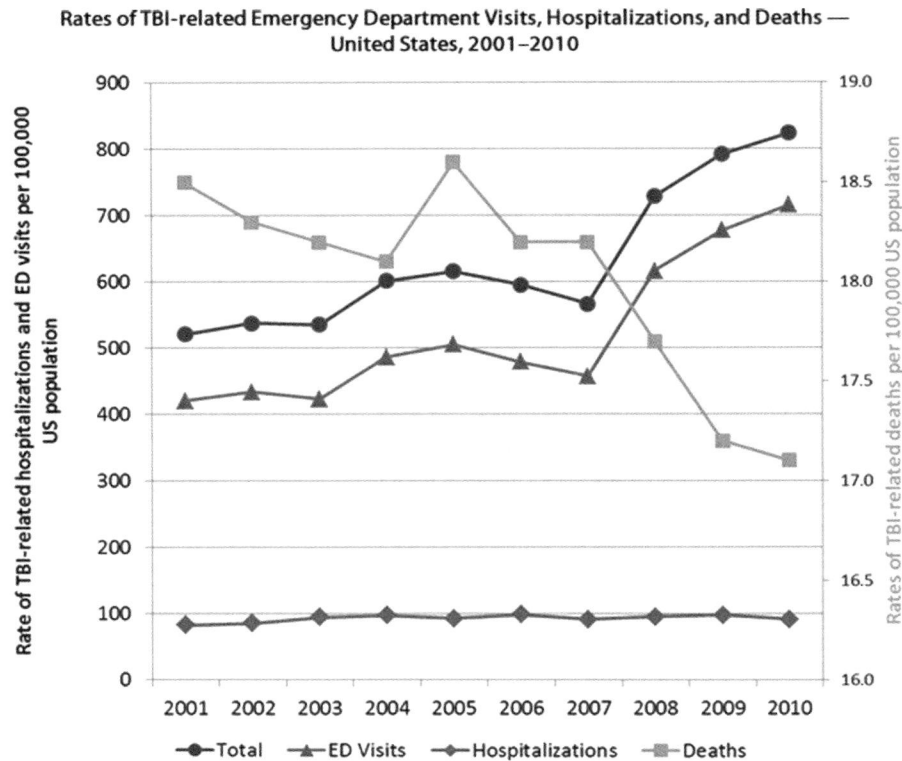

(Source: Centers for Disease Control and Prevention, National Center for Injury Prevention and Control, retrieved 2015 from: http://www.cdc.gov/traumaticbraininjury/data/rates.html)

11. According to Graph 1, which of the following is true?
    a. Deaths due to TBI have more than doubled from 2001 to 2010
    b. Emergency department visits for TBI have increased more than 1.5 times from 2001 to 2010
    c. Hospitalizations for TBI started to increase after 2005, and then decreased from 2005-2010
    d. The total number of people affected by TBI has been steadily decreasing since 2007

12. According to Graph 1, which of the following is true?
    a. More people are choosing to avoid treatment for TBI and are instead dying from their injuries
    b. It appears as though more people are seeking treatment and are being hospitalized for TBI
    c. Although the number of TBIs has increased, the number of deaths due to TBI has decreased
    d. Surgical methods for TBI are improving, which is decreasing the death rates for TBI

13. A health education specialist is asked to find school health resources for physical activity. The most appropriate bibliographic database to search is:
    a. MEDLINE.
    b. EBMR.
    c. CHID.
    d. ERIC.

14. While hiring new employees, the health education specialist should contact the candidates' professional references and validate the employee's degrees. In doing so, discrepancies may be:
    a. revealed prior to hiring.
    b. concealed and are a waste of time.
    c. able to reveal the exact quality of the persons.
    d. complicate the termination process.

15. The health education specialist has core substance abuse prevention coalition members in place and is currently broadening group representation. Some new members only contribute money to the coalition and are categorized as:
    a. occasional participants.
    b. executive participants.
    c. supporting participants.
    d. active participants.

16. A group of health education specialists run into a situation where they need to elicit specialized guidance and expert opinion on a specific health topic in order to aid in decision-making. Of the following, which type of group should be consulted?
    a. Committee-of-the-whole
    b. Task force
    c. Standing committee
    d. Advisory board

17. Consumption, medication compliance, and self-care are considered which type of factors related to health?
    a. Attitudes
    b. Environmental
    c. Behavioral
    d. Genetic

18. Health departments and worksites are implementing a new health education/promotion program to increase influenza vaccine rates for adults in a five county area. What will the project lead focus on to assess the fidelity of implementation?
    a. Location of vaccinations for children
    b. Workers reading materials distributed to all worksites
    c. Amount of vaccine available to the public
    d. Program components being implemented in the correct order

19. When choosing a policy or issue to advocate on with a legislator, which criteria should be considered first?
    a. How receptive the community or target population is to the proposed policy or advocacy effort
    b. If there have been any peer-reviewed articles published on this issue or policy
    c. If advocating on the policy or issue would violate the Code of Ethics for Health Education
    d. If there is potential funding for the proposed policy

20. The health education specialist is working with a local community to institute a smoke free environment in local businesses, agencies, and restaurants throughout the entire community. What type of health strategy would the health education specialist implement in the community?
    a. Position statement
    b. Ordinance
    c. Executive order
    d. Regulation

21. A health education specialist is identifying the types activities to be included in a health education/promotion program. In a logic model, these activities would be included in:
    a. outcomes.
    b. outputs.
    c. inputs.
    d. processes.

22. In the social ecological model, a school or worksite would fall under which factor or level?
    a. Community
    b. Individual
    c. Institutional
    d. Interpersonal

23. A local health department has decided to adopt an evidence-based program for obesity prevention with educational materials that are not completely compatible with the community it serves. In the process of adapting the materials to make them more suitable for the population, the health education specialist should be cautious not to:
    a. change the core elements that make the program effective.
    b. modify materials to fit the population's culture, age, and context.
    c. substitute statistics for other racial or ethnic populations.
    d. tailor instructions, incentives, or activities to audience.

24. If selecting items from an existing instrument, which of the following is the correct procedure?
    a. One cannot select individual or groups of items on an instrument and maintain validity
    b. Keep the instrument short, select one or two items from a scale or subscale, and compile into one instrument
    c. Retain the original language of the question to maintain validity, even when using on a different population
    d. Retain scales to cover an entire domain, rather than select one question for a complex domain

25. With so many changes in health education and health-related policy on a daily basis, it is essential that health education specialists advocate for professional development for the field. Which of the following is a way to advocate for professional development in the field of health education?
    a. Develop a brochure on the diabetes management for patients
    b. Contact a legislator to support a no-smoking policy
    c. Publish articles in peer-reviewed journals on the importance of professional development
    d. Write a grant that would fund a community-based injury prevention program

26. A health education specialist is developing a new Web site as part of an intervention for people with visual disabilities. Which law should the health education specialist review and consider when developing the Web site?
    a. Section 508 of the Rehabilitation Act
    b. Plain Language Act
    c. Title IX Act
    d. Affordable Care Act

27. Which of the following is true about successful partnerships:
    a. Specific indicators related only to the to the program can be used to define success.
    b. Reports, memorandums, and newsletters are the best ways to establish and maintain communication within a partnership.
    c. Constituency relations through uni-directional communication are important to the viability of an organization that values cooperation.
    d. Effective communications should include feedback loops through which intentions, ideas, and information can be exchanged.

28. Which of the following is an example of grassroots advocacy?
    a. Donating money to a political candidate
    b. Contacting a policymaker to set up a meeting
    c. Drafting a position paper for a professional association
    d. Starting a community petition drive

Scenario A: The following scenario is used for questions 29, 30, and 31.
A health education specialist is planning a multilevel program to decrease rates of obesity in an urban community. Community gardens are planned for empty lots, and local convenience stores have agreed to begin selling fresh fruits and vegetables. To assist families, mobile devices will be given out and used to help deliver messages and tips, as well as to collect data. Additionally, community leaders have pledged to focus on making the community safe for physical activity. Volunteers are mapping out walking routes to encourage families to walk together. Partnerships have formed and memorandums of understanding have been drafted.

29. In Scenario A, which of the following would be considered an infrastructure/supply need?
    a. Family participation
    b. Partnerships
    c. Mobile devices
    d. Community leaders

30. In Scenario A, if mobile devices were not given to the priority population, which ethical principle might have been breached, especially in terms of program delivery?
    a. Transparency
    b. Equity
    c. Beneficence
    d. Confidentiality

31. In Scenario A, which of the following could be considered a financial resource for the program?
    a. Partnerships
    b. Family participation
    c. Mobile devices
    d. Community gardens

32. A hospital is expanding outreach services and facilities with a new unit focused on prevention and the treatment of chronic disease. The health education specialist is tasked with gathering local data on these conditions. Which is the most useful rate to use?
    a. Incidence rate
    b. Prevalence rate
    c. Attack rate
    d. Natality rate

33. A foodborne outbreak has closed three local restaurants, and epidemiologists and food safety staff are hoping to identify the outbreak source. Health education specialists and communication specialists plan to use earned media and social media to educate local community members about the outbreak. What should the health education specialists and communication specialists do first?
    a. Pick a theory or model to use
    b. Identify the audience
    c. Check for available funds
    d. Find partners to help

34. A health education specialist notices one of the lessons is not working as planned. What is the appropriate way to proceed?
    a. Stop the intervention and rework the entire program in response to the problematic lesson
    b. Keep implementing the lesson as planned, regardless of whether the learners understand it
    c. Adapt the lesson to the learners' needs so they are able to understand the information or skill
    d. Ignore the lesson and move to the next lesson in the program

35. During flu season, health education specialists often try to promote the flu vaccine to the general public. According to the Elaboration Likelihood Model, a person who does not feel susceptible to the flu might does not pay attention to messages promoting the vaccine. How might a health education specialist craft a message in order to target this person?
    a. Use peripheral stimuli, such as pictures or video to increase attention
    b. Use the 4 Ps of the social marketing to create a campaign
    c. Use messages to trigger memories of previously having the flu
    d. Use social media posts to encourage vaccination

36. In planning a health education/promotion program, a health education specialist needs to develop a timeline for delivery of the intervention. Which of the following accomplishes this task?
    a. SMOG assessment
    b. Logic Model
    c. SWOT analysis
    d. Gantt chart

37. A health educator has just begun his career after graduation. He is trying to make contacts with other professionals so that he can network and share ideas. Which of the following ways is the best way to achieve this?
    a. Subscribe to a health education listserve
    b. Listen to podcasts regarding health issues by experts in the field
    c. Call the state health department to request a mailing list of health educators
    d. Join a professional health education organization

38. The health education specialist would use a prioritization matrix in which phase of the PRECEDE-PROCEED Model?
    a. Social assessment and situational analysis
    b. Epidemiological assessment
    c. Intervention alignment and administrative and policy assessment
    d. Implementation

39. Which of the following is a common way to illustrate alignment of programs with an organization's mission and goals?
    a. Gantt chart
    b. Logic model
    c. Timeline
    d. Evaluation plan

40. A community agency is targeting a variety of social ecological levels to help reduce drug use in the community. Some of the levels will take substantially more time to target. Rather than wait for all aspects of the intervention to be ready, the agency looks to begin with one level and then will add in other levels over time. This is an example of:
    a. phasing in.
    b. pilot testing.
    c. total implementation.
    d. primary strategies.

41. An evaluation of a program has been conducted, and a health education specialist is preparing a report in a very tight timeline. Though all sections of the report are important for clarity and content, on which section should the health education specialist spend the most time since it likely will be read more closely by stakeholders?
    a. Methods
    b. Literature review
    c. Conclusions
    d. Introduction

42. To deal with the greatest drawback to a multilevel strategy intervention, which of the following models should be followed?
    a. RE-AIM
    b. IMB Skills Model
    c. PAPM
    d. CRM

43. A health education specialist would like to use a planning tool that outlines when specific tasks are to be accomplished before, during, and after a program. The health education specialist would also like to track actual accomplishment of these tasks using this same tool. Which of the following method would be most useful?
    a. Progress report
    b. Logic model
    c. Activity log
    d. Gantt chart

44. Which of the following is an example of a behavioral factor that must be considered to assess the root causes of racial and ethnic disparities?
    a. Exposure to toxins
    b. Limited access to quality health care
    c. Lack of seat belt use
    d. Poverty

45. When considering materials to use for a health education/promotion program, which of the following should a health education specialist do first?
    a. Have members of the priority population help develop materials for the intervention
    b. Create materials for the majority of the intervention, and then conduct a literature search to find additional materials
    c. Look for evidenced-based interventions and use existing protocols and materials, if possible
    d. Create an environment conducive to learning, including creating mutual respect between teachers and learners

46. A health education specialist is creating a program and is concerned about sustainability of the program. Which of the following actions creates the greatest likelihood for sustainability?
    a. Identify partners and stakeholders who can help with sustainability during the planning process
    b. Once the program has been evaluated, modify it, and then implement it again before funding ceases
    c. After the program has been evaluated, identify stakeholders or partners who can help with sustainability
    d. Attempt to attain political support with the evaluation results

Graph 2: *New Cases of Infection*

Use for question 47.

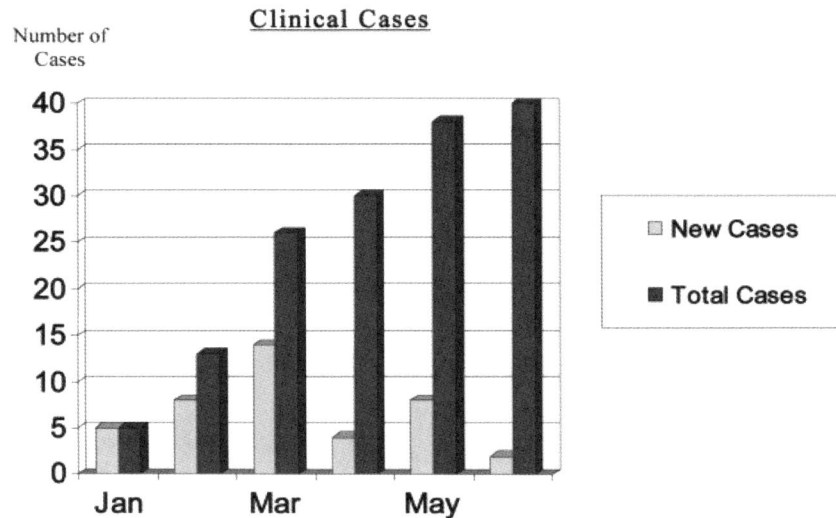

47. To depict the number of infections among a cohort of 113 women, a health education specialist presented existing data in the form of Graph 2. The graph reveals the number of new cases each month of a diagnosed asymptomatic infection and the cumulative number of cases at the end of six months. From the following statements, which is the best account regarding what is represented in the graph?
    a. Incidence is higher every month
    b. Prevalence has risen steadily each month
    c. Prevalence is variable every month
    d. The identified infectious cases appear to have been cured

48. A health education specialist would like to attend a school board meeting to discuss safety issues in the school. Though multiple forms of data will be used, which of the following will cause a more emotional reaction to evidence the necessity of an intervention?
    a. GIS data of the community
    b. National data from the CDC compared to state data regarding safety
    c. Data presented from a survey of high school seniors
    d. Photovoice or story telling from the students' point of view

49. Reach, recall, and media impressions are common metrics used to evaluate:
    a. the impact of messages.
    b. health literacy skills.
    c. Web site traffic.
    d. numeracy skills.

50. A health education specialist has been asked to collect qualitative data from participants. Given a short time period to collect data, which method takes the least amount of time?
    a. Interviews
    b. Focus groups
    c. Delphi technique
    d. Quantitative surveys

51. A health education specialist finds a Web site called The Teen Pregnancy Place, which provides a discussion board where pregnant and parenting teens can obtain advice and make friends online. It is unclear who developed the material or sponsors the site. A fact sheet regarding the weekly development of a fetus is provided, but no references are cited for the information it contains. A links page directs visitors to other Web sites for resources, services, and products related to pregnancy and parenting. Visitors to the Web site should assume that:
    a. the developer has expertise in teen pregnancy.
    b. all of the information could be inaccurate.
    c. the discussion board is a valid source of information.
    d. the developer has expertise in fetal development.

52. The healthy hearts coalition emails all PTA/PTO members and asks them to contact their district school board members to vote for the healthy snacks in school policy. This appeal is considered:
    a. media advocacy.
    b. direct lobbying.
    c. legislative advocacy.
    d. grassroots lobbying.

53. Which one of the following is typically considered a good reason for a public health agency to seek outside help from someone other than a staff member?
    a. To seek someone with specialized skills not available internally
    b. No one within the agency wants to do the task
    c. To reduce costs of program evaluation
    d. To increase bias of program results

54. Which organization is a reliable source for data related to disabilities resulting from automobile crashes that would be used in health education program planning?
    a. National Highway Traffic Safety Administration
    b. American Automobile Association
    c. Occupational Safety and Health Administration
    d. Health Care Financing Administration

55. A client comes to the health education specialist for health counseling and coaching. The client feels stress associated with unresolved conflict and poor coping patterns. The health coach decides to use which of the following approaches/theoretical orientations to counseling in order to meet this specific client need?
    a. Exploratory counseling
    b. Client-centered counseling
    c. Behavioral counseling
    d. Counseling for decision-making

Graph 3: *Estimated New HIV infections in the U.S., 2010*

Use for question 56, 57and 58.

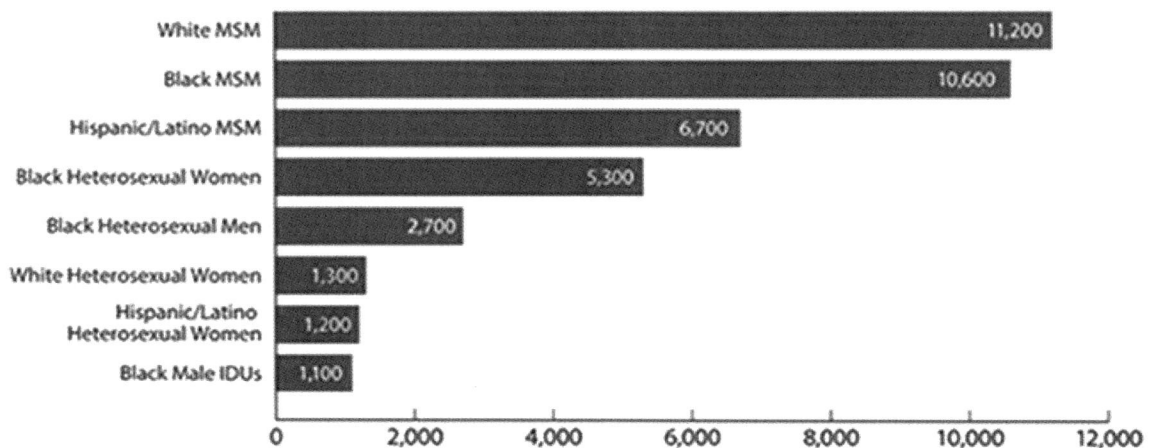

Source: CDC (2014). HIV in the United States: At A Glance. Figure 1: Estimated New HIV Infections in the United States, 2010, for the Most Affected Subpopulations.

56. According to Graph 3, which of the following groups is at greater risk for HIV infection?
    a. Hispanic/Latino MSM
    b. White Heterosexual Women
    c. Black MSM
    d. Black Male IDUs

57. A health disparity illustrated in Graph 3 is:
    a. the prevalence of HIV infection is greatest in injection drug users.
    b. the incidence of HIV infection is greater in men than in women.
    c. heterosexual and homosexual men have the greatest risk for HIV infection.
    d. homosexual women are at greater risk of HIV infection than heterosexual women.

58. A health education specialist is concerned about HIV infection in the community. The health education specialist might use the data on the graph above:
    a. to compare to secondary data in the state to understand community need.
    b. to compare to primary data in the community to understand community need.
    c. to use as a form of primary data to identify the specific community's priority population.
    d. to use as evidence that all populations are at great risk for HIV infection.

59. If a health education specialist is trying to gain support for a program within an organization, which is one way to illustrate a rationale for the program to key stakeholders?
    a. Use a logic model to show how the program aligns with the organization's mission
    b. Create an evaluation plan and show how each variable will be measured
    c. Present a timeline to illustrate how the program will impact the organization
    d. Present secondary data to illustrate program need

60. In the process of selecting the most appropriate educational method to use in a health education program, which of the following guidelines should be used?
    a. Use favorite methods of the person delivering the program
    b. Consider the nature of the audience and the purpose of the program
    c. Find a program delivered to a different audience and deliver it to your audience
    d. In order to be useful, a program must include all of the intervention strategies

61. One of the ways to comprehensively engage the priority population in the program planning, implementation, and evaluation process is to:
    a. develop a partnership between two community organizations.
    b. use community-based participatory research.
    c. use a focus group to assist with the needs assessment.
    d. ask a stakeholder to serve as a consultant for the project.

62. When planning a cardiovascular disease prevention program following the PRECEDE-PROCEED Model, data on high fatty acid intake would fall into which assessment phase?
    a. Educational and ecological assessment
    b. Social assessment and situational analysis
    c. Epidemiological assessment
    d. Intervention alignment and administrative and policy assessment

63. Which of the following statements contains accurate principles to address low health literacy?
    a. Assume that everyone reads at the 12th grade level, since most people graduate from high school
    b. Present many health statistics, as people tend to understand numbers better than words
    c. Try to fit everything on one page, even if it means making the font smaller than desired
    d. Use graphs or charts, rather than tables or numbers, to show rates of illness or injury

64. According to the Centers for Disease Control and Prevention's Framework for Program Evaluation, being "realistic, prudent, diplomatic and frugal" is part of which standard for effective evaluation?
    a. Feasibility
    b. Utility
    c. Propriety
    d. Accuracy

65. Among program participants, smoking rates will decrease by 35 percent in 12 months is an example of a/an:
    a. behavioral objective.
    b. learning objective.
    c. administrative objective.
    d. environmental objective.

66. To help improve intervention fidelity, a health education specialist should create:
    a. an evaluation plan.
    b. an implementation guide.
    c. evidence-based practice.
    d. tailored materials.

67. A health education specialist gives data from an evaluation regarding drug use in a community to a community volunteer to enter. Some of the participants wrote their name on top of the survey. What ethical issue has occurred?
    a. Failure to obtain informed consent
    b. Lack of objectivity
    c. Breach of confidentiality
    d. Failure to discuss benefits and risks

68. Which of the following is a SMART training objective?
    a. Participants will report all cases of sexual misconduct by the end of the session.
    b. Participants will increase their knowledge of sexual misconduct by the end of the session.
    c. Participants will be able to list two types of sexual misconduct.
    d. Training participants will be able to list three resources for patients who report sexual misconduct by the end of the training session.

69. By 2018, volunteers will distribute informational fliers to at least 50% of program participants. This is an example of which type of objective?
    a. Impact
    b. Process
    c. Outcome
    d. Summative

Graph 4: *Injury Deaths Compared to Other Leading Causes of Death for Persons Ages 1–44, United States, 2011*

Use for question 70.

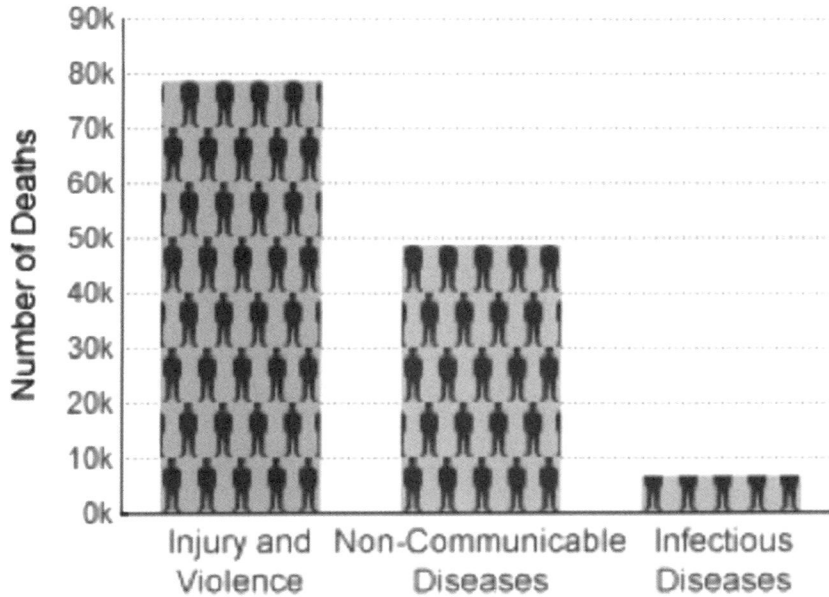

70. Based upon the data in Graph 4, what can a health education specialist infer about the health needs of people ages 1-44?
    a. More people ages 1–44 die from injuries than from noncommunicable and infectious diseases combined
    b. More than 187,000 deaths occur from injury each year, which equates to 1 person every 3 minutes
    c. Infectious diseases kill 10,000 people each year
    d. More people ages 1-15 die from injuries than people ages 20-39

71. A health education specialist is planning a comprehensive community-based strategy to promote physical activity. In the planning process, the health education specialist would like to use the Social Marketing Model. If he/she takes into account the physiological impact of exercise for a sedentary person (such as muscle soreness), which of the 4 Ps is the health education specialist addressing?
    a. Product
    b. Price
    c. Place
    d. Promotion

Certified Health Education Specialist Practice Examination Questions

Scenario B: The following scenario is used for questions 72 and 73.

A health education specialist is working with a community agency to implement an obesity prevention program in the community. They have decided BMI will be measured to assess rates of obesity at baseline and at one year, physical activity recalls and dietary logs to assess behavior weekly during the six month program, and surveys to assess attitudes at the beginning and end of the program. The evaluator will assess fidelity and acceptability of the intervention throughout the intervention.

72. If the health education specialist created a logic model for Scenario B, which outcomes would be considered short-term outcomes?
    a. Attitudes
    b. Physical activity and diet
    c. Feasibility and acceptability
    d. BMI

73. In Scenario B above, which measurements are parts of a formative evaluation?
    a. BMI only
    b. BMI, physical activity, diet and attitudes
    c. Diet and physical activity
    d. Fidelity and acceptability

74. Which of the following are considered "safe" changes to materials or program activities when using a packaged health education program?
    a. Changing theoretical focus
    b. Changing text size or statistics
    c. Shortening the program
    d. Changing the behavioral theory

75. A health education specialist wants to collect ratio data on smoking rates. Which of the following questions would achieve this level of measurement?
    a. Do you smoke?
    b. Do you smoke 1-10, 11-20, or 20-30 cigarettes per day?
    c. How many cigarettes do you smoke per day?
    d. Do you smoke 0, 1-10, or 20+ cigarettes per day?

76. In health education presentations, which of the following is an appropriate guideline to promote learning?
    a. Do not repeat information in any planned learning activity
    b. Use passive learning methods, such as lectures
    c. Establish the relevance of the information to learners
    d. Present information unique to one setting or situation

77. A health education specialist is asked to measure actual use of a walking trail in a local community. Which of the following methods is best to measure actual use of the trail over a period of a week?
    a. Nominal group process
    b. Surveys
    c. Focus groups
    d. Observation

78. As a health education specialist monitors program implementation, he/she finds several lessons were not implemented as originally planned. This illustrates lack of:
    a. reliability.
    b. fidelity.
    c. validity.
    d. assessment.

79. When creating a marketing plan, the health education specialist must segment the audience. How does this occur?
    a. By outlining specific portions of the priority population to focus on
    b. By identifying benefits of the health program for the audience
    c. By developing a communication strategy for the entire priority population
    d. By outlining all components for a solution to the health issue or problem

80. An organization is undergoing restructuring because of budgetary cuts, which in turn impacts health promotion efforts. Which approach to organizational change is occurring?
    a. Revolutionary
    b. Evolutionary
    c. Regulatory
    d. Reactionary

81. Health education specialists in a local health department are trying to understand mental health conditions common in those with chronic illness such as diabetes and cancer. Which of the following resources would be the best database to find mental health research articles?
    a. HaPI
    b. CHID
    c. PsychInfo
    d. Medline

82. The intervention program has been adopted, and the priority population is ready to participate. The implementation team needs to know their tasks and associated due dates, and the health education specialist needs a relatively simple way to track the team's projected and actual task completion progress. To meet both needs, as well as to identify and prioritize all of tasks needed for full implementation, the health education specialist creates a:
    a. CPM chart.
    b. logic chart.
    c. TDTL chart.
    d. Gantt chart.

83. An afterschool program was developed to help overweight and obese adolescents lose weight. In developing the program, the health education specialist considered the adolescents' attitude, beliefs, and values regarding diet and physical activity. Knowing this information, the health education specialist helped to:
    a. develop clear program goals and objectives.
    b. institutionalize the program in the community.
    c. implement new school-based policies for youth.
    d. ensure the program was culturally appropriate and relevant.

84. A health education specialist wants to raise awareness among a general audience of the dangers of second-hand smoke. Which delivery method would reach a broader audience?
    a. Producing a public service announcement for local radio
    b. Organizing a town hall meeting about second-hand smoke
    c. Developing an antismoking workplace wellness campaign
    d. Creating a fact sheet for patients at a health center

85. The social media campaign to change social norms related to teen pregnancy developed by a health education specialist is reviewed by a group of adolescents from the priority population. Their feedback allows the health education specialist to make changes before implementing the campaign. What type of evaluation is this?
    a. Summative
    b. Formative
    c. Impact
    d. Process

86. A health education specialist does not have additional staff to assist with data collection, data entry, or analysis, and has a tight timeline for data collection and analysis. Which of the following is a feasible method for the health education specialist to collect data on attitudes toward antismoking legislation in a region?
    a. A Web-based qualitative survey
    b. A mailed quantitative survey
    c. A Web-based quantitative survey
    d. A telephone survey

87. The lead and radon program at a state health department did not have its funding renewed and is scheduled to end in the next twelve months. A strategic plan, vision, and program evaluation data are available. What other sustainability domain or element should a health education specialist explore for sustaining the program?
    a. Collaborations or partnerships
    b. Creating a new vision
    c. Volunteer or intern staff
    d. Free materials and services

88. An informal channel for communicating information about smoking policies at the work site could include:
    a. posting of smoke-free policies.
    b. in-house smoking cessation seminars.
    c. support groups for smokers in a cessation program.
    d. mandatory in-service programs about the effects of second hand smoke.

89. A health education specialist was asked to provide a school district with accurate Web-based resources for their sexuality education program. What key items would a health education specialist assess?
    a. Political affiliation, committee opinions, and visual presentation of the data
    b. Appropriateness, reading level, and clarity
    c. Form, target audience, and availability
    d. Author's credentials, Web site's purpose, and references

90. A university is working with community health workers, an American-Indian tribe, and the Tribal Health Organization to implement a diabetes prevention program. Two-day training is being planned for the community health workers to ensure proper program delivery. What should the trainers do to create an inclusive learning environment?
    a. Obtain leadership approval to offer the training
    b. Build trust and respect between the learners and instructor(s)
    c. Pay for food and travel to the training for all participants
    d. Offer the training only during the working hours

91. When starting the advocacy process, the health education specialist should develop:
    a. a fact sheet about the issue.
    b. a strategic plan.
    c. SMART objectives.
    d. a program.

92. When facilitating a training workshop on a new electronic medical records system at a clinic, the health education specialist is following the steps for successful training programs. He/she is confident in implementing the training steps, as there is little difference between this process and general health education program implementation, except for the need to:
    a. specify teaching-learning methods.
    b. specify learning needs.
    c. specify job performance.
    d. specify instructional resources.

93. Which of the following questions does NOT help to assess the accuracy of a resource?
    a. What are the funding source(s) of the site?
    b. Is the information compatible with the community context?
    c. Does it cite evidence-based references?
    d. What are the credentials of the content reviewers?

94. The trainer's primary responsibility is to:
    a. select teaching-learning methods.
    b. establish conditions for learning.
    c. ensure program objectives are met.
    d. skillfully conduct the training.

95. The health education specialist must analyze the meaning of the data collected during the assessment and determine health education/promotion needs. If the health education specialist aggregates the data, which cognitive process of qualitative research is he/she focusing on?
    a. Synthesizing
    b. Comprehending
    c. Theorizing
    d. Recontextualizing

96. If a health education specialist wishes to use online surveys because of the ease of data collection, but the priority population struggles with technology. This is a breach of which ethical principle in managing technology?
    a. Equity
    b. Transparency
    c. Beneficence
    d. Confidentiality

97. After his partner was diagnosed with breast cancer, an older citizen of a community is overwhelmed by the amount of information on the topic on the Internet. He asks how to sort through the information to find reputable sources. One way to help him easily limit his search is to tell him to:
    a. only visit sites that end in .gov, .org, or .edu.
    b. review the resources for timeliness and research.
    c. review the intent of the Web site.
    d. find the author contact information.

98. Health education specialists wishing to target subgroups of the priority population should:
    a. create a generic newsletter and send it to the entire community.
    b. always begin with social media, as word can spread quickly using this type of media.
    c. advertise in the newspaper because this is a form of mass media.
    d. first consider how the priority population prefers to get their information.

99. In a community-based heart disease intervention, mass hypertension screenings at the shopping mall were used as the "kick-off" activity. Which level of prevention are the screenings?
    a. Diagnostic
    b. Primary
    c. Tertiary
    d. Secondary

100. Which of the following is an example of a correctly written learning objective?
    a. "Individuals in the program will increase their level of physical activity by 25 percent by the 6th week of the program"
    b. "Individuals participating in the health education program will be able to identify three ways to protect their skin from the sun by the end of the program"
    c. "Seventy-five percent of individuals participating in the program will increase their knowledge of the dangers of smoking over the following three months"
    d. "There will be a 20% decrease in heart disease death rates among individual living in Brockport by the end of the first year of the program"

101. Goals, organizational considerations, constituents, allies, opponents, targets, and tactics are all elements of:
    a. interpersonal communication channels.
    b. SMART goals and objectives.
    c. an advocacy plan.
    d. social marketing.

102. Advocacy evaluation often involves careful tracking of implementation throughout the advocacy effort. What type of program evaluation is this considered?
    a. Impact
    b. Process
    c. Outcome
    d. Summative

103. Forgetting to inform participants about the risks associated with physical activity before having the participants begin a program is an example of:
    a. commission.
    b. negligence.
    c. deregulation.
    d. beneficence.

104. Conducting a capacity assessment focuses on identifying community:
    a. resources.
    b. health problems.
    c. weaknesses.
    d. needs.

105. Before implementing a program, a health education specialist should develop "how-to" materials for implementing the program. This is called a:
    a. environmental scan.
    b. literature review.
    c. procedural manual.
    d. adapted pilot test.

106. The organization that accredits undergraduate teacher preparation programs is:
    a. NCHEC.
    b. SOPHE.
    c. APHA.
    d. CAEP.

107. A health education specialist needs to conduct training for individuals who will be delivering the intervention. Which of the following is a critical consideration when conducting trainings?
    a. Personal characteristics of the instructor
    b. Costs associated with the program
    c. Maintenance of the training program
    d. Social norms for the organization

108. The videos and accompanying workbook activities chosen for an intervention are pretested then revised and improved right before the start of the intervention. This type of evaluation is called:
    a. impact.
    b. summative.
    c. formative.
    d. process.

109. When writing objectives for the worksite exercise promotion intervention, the health education specialist wishes to measure any morbidity, mortality, and health status change occurred as a result of the intervention. He/she would write which type of objective?
    a. Process
    b. Outcome
    c. Impact
    d. Environmental

110. Which method represents a secondary source for a needs assessment?
    a. Interviews with key informants
    b. Focus groups with a priority population
    c. Published data from a CDC article
    d. Internet survey of program participants

111. Using a written questionnaire, a cross-sectional survey about personal alcohol, tobacco, and other drug use behaviors was administered to a priority population. The priority population for the survey did not respond. The health education specialist would then need to find other evidence that the behaviors occurred or did not occur using:
    a. proxy measures.
    b. multistep written surveys.
    c. self-assessments.
    d. telephone interviews.

112. The school wellness committee placed speed bumps on all school parking lots bordering school playgrounds. This is an example of which type of intervention strategy?
     a. Health education change
     b. Environmental change
     c. Communication change
     d. Health policy change

113. A health education specialist is managing a mobile health intervention collecting demographic and behavioral information about its participants. After discovering a breach in the program's data storage system, what is the manager's most pressing ethical issue?
     a. Equity
     b. Beneficence
     c. Transparency
     d. Confidentiality

114. When creating a marketing plan for a program, which of the following should be identified first?
     a. Communication methods
     b. Message
     c. Audience
     d. Financial resources

115. A health education specialist is developing a tobacco prevention program. The health education specialist is looking for evidence-based interventions as part of his/her planning process. The least helpful resource would be:
     a. U.S. Census databases.
     b. Cochrane reviews.
     c. community guide to preventive services.
     d. research-tested interventions programs.

116. A nonprofit agency can perform lobbying as long as that lobbying:
     a. is performed only during the lunch hour, when employees are on break.
     b. involves asking policy makers to pass or dismiss a certain piece of legislation in one legislative session.
     c. is performed while "on" organizational time, not on personal time.
     d. meets federal guidelines and does not exceed a certain percentage of the nonprofit's activities.

117. A hospital would like to post information throughout the facility to increase awareness of the potential dangers, spread, and prevention of influenza. Which format would best accomplish this?
    a. An infographic with data and short messages
    b. A pamphlet containing detailed information
    c. Data printed from the CDC's Web site regarding influenza
    d. Graphics showing proper hand washing procedures

118. During delivery of a health promotion program, it becomes apparent the amount of time allotted to each lesson or activity is not sufficient. The person delivering the program decides to delete some content to make the lesson fit. This action could result in a lack of:
    a. evaluation.
    b. fidelity.
    c. validity.
    d. reliability.

119. In a health education program, participants are asked about their readiness for change so that content in a message can be personalized. This is an example of:
    a. tailoring a message.
    b. conducting a needs assessment.
    c. identifying a message source.
    d. analyzing message content.

120. During a health education program, questions about whether the participants like the instructional materials and if instructors find them easy to use are examples of:
    a. summative evaluation.
    b. process evaluation.
    c. impact evaluation.
    d. outcome evaluation.

121. When developing and preparing to implement an intervention, which of the following practices is most pedagogically sound?
    a. Change the strategy every five minutes to keep the learner engaged
    b. Use mostly presentation software to deliver content
    c. Use a mix of strategies to involve the learner
    d. Use the latest technology to deliver content

122. To determine the immediate effects of a health education program, the health education specialist should use which type of evaluation?
    a. Formative evaluation
    b. Process evaluation
    c. Impact evaluation
    d. Outcome evaluation

123. *Healthy Children in Healthy Communities* is an example of:
    a. a goal.
    b. an objective.
    c. a mission statement.
    d. a vision statement.

124. When reporting a program's evaluation results to community members, the most important aspect to highlight is:
    a. the extent to which program objectives were achieved through advanced statistics.
    b. the participants' perceived benefits of the program.
    c. the results indicating which activities within the program intervention were most successful.
    d. details of the program's history and IRB protocol.

125. Print material was selected as the appropriate way to provide a take-home message to reinforce concepts presented during a behavior change intervention. The first step in planning the specific materials to be developed is to:
    a. define the audience for the material.
    b. develop goals and objectives for the material.
    c. develop material content and graphics.
    d. gather information about the audience for the material.

126. Which represents primary sources that could be used for a community needs assessment?
    a. Published scientific studies and reports
    b. United States census data, vital records, disease registries
    c. State health data from the health department
    d. Informal interviews, observations, and surveys

127. A health education specialist collects data with a "yes" or "no" response option. This is what type of data?
    a. Ordinal
    b. Nominal
    c. Interval
    d. Ratio

128. In a community, twice as many people died over the course of one year in house fires than in car crashes. Community members demand the health education specialist immediately create a fire prevention intervention. Before planning the fire prevention intervention, the health education specialist should first determine the:
    a. population at risk.
    b. life expectancy in the community.
    c. point source epidemic curve.
    d. odds ratio.

129. A health education specialist would like to present visual data regarding community assets. Which of the following can be used to achieve this?
    a. GIS mapping
    b. Prevalence rates
    c. Assets listed by address
    d. Presentation of public records

Scenario C: The following scenario is used for question 130.
A health education specialist is working with a community agency on an obesity prevention program in the community. They have decided to use BMI to measure rates of obesity at baseline and at one year, physical activity recalls and dietary logs to assess behavior weekly during the six month program, and surveys to assess attitudes at the beginning and end of the program. The evaluator will assess fidelity and acceptability of the intervention throughout the intervention.

130. In Scenario C, which measurements are parts of the summative evaluation?
    a. BMI only
    b. BMI, physical activity, diet, and attitudes
    c. Fidelity and acceptability
    d. Diet and physical activity

131. If a health education specialist is designing an intervention to be delivered using an emerging technology, which preliminary planning question is most important?
    a. Which journal will publish a paper about a health intervention using this technology?
    b. How much will it cost to conduct staff training on this technology?
    c. Does the priority population of interest use this type of technology?
    d. What other health organizations are using this type of technology?

132. A health education specialist has a limited budget and is looking for baseline data. Which of the following may be a secondary data option to consider?
    a. Randomly sampling the priority population
    b. Conducting a survey with the priority population
    c. Pilot testing an interview with family members and co-workers
    d. Searching federal, state, city, and county open data portals

133. A process that is used in organizations, similar to a needs assessment, assesses assumptions and values related to health education /promotion. This is a:
    a. cultural audit.
    b. strategy assessment.
    c. strategic plan.
    d. asset map.

134. The most critical step in the implementation process is to:
    a. field test the program.
    b. establish a management system.
    c. get the priority population to accept the program.
    d. evaluate the program.

135. After conducting a needs assessment, a health education specialist finds the community lacks the infrastructure to support physically active lifestyles. However, community members are more concerned about drug use in the community. In this example, drug use is a:
    a. normative need.
    b. actual need.
    c. perceived need.
    d. political need.

136. When working with consultants or contractors, it is necessary to secure:
    a. a signed ethics agreement from the consultant or contractor.
    b. extra funds to cover the cost of unexpected expenditures.
    c. an implementation plan from the consultant or contractor.
    d. a written agreement outlining the work needed.

137. A large group of tourists traveled on an ocean liner to a tropical island and developed an acute, flu-like illness. The suspected cause of illness is associated with cruising on this ocean liner. Health authorities need to know the number of all passengers who became ill, as well as those who traveled on the ocean liner. Which rate should the health education specialist calculate to provide information to health authorities?
    a. Prevalence rate
    b. Attack rate
    c. Fatality rate
    d. Cause-specific mortality rate

138. Following the PRECEDE-PROCEED Model, which type of factor in the educational and ecological assessment would assess whether community members have adequate access to oral health care services?
    a. Predisposing
    b. Enabling
    c. Reinforcing
    d. Motivating

139. When creating a partnership, which of the following tasks should be completed first?
    a. Create partnership mission, goals, and outcomes
    b. Begin program development
    c. Create a memorandum of understanding
    d. Create a shared budget for the program

140. In a meeting, community members offer suggestions for curbing the community's obesity problem. They focus on the behaviors of individuals in the community, thinking if community members change their dietary behaviors, then the obesity problem will be solved. A health education specialist explains the solution is not this simple because:
    a. sometimes behaviors are influenced by other factors, such as lack of access to healthy food, that are out of a person's control.
    b. attitudes are the only important factor to consider when designing obesity prevention or treatment programs.
    c. access to healthcare is more important than behaviors when weighing factors related to obesity treatment or prevention.
    d. there are other behaviors more important when trying to decrease rates of obesity in the community.

141. After the end of a year-long program, a partnership is being evaluated. The evaluation reveals that the results of the program are minimal, and the expense high for both partners. However, the community supports the partnership, and both agencies enjoy working together on the program. What is likely to be the finding of the evaluation report?
    a. Because both agencies enjoy working together, the program should continue
    b. Because the community supports the partnership, it should be continued
    c. The partnership is not cost effective, and should be reexamined
    d. The program should be repeated to see if it is more successful the second time

142. A health education specialist is assessing which resources to use in a smoking prevention campaign for a community. Because the health education specialist wishes to focus on primary prevention, which strategy is likely to reach the intended audience?
    a. News outlets
    b. Community intervention
    c. Billboards
    d. Social media

143. One use of logic models is to:
    a. outline the lesson plan scope and sequence.
    b. track if activities produce outputs that lead to outcomes.
    c. identify the timing of when all of the planning should occur.
    d. outline evaluation stages for the program.

144. Which of the following is the first step in designing a survey?
    a. Determining the objectives of the survey
    b. Determining the questions to be used
    c. Determining the types of scales to be used
    d. Determining the specific data to be collected

145. Program planning begins with:
    a. a measurement of social marketing process.
    b. an identification of the specific focus of an intervention.
    c. an assessment of existing health needs and problems.
    d. the creation of program and learning objectives.

146. A community coalition is seeking more information to understand the complexities of promoting the human papilloma virus (HPV) vaccine among teenagers to prevent cervical cancer. The health education specialist should refer them to which type of source for the most accurate information that is also relevant and useful to the coalition?
    a. A Web site of a commercial pharmaceutical manufacturer
    b. A systematic review of the scientific literature
    c. Fact sheets from a federal health agency
    d. A blog from a social advocate

147. Health illiteracy, economics, and poverty are considered which type of factors that cause racial and ethnic health disparities?
    a. Societal
    b. Environmental
    c. Individual
    d. Medical care

148. If a health education specialist wished to use the application level of Bloom's taxonomy in an intervention aimed at decreasing saturated fat consumption, what might the health education specialist have the priority population do?
    a. Outline the health benefits of decreasing fat intake
    b. List foods containing saturated fats
    c. Compare saturated and unsaturated fats
    d. Demonstrate how to prepare a healthy meal

149. A health education specialist is developing health literature about symptoms of stroke and what to steps are necessary to take action for adults in the community. What is the most valid source of information to use?
    a. Prevention Institute
    b. American Heart Association
    c. Centers for Medicare and Medicaid Services
    d. American Diabetes Association

150. A new HIV testing intervention is being planned to support efforts to increase screening rates. The intervention is planned to start in six months. Which of the following is a proven method to create a timeline and plan for the intervention?
    a. Critical Path Method
    b. Epidemiology curve
    c. Weekly program meetings
    d. Strategic plan

151. The community heart health coalition was formed about one year ago, and it is now in the process of collecting needs assessment data and creating a strategic plan. This coalition is cycling through which stage of coalition development?
    a. Outcome
    b. Maintenance
    c. Implementation
    d. Formation

152. A health education specialist has collected some resources on drug use and prevention for various audiences. The CEO of a company would like to see information regarding prescription drug abuse. What is the best way to present this information to the CEO?
    a. An infographic
    b. A pamphlet produced by NIDA
    c. A formal presentation
    d. A literature review

153. A health education specialist needs to determine specific alcohol, tobacco, and other drug use prevention needs and immediately prioritize those needs with a few experts from the priority population. Which primary data collection technique would be the <u>best</u> to use in this scenario?
    a. Nominal group process
    b. Focus group
    c. Community forum
    d. Electronic interviews

154. A health education specialist schedules a panel to discuss issues with program staff related to an emerging disease. This is an example of what kind of strategy?
    a. Policy
    b. Health Engineering
    c. Communication
    d. Educational

155. When implementing well designed health education class lessons for adult learners, the health education specialist should incorporate which of the following adult learning principles?
    a. Progressing from unknown to known material through the lesson
    b. Moving from complex to simple concepts throughout the lesson
    c. Moving as quickly as possible through the lesson
    d. Stating the purpose of the lesson

156. Within the healthcare system, the primary function of the health education specialist is to:
    a. ensure appropriate client clinical services are being offered.
    b. conduct research and implement surveys regarding the availability of health services.
    c. provide educational services and professional development to other clinicians.
    d. help the client identify and understand their options.

157. While working with a tight timeline, a health education specialist chooses to modify an existing instrument to measure self-efficacy in high school students. However, the original instrument was used in a college population. In order to use the instrument, the health education specialist must:
    a. establish validity and reliability for the modified instrument in the high school population.
    b. modify the instrument and then proceed with data collection for evaluation.
    c. not modify the instrument, since the two populations are similar.
    d. realize modifying an instrument makes it invalid, and this is not a proper procedure for data collection.

158. In order for partnerships to be effective, their composition needs to reflect members that are knowledgeable about the populations they serve, reflect multiple domains in consideration of relative risks and protective factors, and possess a diverse representation. A model that facilitates this selection process is:
    a. the essential public health services.
    b. communications feedback loops.
    c. an ecological model of health.
    d. a continuous quality improvement process.

159. Communication aimed at patients with non-life-threatening medical conditions is primarily developed to:
    a. promote open discussion of the condition with significant others.
    b. provide motivation to seek medical help immediately.
    c. increase awareness of the potential effects of the condition.
    d. encourage consideration of nonmedical opinions.

160. Stakeholders are typically involved in the program planning process in many ways, except:
    a. monitoring program operations.
    b. deciding on salary of key personnel.
    c. serving as primary users of the program.
    d. ensuring implementation proceeds smoothly.

161. In working with a community that has a large Spanish-speaking population, a health educator engages a lay-health worker early in the planning process to be sure that the program is planned, implemented, and evaluated appropriately. An advisory group is formed to assess the relevance of the program activities. These important steps are a way to help improve:
    a. Cultural competency
    b. Cultural identification
    c. Cultural norms
    d. Cultural assimilation

162. One of the first considerations when determining the potential appropriateness of an external organization for collaboration is an alignment of:
    a. mission, vision, and values.
    b. an operational budget.
    c. a staffing pattern.
    d. an organizational structure.

163. A health education specialist is working with several agencies to develop an intervention. When selecting strategies, which of the following should the health educator do first?
    a. Do a literature search to find the best program regardless of audience
    b. Know their audience and what they have access to
    c. Use social media and other popular technologies
    d. Convene the agencies to discuss what strategies they think are best

164. A health education specialist needs to find an instrument to measure program impact. Which database is best for this?
    a. SAMSHA
    b. HRSA
    c. HaPI
    d. MEDLINE

165. A health education specialist is trying to decide how to collect data for program evaluation in a program to improve nutrition in a low-income community sample. The health educator is looking to randomly select a small number of participants and assess their individual attitudes toward dietary behavior change and their dietary behavior. Which of the following data collection methods would be best to get the largest response rate in this sample?
    a. Surveys administered in person
    b. Web-based surveys
    c. Mailed surveys
    d. Nominal Group Process

CHES PRACTICE EXAM ANSWER KEY

1.	c	Area III	35.	a	Area VII	69.	b	Area II	103.	b	Area III	137.	b	Area I
2.	b	Area III	36.	d	Area II	70.	a	Area II	104.	a	Area I	138.	b	Area III
3.	d	Area I	37.	d	Area VII	71.	b	Area VII	105.	c	Area III	139.	a	Area V
4.	a	Area V	38.	b	Area II	72.	a	Area III	106.	d	Area VII	140.	a	Area I
5.	d	Area VII	39.	b	Area V	73.	d	Area IV	107.	a	Area III	141.	c	Area V
6.	c	Area II	40.	a	Area III	74.	b	Area VI	108.	c	Area II	142.	d	Area III
7.	b	Area IV	41.	c	Area IV	75.	c	Area IV	109.	b	Area II	143.	b	Area III
8.	b	Area III	42.	a	Area III	76.	c	Area II	110.	c	Area I	144.	a	Area I
9.	b	Area I	43.	d	Area III	77.	d	Area I	111.	a	Area I	145.	c	Area II
10.	a	Area VII	44.	c	Area II	78.	b	Area III	112.	b	Area II	146.	c	Area VI
11.	b	Area I	45.	c	Area III	79.	a	Area II	113.	d	Area V	147.	a	Area II
12.	c	Area I	46.	a	Area III	80.	a	Area V	114.	c	Area III	148.	d	Area I
13.	d	Area VI	47.	b	Area I	81.	c	Area VI	115.	a	Area VI	149.	b	Area VI
14.	a	Area V	48.	d	Area V	82.	d	Area II	116.	d	Area VII	150.	a	Area III
15.	c	Area II	49.	a	Area VII	83.	d	Area III	117.	a	Area VI	151.	c	Area II
16.	d	Area II	50.	b	Area I	84.	a	Area VII	118.	b	Area III	152.	c	Area VI
17.	c	Area I	51.	b	Area VI	85.	b	Area III	119.	a	Area III	153.	a	Area I
18.	d	Area III	52.	d	Area II	86.	c	Area IV	120.	b	Area IV	154.	d	Area II
19.	a	Area VII	53.	a	Area III	87.	a	Area III	121.	c	Area III	155.	d	Area II
20.	b	Area I	54.	a	Area VI	88.	c	Area VII	122.	c	Area IV	156.	d	Area VII
21.	c	Area II	55.	d	Area III	89.	d	Area VI	123.	d	Area II	157.	a	Area IV
22.	c	Area III	56.	c	Area I	90.	b	Area III	124.	b	Area IV	158.	c	Area V
23.	a	Area VI	57.	b	Area I	91.	a	Area VII	125.	a	Area I	159.	c	Area VII
24.	d	Area IV	58.	b	Area I	92.	c	Area III	126.	d	Area I	160.	b	Area II
25.	c	Area VII	59.	a	Area V	93.	b	Area VI	127.	b	Area IV	161.	a	Area VII
26.	a	Area III	60.	b	Area II	94.	c	Area III	128.	a	Area I	162.	a	Area V
27.	d	Area V	61.	b	Area V	95.	a	Area I	129.	a	Area V	163.	b	Area III
28.	d	Area VII	62.	c	Area II	96.	c	Area V	130.	b	Area IV	164.	c	Area VI
29.	c	Area V	63.	d	Area VII	97.	a	Area VI	131.	c	Area V	165.	a	Area IV
30.	b	Area V	64.	a	Area IV	98.	d	Area III	132.	d	Area III			
31.	a	Area V	65.	a	Area II	99.	d	Area II	133.	a	Area V			
32.	b	Area I	66.	b	Area III	100.	b	Area II	134.	c	Area III			
33.	b	Area III	67.	c	Area IV	101.	c	Area VII	135.	c	Area II			
34.	c	Area III	68.	d	Area III	102.	b	Area VII	136.	d	Area III			

This page was
intentionally left blank

Master Certified Health Education Specialist Practice Examination Questions

The following practice examination questions address Sub-competencies identified as entry-, advanced 1-, and advanced 2-levels as defined by the Health Education Specialist Practice Analysis (refer to pages 6 and 235) and outlined and addressed within this study companion. The practice questions, written by health education specialists, may assist the user in preparing for the Master Certified Health Education Specialist (MCHES) examination and/or to identify areas of concentration for professional development and training of practicing health education specialists. The questions are not on the current certification examination. Some of the questions have been altered from discarded certification examination questions. The practice questions in this publication have not been subjected to the same rigorous psychometric testing procedures as questions appearing on the CHES or MCHES examinations. Specifically, a passing score on the practice examination questions does not in any way predict or guarantee a passing score on the CHES/MCHES examinations. The practice questions should only be used to direct study efforts.

The practice questions are meant to be challenging. Initially, the user may find that more than one answer appears to be correct. In these instances, the user is encouraged to conduct careful analysis of the questions and possible answers to identify the correct responses. It might be helpful to use the practice examination MCHES examination is officially administered. For example, the user would be allowed no more than three hours to complete the examination. The user would not utilize or depend on resources such as the study guide, textbooks, publications, or calculators to complete the examination.

An answer key is provided at the end of the practice examination questions. In addition to providing the user with the correct answer, the user will find at least one Area of Responsibility that aligns with the question identified. A review of the number of incorrect answers from any particular Area of Responsibility may help the user to target areas of weakness where more study would be beneficial. ***It is strongly recommended that resources beyond the use of this study companion are used to adequately prepare for the certification examination.***

In closing, feedback from candidates who were successful in passing previous certification examinations and previous study guide users indicates that being part of a small group that allowed participants to "work through" the practice examination questions and discuss why answers are were correct or incorrect can be beneficial.

Master Certified Health Education Specialist Practice Examination Questions

Select the *best* answer.

1. The health education specialist is organizing a summative evaluation. Which evaluation design offers the most control over confounding variables?
   a. Time-series
   b. Quasi-experimental
   c. Non-experimental
   d. Experimental

2. For people with less than 12 years of education, the infant mortality rate and overall death rate is almost twice as high as people with 13 or more years of education. These are examples of:
   a. health inequities.
   b. health disparities.
   c. social determinants of health.
   d. health equity.

3. A health education specialist is meeting with a college campus community to try to make the campus a smoke free. In order to gain support from key stakeholders in the first meeting, which of the following should be the focus of the health education specialist's message?
   a. The necessity for the change in policy
   b. The specific enforcement plan
   c. The health communication strategy to be used
   d. The incentive program could be used

4. An outbreak of dysentery occurred in a community over the course of a week. The number of cases and time of onset of symptoms was determined. All who displayed symptoms ate sprouts at the same restaurant. For this outbreak, which type of epidemic curve can be prepared for the descriptive study?
   a. Single
   b. Seasonal
   c. Secular
   d. Propagated

5. The intervention program is doing so well it needs to be expanded; however, the sponsoring agency has limited funding for expansion. The health education specialist found another agency willing to provide a larger venue in exchange for access to the sponsor's educational library. This method of financing the program is called:
   a. organizational sponsorship.
   b. cost-sharing.
   c. third-party support.
   d. cooperative agreements.

6. Measuring program reach and response is an element of which type of evaluation?
    a. Outcome
    b. Impact
    c. Process
    d. Summative

7. The health education specialist's advocacy efforts are starting to be successful. The city council has voted 4-1 to hold a town hall meeting to discuss a clean indoor air ordinance. Which type of advocacy benchmark is this?
    a. Shift in critical mass
    b. Community or individual behavior
    c. Changing definitions/reframing
    d. Institutional policy

8. A health education specialist wishes to use the ecological model in a needs assessment. Which of the following is an example of a way to assess levels of this model?
    a. Assessing use of intrapersonal behavior change constructs in the community
    b. Assessing health and quality of life of community members and evaluating current programs
    c. Assessing community norms and behaviors related to health issues
    d. Assessing attitudes, behaviors, policies, and social norms in a community

9. The agency administrator wants the big picture or summary of an intervention's resources, activities, and results. The health education specialist creates which of the following to put in his/her report to the administrator?
    a. Marketing mix
    b. Logic model
    c. Instructional design framework
    d. Unit of study

10. When planning an adult audience training, the health education specialist should include adult learning theory principles. Which of the following is an example of an adult learning principle to use when planning the training?
    a. Adults should only be involved in pilot testing activities
    b. Adults should not be involved in planning and evaluation
    c. Adults should be actively involved in planning and evaluation
    d. Adults should only be involved in planning activities

11. Working as a health coach to increase a client's physical fitness level, the health education specialist uses an intervention based on the Transtheoretical Model. He/she emphasizes behavioral activities including counter-conditioning and reinforcement using which core construct?
    a. Processes of change
    b. Stages of change
    c. Decisional balance
    d. Self-efficacy

Use Figure 1 to answer question 12.

Figure 1.

Trends in Homicide Rates among Persons Ages 10-24 Years, by Race/Ethnicity, 1994–2010

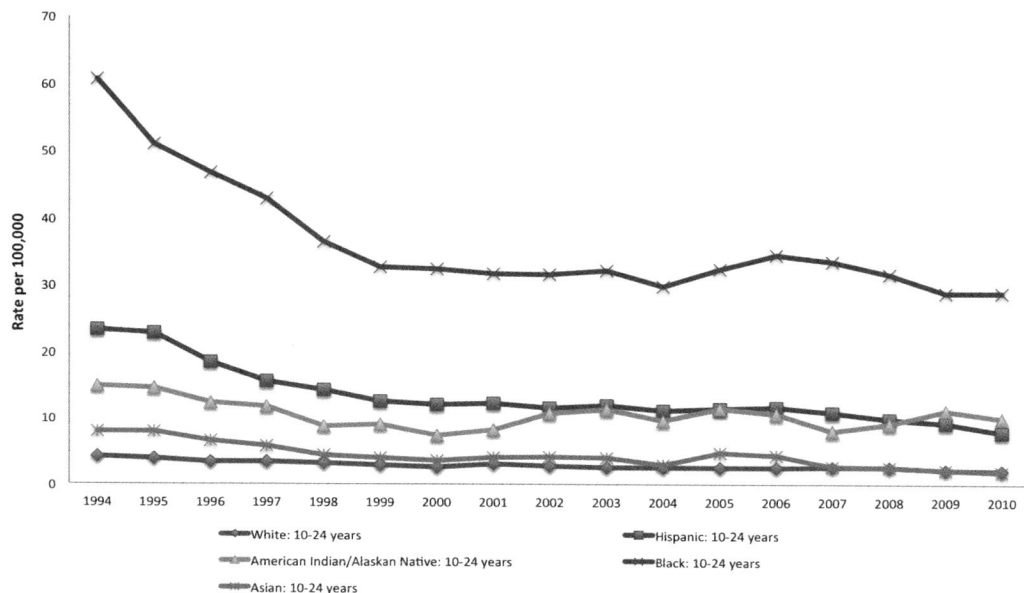

Taken from: CDC Injury Center. (2013). Violence prevention: Trends in homicide rates among persons ages 10-24 years, by race and ethnicity, 1994-2010.

12. According to the Figure 1, Trends in Homicide Rates graph, what programming decisions might be made?
    a. Because homicide rates are second highest in American Indian/Alaskan Native 10-24 year olds, it may be that further data collection is needed to determine program needs
    b. Because rates of homicide among Hispanic 10-24 year olds have doubled since 1994, there is an increased need for programming to reduce violence
    c. Because rates of homicide among Black 10-24 year olds have decreased by 25% since 1994, there is no need for more programming to reduce violence
    d. Because rates of homicide among Asian 10-24 year olds have slightly increased since 1994, there is an increased need for programming to reduce violence

13. A health education specialist is planning to train staff from partners and community members to help implement a healthy food access initiative with corner stores and convenience stores. A needs assessment is being planned to identify trainee knowledge on the subject. What should the assessment focus on?
    a. Availability to attend training(s)
    b. Training methods preferred
    c. Desired learning outcome(s)
    d. Previous knowledge or experience

14. The Healthy Families Network holds an annual conference. In order to evaluate the conference and gather information from the participants, what is the best way for the health education specialist to collect this information?
    a. Archival review of documents
    b. Surveys or feedback forms
    c. Observations of participants
    d. Pre and post test

15. In the correct order, what are the "six steps" of the CDC's framework for Program Evaluation?
    a. Describe program; engage stakeholders; gather credible evidence; focus on the evaluation design; justify conclusions; ensure use and share lessons learned
    b. Describe the program; gather credible evidence; focus on the evaluation design; justify conclusions; ensure use and share lessons leaned; engage stakeholders
    c. Engage stakeholders; describe program; focus on the evaluation design; gather credible evidence; justify conclusions; ensure use and share lessons learned
    d. Gather credible evidence; engage stakeholders; describe program; justify conclusions; focus on the evaluation design; ensure use and share lessons learned

16. From a fiscal perspective, which funds represent the portion of a project the applicant's agency or organization is providing?
    a. Petty funds
    b. Compliance assurances
    c. Cash contributions
    d. Matching funds

Master Certified Health Education Specialist Practice Examination Questions

17. A health education specialist is collaborating with the state health department on a training effort to implement effective physical activity programs. The training team has completed the first step, which was to determine training needs. What is the next step to advance the training?
    a. Prepare audiovisuals
    b. Set objectives
    c. Select participants
    d. Determine subject content

18. The health education specialist overhears two employees in a verbal debate about which department should receive the budget surplus generated this fiscal year. What is the best first step in conflict resolution in this situation?
    a. Analyze the conflict
    b. Estimate the parties' positions
    c. Determine the management strategy
    d. Create options for both parties

Scenario A - The following scenario is used for questions 19 to 20.
The health education specialist has limited resources available for an immunization program to be implemented in the large urban community. Input from stakeholders will be solicited. Two possible options under consideration include: (a) implement a new program, a drive through clinic available during the weekend or (b) stay with the old program, hiring additional nurses to be employed at the health clinic during regular business hours.

19. In Scenario A, which of the following analyses would be used to determine the option that provides the greatest number of immunizations to community members at the least cost?
    a. Cost benefit analysis
    b. Cost-effectiveness analysis
    c. Cost utility analysis
    d. Cost verification analysis

20. In Scenario A, what can the health education specialist use to facilitate stakeholder collaboration in the immunization project to outline predetermined objectives agreed upon by all partners?
    a. Budget reconciliation sheet (BRS)
    b. Memorandum of Understanding (MOU)
    c. Willingness to Pay (WTP)
    d. Contingent Valuation (CV)

21. When identifying root causes of health issues, it is important to consider multiple factors. If a community would rather ignore a drug problem than address it, this is an example of which type of factor?
    a. Medical care
    b. Societal
    c. Individual
    d. Environmental

22. Performance appraisals of staff members and volunteers will normally:
    a. focus on skills and knowledge.
    b. be performed on those who have recently joined the organization/agency.
    c. focus on strengths and areas for improvement.
    d. be performed on those who are having problems.

23. A health education specialist visits elected officials to advocate for an evidence-based nutrition program. The health education specialist prepares a packet that summarizes the position statement that will be given during the visit. This is an example of influencing public policy in what way?
    a. Identifying the players
    b. Responding quickly
    c. Reinforcing the message
    d. Crafting your position

Scenario B - The following scenario is used for questions 24 and 25.
In collecting primary data to determine a community's health needs, the local health department found the following in regards to CVD and cancer deaths:

Total Midyear Population	20,000
CVD-related deaths	500
Female CVD deaths	200
Male CVD deaths	300
Cancer deaths	450
Female cancer deaths	300

24. In Scenario B, how would a health education specialist calculate the crude cancer death rate (assume per 1000)?
    a. 500*1000/20,000
    b. 450/20,000 *1000
    c. (500/20,000) /1000
    d. 20,000/450 * 1000

25. What would a health education specialist need to know to calculate age-specific death rates from cardiovascular disease?
    a. The total number of deaths for each specific cause by age
    b. The total mid-year female population in the community
    c. The total mid-year male population in the community and the number of deaths for each age group
    d. The breakdown of deaths by age group and the midyear population by age

26. A researcher is coding data to categorize individuals based on sex, race, and political party affiliation. What type of scale is the researcher using?
    a. Nominal scale
    b. Ordinal scale
    c. Likert scale
    d. Interval scale

27. Providing access to fruit and milk in a school vending machine is an example of which of the following strategies?
    a. Health communication
    b. Community mobilization
    c. Health engineering
    d. Health policy and enforcement

28. A health education specialist is searching for a valid information source specifically addressing a population's health status, health questionnaires, and health care delivery trends. The best source to use would be:
    a. HON.
    b. NCHS.
    c. FDA.
    d. EPA.

29. The health education specialist is having difficulty in segmenting the priority population when designing a marketing strategy for a health promotion intervention. Building the strategy on which of the following theories would help him/her segment the audience and assist with a marketing mix decision?
    a. Diffusion Theory
    b. Health Belief Model
    c. Theory of Reasoned Action
    d. Theory of Planned Behavior

30. When a researcher is conducting a study, it is important to remain _____ to reduce _____.
    a. uninvolved; bias
    b. biased; error
    c. involved; threats to validity
    d. neutral; error

31. The local health promotion coalition elected to implement a single strategy intervention for a complex health problem because of its ease of implementation and lower cost. The health education specialist advises the use of a multistrategy intervention in hopes that at least one or a combination of the strategies makes a difference; however, he/she understands that the greatest drawback to the multistrategy intervention is:
    a. priority population segmentation is complex.
    b. multiple levels of influence send mixed messages.
    c. it is difficult to separate the effects of each strategy in evaluation.
    d. the settings approach is not addressed.

32. Which of the following is a major health policy question faced at the national government (U.S. Federal) level?
    a. What population groups should receive subsidized coverage from tax revenues?
    b. What should be the state's role in subsidizing care for the uninsured?
    c. What efforts should be undertaken to encourage local emergency planning?
    d. What services should be provided in addition to those normally provided by one's specialty?

33. A researcher is analyzing a data set. The researcher computes the absolute difference between the highest and lowest score on a particular variable in the sample. The researcher has computed which statistic for this data set?
    a. Variance
    b. Mean
    c. Range
    d. Standard deviation

34. A health education specialist has completed a quick assessment of the Stages of Change in the priority population. According to the assessment, most individuals are not quite ready to take action, but are beginning to think about taking action. They do not have any immediate plans, but are willing to listen to what the health education specialist has to say. What is the likely stage of participants?
    a. Preparation
    b. Action
    c. Precontemplation
    d. Contemplation

Master Certified Health Education Specialist Practice Examination Questions

35. A health education specialist serves as a patient educator at a hospital. Part of his/her job is to work with patients who have recently suffered a heart attack. This is an example of:
    a. primary prevention.
    b. tertiary prevention.
    c. secondary prevention.
    d. intermediary prevention.

36. The health education specialist hypothesizes a certain skin disease is more common in men who swim than men who do not swim. To study this specific disease-exposure relationship in order to determine if an association exists for further study, the health education specialists conducts which type of study?
    a. Randomized study
    b. Descriptive study
    c. Case/control study
    d. Probability study

37. When creating the budget for a grant application, contributed income can be classified into which two categories?
    a. Cash and in-kind
    b. Earned and cash
    c. Sales and in-kind
    d. In-kind and earned

38. When using the NREPP to inform program decision making, the health education specialist must recognize that although the quality of the research supporting intervention outcomes and the quality and availability of training and implementation materials has been rated, users should:
    a. make a curricular decision because the list is exhaustive.
    b. carefully read and understand the research results for each outcome.
    c. understand that NREPP has reviewed all interventions.
    d. be limited to selecting only among NREPP interventions.

39. Which of the following contains the correct steps in the generalized model of program planning and evaluation?
    a. Write goals and objectives, understand and engage the population, create a needs assessment, create intervention, implement the program, and evaluate intervention
    b. Understand and engage the population, create a needs assessment, write goals and objectives, create intervention, implement the program, and evaluate intervention
    c. Create a needs assessment, understand and engage the population, write goals and objectives, create intervention, implement the program, and evaluate intervention
    d. Create a needs assessment, write goals and objectives, understand and engage the population, create intervention, implement the program, and evaluate intervention

40. When attempting to get people to quit smoking, a health education specialist has to work through several adopter groups according to the Diffusion of Innovations. Many smokers have adopted the behavior change, but one group is particularly difficult to reach and is quick to dismiss efforts to change. This characterizes which group?
    a. Latent adopters
    b. Late majority
    c. Innovators
    d. Laggards

41. Which type of literature review typically identifies current gaps in the literature after comprehensively reviewing the literature on a topic?
    a. Systematic review
    b. Meta-analysis
    c. Pooled analysis
    d. Computerized review

42. A health education specialist has a request to develop a worksite training to be implemented with a company that focuses on technology security. Management within the company is trying to find a time to schedule a series of training sessions that may change dietary behaviors, but one common meeting time for all employees is not feasible. What is the health education specialist's *best* option, based upon the content and needs of the company?
    a. Create a pamphlet with tips for eating healthy to hand out to employees
    b. Conduct a series of seminars at the company, with make-up sessions for those who cannot make the meetings
    c. Create an interactive distance learning module that employees can complete as they have time
    d. Create a cookbook with healthy recipes for the employees to use

43. A university health education specialist is implementing a program for females on campus about the HPV vaccine. Which statement would be reflective of Preparation in the Stages of Change?
    a. I have already been vaccinated
    b. I was not aware of the vaccine
    c. I have not thought much about the vaccine
    d. I have decided to get the vaccine next week

44. When presenting data to stakeholders or superiors in an organization, which of the following would *best* represent how percentages relate to each other as a whole?
    a. Graphs
    b. Charts
    c. Maps
    d. Tables

Master Certified Health Education Specialist Practice Examination Questions

Scenario C - The following scenario is used for questions 45 and 46.
A health education specialist is developing a program to help reduce rates of cardiovascular disease in employees at a worksite. There are multiple layers of intervention, including increasing awareness of cardiovascular disease risk factors, physical activity programming, increasing the lunch hour to allow for physical activity, encouraging walking meetings, and increasing healthy foods served in the cafeteria, among others.

45. In Scenario C, increasing awareness of risk for cardiovascular disease occurs at which level?
    a. Intrapersonal
    b. Institutional
    c. Organizational
    d. Policy

46. In Scenario C, increasing the lunch hour to allow for physical activity occurs at which level?
    a. Community
    b. Intrapersonal
    c. Interpersonal
    d. Policy

47. The health education specialist called their state legislator and asked them to specifically support a bill to require 60 minutes of physical activity in school. Which of the following terms would describe this activity?
    a. Direct advocacy
    b. Indirect advocacy
    c. Lobbying
    d. Educational advocacy

48. According to a 4-level training evaluation, during which level does the evaluator measure participant satisfaction with the training?
    a. Learning
    b. Reaction
    c. Behavior
    d. Results

49. The sequence for pretesting health education messages focused on knowledge is:
    a. concept development, partially completed materials testing, alternative materials testing, and final product.
    b. concept development, alternative materials testing, partially completed materials testing, and final product.
    c. alternative materials testing, partially completed material testing, concept development, and final product.
    d. alternative materials testing, concept development, partially completed materials testing, and final product.

50. An objective that is concerned with increasing social support is what type of objective?
    a. Behavioral
    b. Learning
    c. Outcome
    d. Process

51. The health education specialist is questioning whether pre-post health behavior changes recorded by trained observers over a long period of time can be directly attributed to his/her intervention. He/she is questioning which type of threat to the internal validity of evaluation?
    a. Selection
    b. Statistical regression
    c. Diffusion of treatments
    d. Instrumentation

52. A person's environment can help or hinder their physical activity behavior, even when a person is highly motivated to be active. This illustrates the concept of:
    a. locus of control.
    b. emotional-coping response.
    c. reciprocal determinism.
    d. efficacy expectations.

53. What is the best first step in developing a health education program budget?
    a. Review budget requests
    b. Prepare a budget calendar
    c. Define administrative roles in budget preparation
    d. Establish program goals

54. Understanding why participants drop out of a program is important for establishing:
    a. validity.
    b. consistency.
    c. reliability.
    d. organization.

55. A local health agency matches senior staff to new hires during their first year. A health education specialist is considering ways to mentor new staff. Which of the following mentoring strategies is most likely to help new hires adjust to the job?
    a. The health education specialist gives the new hire large tasks to see how well they do managing them
    b. New hires pair up with other new hires to help each other
    c. The health education specialist has a new hire join an ongoing project to see how it is currently being handled
    d. The senior staff delegate the small projects to the new hires to protect them from the bigger, more involved projects as they adjust

56. During a physical activity intervention session, a health education specialist asks participants to brainstorm ways to overcome barriers to physical activity. This session is focusing on which construct from Social Cognitive Theory?
    a. Self-control
    b. Self-efficacy
    c. Social support
    d. Reciprocal determinism

57. A health education specialist finds there are more people requesting a smoking cessation program than can be accommodated. This is an example of which type of need?
    a. Normative need
    b. Expressed need
    c. Perceived need
    d. Relative need

58. A health education specialist successfully implemented a smoking cessation intervention for tenants in public housing. To maintain the work, what ecological level should the health education specialist focus on to help tenants sustain their smoking cessation?
    a. Organizational
    b. Individual
    c. Interpersonal
    d. Public policy

59. A health education specialist is trying to find data on emergency room visits and hospitalizations in the community. Which of the following secondary sources is the best source of this data?
    a. NHCS
    b. NHIS
    c. NHANES
    d. BRFSS

60. The Cancer Control Coalition has decided that they have the capacity for and interest in planning for an advocacy campaign. Generally, the first step in *advocacy* planning is to address:
    a. resources/assets.
    b. goals.
    c. extent of community support.
    d. targets of change.

61. In a behavior change intervention for weight management following social cognitive theory, participants are asked to list both positive and negative environmental influences on their snacking behavior. The concept applied in this type of exercise is called:
    a. relative advantage.
    b. behavioral capability.
    c. reciprocal determinism.
    d. observational learning.

62. When the health education specialist needs to measure the severity of a disease related to the degree of pathogenicity of the disease organism, he/she calculates the:
    a. proportionate mortality rate.
    b. case fatality rate.
    c. cause-specific mortality rate.
    d. crude death rate.

63. When planning a smoking prevention program following the PRECEDE-PROCEED Model, data regarding self-efficacy to avoid smoking in an adolescent population would fall into which assessment phase?
    a. Educational and ecological assessment
    b. Social assessment and situational analysis
    c. Epidemiological assessment
    d. Intervention alignment and administrative and policy assessment

64. Advocacy evaluation is typically an ongoing activity, given social and political environments are constantly changing. What type of health program evaluation is this similar to?
    a. Impact
    b. Summative
    c. Process
    d. Outcome

65. Which of the following is an important learning principle for andragogy?
    a. Use examples that could be used with a variety of audiences
    b. Focus on technology and gaming to make learning fun
    c. Use mostly traditional formats, as this is what adults are accustomed to
    d. Focus on problem solving skills rather than learning content

66. Health risk appraisals are which type of intervention strategy?
    a. Health related community service strategy
    b. Health policy and enforcement strategy
    c. Health communication strategy
    d. Health engineering strategy

67. To understand the three human subjects protection guidelines of "respect for persons," "beneficence," and "justice," one would look to the:
    a. Belmont report.
    b. CNHEO code of ethics.
    c. Informed consent procedures.
    d. Geneva Convention Treaty.

68. A health education specialist has been charged to develop a comprehensive childhood obesity intervention in a community identified as having a high prevalence of childhood obesity. What planning model would *best* assist the health education specialist in developing the program?
    a. Community Model
    b. PRECEDE-PROCEED Model
    c. Logic Model
    d. Health Belief Model

69. A current problem faced by organizations relying on volunteers is retention rate. In order to increase retention of volunteers, an organization might focus on which of the following?
    a. Recruiting
    b. Supervision
    c. Training
    d. Recognition

70. Which of the following is an effective strategy for a health education specialist to determine the training needs of parents of preschool children regarding infectious disease prevention?
    a. Collect immunization records for the children in the community ages five and younger
    b. Survey parents of preschool aged children regarding their knowledge of infectious disease prevention
    c. Compile a list of the five most frequently reported infectious diseases reported by child care providers
    d. Review infectious disease rates for the community over the last five years

71. Which level of training evaluation is the extent to which participants are employing the skills on the job?
    a. Results
    b. Behavior
    c. Knowledge
    d. Reaction

72. During a needs assessment, the priority population identifies the desire for safe places to exercise in the community. They have identified:
    a. a perceived need.
    b. a normative need.
    c. an expressed need.
    d. a relative need.

73. The health department notices a spike in drug use of high school students in the county and wishes to predict which students could be at high risk in order to target an intervention program. They would like to determine the relationship between drug-use and demographic, as well as health behavior variables, and then determine which of these variables or combination of these variables best predicts drug use risk. They would conduct which two types of studies?
    a. Clinical control trial and then case study
    b. Causal comparative and then correlational
    c. Correlational and then multiple regression
    d. Causal comparative and then ex post facto

74. The health education specialist is directing a local youth health advisory group and a statewide youth coalition. In this role, the health education specialist is acting as a:
    a. planner.
    b. coordinator.
    c. implementer.
    d. resource person.

75. When evaluating training, a health education specialist is investigating the impact of reduced turnover in a company. Which level of training evaluation is this?
    a. Reaction
    b. Behavior
    c. Learning
    d. Results

76. A university cooperative extension service program is focusing on health injury prevention and increased safety helmet use. The cooperative extension service program is providing technical assistance to cub scouts and boy scouts to implement individual counseling and small or large demonstrations at skate parks. What is the greatest challenge the cooperative extension service staff might experience when attempting to provide technical assistance?
    a. Readiness to receive technical assistance
    b. Understanding of the program and topic
    c. Engaging enough cub scouts and boy scouts
    d. Participation in the entire program

77. What is the main difference between quasi-experimental and experimental study design?
    a. Quasi-experimental designs manipulate more than one independent variable
    b. Random assignment of participants occurs in an experimental design
    c. Comparison groups are used in experimental designs
    d. Experimental designs are only used for drug trials

78. When calculating mortality statistics in a population, the health education specialist needs to weigh deaths of the very young more than deaths of the very old. Which of the following would he/she calculate?
    a. DALYs
    b. YPLL
    c. CSMR
    d. HALE

79. During program planning for a behavior-change intervention, awareness, knowledge, attitude, and skill objectives are written. This hierarchy of objectives is categorized under:
    a. learning objectives.
    b. behavioral objectives.
    c. environmental objectives.
    d. process objectives.

80. "The Moving Mommas Program will reduce risk of preeclampsia in Shelbyville" is an example of:
    a. a vision statement.
    b. a mission statement.
    c. a goal statement.
    d. an objective statement.

81. A process to ensure the readability of intervention materials and items used to collect data is:
    a. Test Re-test.
    b. split forms.
    c. pilot testing.
    d. SMOG.

82. In a community, twice as many people died over the course of one year in house fires than in car crashes. Community members demand the health education specialist immediately create a fire prevention intervention. Before planning the fire prevention intervention, the health education specialist should first determine:
    a. life expectancy in the community.
    b. population at risk.
    c. point source epidemic curve.
    d. odds ratio.

83. In the strategic planning process, after an organization defines or refines its mission statement, the next step is to:
    a. list internal and external strengths and opportunities.
    b. list mandates and resources.
    c. identify key stakeholders.
    d. write the initial report

84. An instrument measuring what it purports to measure is said be _____, while an instrument repeatedly producing the same results is said to be _____.
    a. reliable; valid
    b. valid; reliable
    c. relevant; dependable
    d. dependable; relevant

85. Effect sizes describe the magnitude of difference between two groups and allow researchers to determine the _____ of the research findings.
    a. strength of association
    b. statistical significance
    c. political context
    d. practical significance

86. When inferring needs of a priority population, the health education specialist:
    a. must remain unbiased and ignore political or cultural influences on health issues of great importance in the community.
    b. creates a program based solely upon the data collected from surveys and hospitals in the area.
    c. considers feedback from the priority population along with data collected on health issues in the population.
    d. focuses only on behavioral issues in the priority population because these issues are the most changeable.

87. The health education specialist would use a prioritization matrix in which phase of the PRECEDE-PROCEED Model?
    a. Epidemiological assessment
    b. Social assessment and situational analysis
    c. Intervention alignment and administrative and policy assessment
    d. Implementation of the program

88. Which type of reliability is important for ensuring any changes detected at the end of an intervention are due to the intervention itself, and not random fluctuation?
    a. Interobserver reliability
    b. Test-retest reliability
    c. Internal consistency reliability
    d. Content reliability

89. When facilitating a training workshop on a new electronic medical records system at a clinic, the health education specialist is following the steps for successful training programs. He/she is confident in implementing the training steps as there is little difference between this process and general health education program implementation except for the need to specify:
    a. learning needs.
    b. job performance.
    c. teaching-learning methods.
    d. instructional resources.

90. A health education specialist developed materials for the behavioral strategies in a multilevel intervention. He/she pilot-tested the strategies with adolescents in the priority population. After the pilot test, it was found that two of the lessons were difficult for adolescents to understand. What is the best way for the health education specialist to proceed?
    a. Use feedback to modify the lessons so adolescents will better understand them
    b. Change a few difficult words in the lessons, but keep the majority of the lessons the same
    c. Revisit the entire behavioral intervention to modify all lessons
    d. Do not make any changes, because adaptation would impact implementation fidelity

91. The grantor has requested a grant progress report from the grantee agency. The health education specialist was assigned the task of report preparation to maintain support for this project. Which of the following is the best first step in report preparation?
    a. Writing the rough draft
    b. Outlining the report
    c. Gathering the data
    d. Analyzing the results

92. An evaluator is considering using a previously developed instrument to measure an intervention designed to improve constructs predicted to influence text messaging while driving behavior. The following table was provided to the evaluator, along with a copy of the instrument:

| | Range | | | | |
Construct	Possible	Observed	M	SD	Cronbach's
Perceived Susceptibility of Texting While Driving	6 – 30	9 – 30	19.40	4.94	0.865
Perceived Severity of Texting While Driving	4 – 20	6 – 20	20.00	15.35	0.918
Perceived Benefits of Texting While Driving	4 – 20	4 – 20	9.11	3.76	0.903
Perceived Barriers of Texting While Driving	4 – 20	4 – 20	13.61	3.89	0.829

Notes: Combined, constructs predicted 45% variance in text messaging while driving behavior

Based on the information provided by the table, the instrument can be considered:
    a. valid.
    b. invalid.
    c. unreliable.
    d. reliable.

93. The researcher needs to select a probability sample of smokers and nonsmokers and wishes to randomize participant selection. He/she divides the population by those two characteristics and then randomly selects subjects from the two groups. This type of sampling procedure is called:
    a. nonproportional.
    b. systematic.
    c. proportional stratified.
    d. matrix.

94. The health education specialist chose the PRECEDE-PROCEED Model as the organizational framework for the needs assessment of a childhood obesity intervention. Which of the following best represents the Behavioral and Environmental Factors phase?
    a. The school districts are institutions with agents that can make change
    b. Childhood obesity is strongly linked to adult overweight and obesity
    c. The highest rates of childhood obesity are found in the southeastern states
    d. Social norms, self-efficacy, and attitudes are most related to obesity rates

95. When forming coalitions, which of the following should occur *first?*
    a. Create awareness of the issue in the community
    b. Analyze the issue or problem that will be the focus of the coalition
    c. Conduct initial coalition planning and recruitment
    d. Develop resources and funding for the coalition

96. A physical fitness assessment was given after a physical activity and exercise intervention was conducted with upper elementary, middle, and high school student groups. To determine if there was a statistically significant difference between the groups, which type of bivariate data analysis should be conducted?
    a. Correlation
    b. T-test
    c. Chi-square
    d. ANOVA

97. Following the PRECEDE-PROCEED Model, assessing if community members have adequate access to oral health care services is which type of factor in the educational and ecological assessment?
    a. Motivating
    b. Predisposing
    c. Reinforcing
    d. Enabling

98. A researcher did not select a random sample of high school students across three high schools in a district, but instead selected only intact classrooms in one high school. The researcher is concerned that the results of the anti-drug intervention the research will be used for cannot be generalized to other high schools in the district. The researcher is concerned about which threat to external validity?
    a. Setting treatment interaction
    b. Selection treatment interaction
    c. History treatment interaction
    d. Statistical treatment interaction

99. A health education specialist conducted an evaluation of the impact of a no-smoking policy on the smoking rate in a county using a pretest, posttest, comparison group design. If the smoking rate were lower in the intervention group and there were a statistical significance between the groups, which level of probability would indicate the results were *least* likely due to chance?
    a. $p=.01$
    b. $p=1.0$
    c. $p=.001$
    d. $p=.10$

100. A hospital is expanding outreach services and facilities with a new unit focused on prevention and the treatment of chronic disease. The health education specialist is tasked with gathering local data on these conditions. Which of the following is the most useful rate to use related to chronic conditions?
    a. Prevalence rate
    b. Incidence rate
    c. Attack rate
    d. Natality rate

101. A health education specialist is planning a training to improve cancer education skills for lay health workers to educate minority communities. What is the second task he/she should complete to accomplish this goal?
    a. Assess training needs of potential participants
    b. Identify resources to conduct the training
    c. Develop a plan for conducting the training
    d. Implement planned training

Master Certified Health Education Specialist Practice Examination Questions

102. A researcher is studying the effects of a health education intervention on reducing obesity rates of employees at Company X. The researcher requires employees have a BMI of 30 or higher to participate in the study. The researcher is applying which type of criteria to restrict enrollment?
    a. Inclusion
    b. Fundamental
    c. Sub-analysis
    d. Observation

103. A national health education organization has developed a broad, long-term economic strategy to ensure program sustainability and expansion. What term *best* describes this strategy?
    a. A grant proposal
    b. A budget
    c. A strategic plan
    d. A financial plan

104. What is an important purpose of a pilot test for data collection instruments?
    a. Gathering a first round of data
    b. Ensuring the consistency of measures
    c. Creating data collecting protocol
    d. Stakeholder engagement

105. A local group was interested in identifying evidence-based interventions to guide the development of a community wide effort to increase physical activities. Participants would be included in decision-making. Which of the following tools might be most useful?
    a. The Community Guide to Community Preventive Services
    b. The Program to Analyze, Record, and Track Networks to Enhance Relationships
    c. The Community Engagement Continuum
    d. Delphi Method

106. The health education specialist must analyze the meaning of the data collected during the assessment and determine health education/promotion needs. If the health education specialist aggregates the data, which cognitive process of qualitative research is he/she focusing on?
    a. Theorizing
    b. Synthesizing
    c. Comprehending
    d. Recontextualizing

Scenario D - The following scenario including Figure 2 is used for questions 107 to 111.
Each program manager submits preliminary budget requests to the health education specialist before the end of the fiscal year, as the health education specialist is charged with preparing an annual, short-term budget for the entire department. The health education specialist chooses a line-item budgeting system for simplicity and ease of accounting. During January, the Fitness/Physical Activity Program Area budgets for only one new exercise class. However, two were added in order to accommodate large numbers of potential participants placed on a waiting list. This was problematic because the additional expense for those two classes was not in the approved budget.

Figure 2.
Use for questions 107 to 111.

Program: Fitness/Physical Activities				January 2015
Category	Description	Jan. Actual	Jan. Budget	Jan. Variance
Salaries	Health Promotion Mgr.	1000.00	1000.00	0
	Exercise Instructors	1500.00	500.00	(1000.00)
	Office supplies	100.00	100.00	0
Operations	Telephone	500.00	400.000	(100.00)
	Printing/copying	500.00	400.00	(100.00)
	Travel/meals	0	0	0
	Advertising	100.00	100.00	0
Equipment	-------------------	100.00	200.00	(100.00)
	Total	3800.00	2700.00	(1300.00)

107. In Figure 2, the budget development strategy used is referred to as:
    a. top-down budget.
    b. bottom-up budget.
    c. functional budget.
    d. line-item budget.

108. In Figure 2, a disadvantage of maintaining the above department's budget categories at the organizational level is:
    a. the cost-effectiveness of each program is difficult to determine.
    b. overall analysis of department effectiveness is more difficult to determine.
    c. capital outlays are more difficult to determine.
    d. sources of funding are more difficult to determine.

109. Figure 2, the expenditure for hiring more part time exercise instructors due to increased participation in the new exercise class is which type of expense?
    a. Linear
    b. Fixed
    c. Variable
    d. Semi-variable

110. In Figure 2, variations between the approved budget amounts and actual costs should be examined and explained. To assure the approved amounts are monitored and used for the specified categories, a budget efficiency ratio is calculated. The percent budget variance for the month of January in the Exercise Instructors line item is:
    a. 3.0.
    b. 0.5.
    c. 2.0.
    d. 4.5.

111. In Figure 2, January's written budget report is past the due date for submission to the health administrator. The most important information to include in this budget report is the:
    a. identification and list of expenses.
    b. detailed cash-flow projections.
    c. explanation of variance and recommended actions.
    d. creation of the working papers for each line item.

112. A health education specialist is conducting a training session and wants to collect qualitative and quantitative data to evaluate the training session. Which of the following is the most appropriate use of a qualitative data collection technique to collect this evaluation data?
    a. Asking participants to provide their opinions regarding the usefulness of their training on a feedback form
    b. Asking participants to complete a Likert scale to rank their opinions regarding the usefulness of the training from 0-3 (not useful, neutral, useful)
    c. Assessing knowledge of the training topic on a scored pretest and posttest
    d. Asking participants to "teach back" the knowledge gained in the training

113. In the strategic planning process, a health education specialist is charged with analyzing assets and areas of weakness in an organization's activities. Which of the following stages of strategic planning would allow for this analysis?
    a. Strategy formulation
    b. Needs assessment
    c. SWOT analysis
    d. Identification of mandates

114. Which of the following is an example of a targeted law?
    a. City-wide smoking laws in public places including restaurants and bars
    b. Laws regarding child safety seats, specifically rear-facing infant seats
    c. Blood pressure screenings that are part of a required physical exam for school
    d. Lead disclosure forms required by a real estate agency

115. The health education specialist, employed at a university, is preparing a grant proposal. Generally, in which category would one find costs associated with facilities and administration?
    a. Fringe
    b. Direct
    c. Indirect
    d. Salaries

116. When pilot testing materials for an intervention, which of the following should be assessed before implementation of the program?
    a. Comprehension and acceptability of the intervention and materials
    b. Potential impact of the intervention on a health behavior
    c. Increases in knowledge of the priority population after the program
    d. Potential costs for development and delivery of the intervention

117. Which analysis measure assesses the economic efficiency of health education programs when the health outcomes are disparate?
    a. Cost verification analysis
    b. Cost-effectiveness analysis
    c. Cost utility analysis
    d. Cost benefit analysis

118. Which section of a government grant proposal would most likely request the provision of a logic model?
    a. Other funding/sustainability
    b. Methods/strategies
    c. Needs statement
    d. Goals/objectives

Master Certified Health Education Specialist Practice Examination Questions

119. When applying the ecological perspective to behavior change, the health education specialist bases his/her smoking cessation intervention on the Precaution Adoption Process Model. At what level of influence is this intervention addressing?
    a. Interpersonal
    b. Intrapersonal
    c. Community
    d. Public policy

120. Administrative support was secured and a program planning committee was formed for a school-based health promotion program. Which of the following should the committee members identify next before advancing the needs assessment process?
    a. Planning committee services
    b. Program rationales
    c. Planning parameters
    d. Preplanning supports

121. A benefit of asynchronous training is:
    a. the instructor and participants can communicate in real time.
    b. busy adults can fit the training into their schedules.
    c. it allows the instructor to reach low income populations.
    d. it allows the instructor to answer questions as they arise.

122. When designing audience-centered, culturally appropriate health education materials, it is essential to:
    a. involve the intended audience in development of materials.
    b. outsource the publishing to another agency.
    c. determine education level of the target audience.
    d. keep production costs reasonable.

123. For this objective, "Women in the program will increase their physical activity rates by the 4th week of the program," what is missing?
    a. It is neither realistic nor time-sensitive
    b. It is neither attainable nor realistic
    c. It is neither specific nor measurable
    d. It is neither specific nor time-sensitive

124. Informing participants in a training program of both the benefits and risks associated with training typically occurs within which procedure?
    a. Informed consent
    b. Parental assent
    c. IRB submission
    d. Beneficence consent

125. Using a socio-ecological model in a school setting, the school would be considered as which level?
    a. Policy
    b. Community
    c. Institutional
    d. Interpersonal

126. What is the main function of an Institutional Review Board (IRB)?
    a. To protect human subjects involved in the research
    b. To make sure the study is valid and reliable
    c. To critique methodology or instrumentation
    d. To make sure not to duplicate studies

127. The questions, "What steps are necessary to move the organization towards the desired future? What progress is being made?" are used during what process?
    a. SWOT analysis
    b. Needs assessment
    c. Program planning
    d. Strategic planning

128. The health education specialist entered into a consulting relationship that required a contract between the consultant and client. This contract is considered:
    a. internal.
    b. external.
    c. technical.
    d. informal.

Master Certified Health Education Specialist Practice Examination Questions

129. The health education specialist is charged with establishing collaborative relationships with organizations to gain access to data for county wide community needs assessments. Which of the following is the best approach to secure the data needed?
    a. Determine the level of relationship needed with each organization to obtain data
    b. Identify key individuals and stakeholders within the various organizations to build a relationship
    c. Establish a data sharing agreement including the outcome, purpose, data ownership, and conditions of release
    d. Establish a network of organizations with data needed for county wide community needs assessment

130. Due to financial constraints, a research team is only recruiting participants from three hospitals in the local metropolitan area. In doing so, the researchers have established:
    a. eliminations.
    b. limitations.
    c. delimitations.
    d. assumptions.

131. A health education specialist is serving as a consultant to a local community-based organization. The client's needs have been identified. What should his next step be?
    a. Consultant selection
    b. Engagement
    c. Issue definition
    d. Resolution pathways

132. The executive director of an organization has returned the health education department's annual budget request. The director is asking for additional information about the proposal. All of the following information should be included in the responding budget justification except:
    a. a literature review verifying the importance of the program and proposed budget.
    b. an outline of the department's specific expense categories (e.g., personnel, supplies, etc.).
    c. a list of detailed formulas which explicitly show how expenses were calculated.
    d. a clear description of the need for each expense category or line item in the budget.

133. A nonprofit health association would like to hire the health education specialist in a formal consulting arrangement to implement and deliver direct services. The next step in the consulting project that the health education specialist needs to perform is:
    a. diagnosis.
    b. action.
    c. recommendations.
    d. evaluation.

134. A health education specialist working in the medical clinic has just demonstrated how to correctly use a peak flow meter to staff. Which technique should be used to ensure the client understands the demonstration?
    a. Analogies
    b. Technical review
    c. Take a test
    d. Teach back

135. An agency needs volunteers at a local health awareness event. Before the recruitment campaign can begin, the best first step is to:
    a. plan the volunteer recognition banquet.
    b. create the volunteer newsletter.
    c. determine the volunteer reward/incentive system.
    d. develop a volunteer job description.

136. The Multi-level Approach to Community Health, or MATCH, refers to a:
    a. model to help guide the delivery of a health education/health promotion program.
    b. sustainability framework to determine if programs can be maintained over time.
    c. timeline tool to help all parties involved to keep track of program implementation.
    d. strategy to determine if a program incorporates principles of cultural competency.

137. In a needs assessment for a drug prevention program in a community with high rates of prescription drug abuse, the following data was gathered: state data regarding prescription drug abuse, rates of prescription drug use in the community, trends in prescription drug abuse nationally, and costs of drug abuse. Which of these is a form of primary data?
    a. Trends in prescription drug abuse nationally
    b. State data regarding prescription drug abuse
    c. Rates of prescription drug use in the community
    d. Costs of drug abuse

138. A practicing health education specialist has entered into a helping process initiated by a client in order to establish an assistive relationship. This relationship is considered:
    a. an evaluation.
    b. an assessment.
    c. a consultation.
    d. a reflection.

Master Certified Health Education Specialist Practice Examination Questions

139. In general, at what grade level should materials be written to account for the health literacy of most adults?
    a. Sixth grade
    b. Twelfth grade
    c. Ninth grade
    d. Eighth grade

140. Because a budget is aligned to resources and elements of the strategic plan, the health education specialist must develop the budget during the:
    a. program support process.
    b. needs assessment process.
    c. annual evaluation process.
    d. planning process.

141. Which of the following provides direct support which builds capacity to complete prevention tasks?
    a. Coalition
    b. Technical assistance
    c. Professional development
    d. Networking

142. Conflict may occur in a community health coalition. Which of the following is the most appropriate order for implementing the steps in the conflict resolution process?
    a. Clarify perceptions, build shared positive power, create options, create goals and objectives, and assure benefit of both parties involved
    b. Assure benefit of both parties involved, build shared positive power, create options, clarify perceptions, and create goals and objectives
    c. Build shared positive power, create options, clarify perceptions, assure benefit of both parties involved, and create goals and objectives
    d. Create goals and objectives, clarify perceptions, create options, assure benefit of both parties involved, and build shared positive power

143. Although the mortality rates of children have declined over the years, the leading cause of mortality in children is:
    a. homicide.
    b. infectious diseases.
    c. malignant neoplasms.
    d. unintentional injury.

144. In an urban area with high childhood obesity rates, first and second grade children were not able to identify more than five of ten fruits and vegetables. Many were from lower income families, where one or more adults in the household worked multiple jobs. There are no grocery stores in the area, and most families shopped for food at convenience stores. Though no one strategy is going to decrease obesity rates by itself, which would likely be most efficacious in decreasing rates of childhood obesity?
    a. Increasing fresh fruits and vegetable options at the convenience stores
    b. Educating children on the importance of eating fruits and vegetables
    c. Teaching parents how to prepare fresh fruits and vegetables
    d. Teaching children how to prepare fresh fruits and vegetables

145. A health education specialist creates a draft fact sheet about asthma. She recruits a group of 6 parents to read the fact sheet and answer a series of questions. This is an example of:
    a. tailoring.
    b. readability testing.
    c. pilot testing.
    d. cultural competency.

146. In the study of acute diseases, which morbidity rate is important to calculate?
    a. Prevalence rate
    b. Incidence rate
    c. Proportionate mortality ratio
    d. Case fatality rate

147. The health education specialist is meeting with a school health advisory council (SHAC) which is trying to encourage the district to adopt an evidence-based sexuality education curriculum. In preparing his/her presentation to the SHAC, the statistical health data related to STIs and teen birth rates is most likely to be effective if presented:
    a. as a regression analysis.
    b. with advanced statistical measurements.
    c. as tabulations.
    d. graphically.

148. Of the following educational techniques, which is more likely to enhance the retention of people participating in a program?
    a. Meet in a classroom setting to help participants contextualize the learning process
    b. Use Powerpoint to create visuals for a lecture
    c. Cover a different issue/idea in each session to reduce overlap between issues/ideas
    d. Involve them in an activity during a session

Master Certified Health Education Specialist Practice Examination Questions

149. A weight management intervention was delivered as a face-to-face class and as an online module. To compare costs for all program materials, trainings, and staff time between the two delivery methods, which type of analysis should be conducted?
     a. Cost-benefit
     b. Cost-identification
     c. Cost-effectiveness
     d. Cost justification

150. Prior to meeting with a legislator or policy maker, what would be the likely first step?
     a. Conduct research on the legislator
     b. Develop an advocacy toolkit
     c. Develop talking points
     d. Send a letter requesting a meeting

151. Which of the following are elements of conducting an effective employee/staff appraisal?
     a. Present the appraisal verbally and in writing and allow opportunities for discussion
     b. Present the appraisal in writing without allowing opportunities for discussion
     c. Present the appraisal verbally and in writing without allowing opportunities for discussion
     d. Present the appraisal verbally and in writing when employee misconduct occurs

152. Which question would be the most appropriate for the health education specialist to ask in the formative evaluation level of a consulting relationship?
     a. What are the recommendations for improvement based on the results?
     b. What were the results of the consultation?
     c. What progress has been made to-date?
     d. What are the implications to the organization?

153. A health education specialist is interested in attempting to change norms which encourage teenage pregnancy. What strategy should the health education specialist employ?
     a. Legislative advocacy
     b. Media advocacy
     c. Grassroots organization
     d. Policy Analysis

154. One of the influences on health behaviors is the pressure to conform to what others in the priority population are doing. According to the Theory of Planned Behavior, which construct describes this phenomena?
    a. Perceived behavioral control
    b. Subjective norm
    c. Intention
    d. Attitudes

155. When establishing the reliability and validity of an existing measurement tool, the evaluator should conduct:
    a. a semantic differential survey.
    b. a norm-referenced test.
    c. an item analysis.
    d. a criterion-referenced test.

156. In a worksite health promotion program for weight management, better results for behavior change were found when the program was more client-centered. To balance client autonomy and health education specialist direction, which specific behavior modification technique should be applied?
    a. Respondent conditioning
    b. Response-contingent
    c. Self-monitoring
    d. Satiation and restraint

157. A health education specialist is working with populations with low health literacy levels. In creating materials for this population, which of the following is essential in resource development?
    a. Use simple terms
    b. Present statistics
    c. Focus on detailed action
    d. Use few headings

158. The health education specialist signed a consulting contract to work with a 350-employee health care facility located in a large suburban location. Administrators requested an analysis of the high turnover among allied health professionals. Employee burnout may be related, and a program for employee stress management may be needed. The type of consultation the health education specialist has entered into would be defined as which of the following?
    a. Contracted consultation
    b. Service consultation
    c. Resource consultation
    d. Formal consultation

Master Certified Health Education Specialist Practice Examination Questions

159. During a teen pregnancy program, the health education specialist discusses confidence so participants can talk to their partners about using a condom. The construct he/she is focusing on is:
    a. self-liberation.
    b. consciousness-raising.
    c. self-efficacy.
    d. contemplation.

160. A health education specialist receives four requests for training. Company One is a large company where employee health is relatively good. Company Two is a smaller company that has high health care costs and high absenteeism among employees. Company Three wants a training seminar on any health topic in order to fulfill policy requirements for employee training. Company Four wants to train three employees to do breast cancer screenings. Based on the urgency of the need for education and the potential impact on the organization, which company should be top priority for training from the health education specialist?
    a. Company One
    b. Company Two
    c. Company Three
    d. Company Four

161. The health education manager in charge of career development wishes to provide career development activities and resources to employees. Of the following, which are the most appropriate activities for career development?
    a. Job rotations
    b. Having an assigned mentor
    c. Quality incentives
    d. Job analysis

162. The health education specialist is measuring the incidence of breast cancer in Texas in January 2015, which women would be counted for the numerator of the incidence measure?
    a. All women with breast cancer from January 1, 2013 to January 1, 2014
    b. All women in Texas who currently have breast cancer in January 2014
    c. Women in Texas diagnosed with breast cancer in January 2015
    d. The number of women living in Texas in January 2014

163. When the results of a second survey instrument reinforce the findings of the first survey instrument, the second is said to have:
    a. criterion validity.
    b. construct validity.
    c. content validity.
    d. internal validity.

164. A health educator is trying to decide how to collect data for program evaluation in a program to improve nutrition in a low-income community sample. The health educator is looking to randomly select a small number of participants and assess their individual attitudes toward dietary behavior change and their dietary behavior. Which of the following data collection methods would be best to get the largest response rate in this sample?
    a. Surveys administered in person
    b. Web-based surveys
    c. Mailed surveys
    d. Nominal Group Process

165. Which question below would help a health education specialist with *policy development*?
    a. What were the sources of the policy content?
    b. Were the right stakeholders engaged in the problem identification?
    c. Who enacted the policy?
    d. What were the barriers and facilitators to implementation?

MCHES PRACTICE EXAM ANSWER KEY

1. d. Area IV	34. d. Area III	67. a. Area III	100. a. Area I	133. b. Area VI
2. b. Area I	35. b. Area II	68. b. Area I	101. c. Area VI	134. d. Area VI
3. a. Area II	36. c. Area IV	69. d. Area V	102. a. Area IV	135. d. Area V
4. c. Area IV	37. a. Area V	70. b. Area III	103. d. Area V	136. a. Area II
5. d. Area V	38. b. Area VI	71. b. Area VI	104. b. Area IV	137. c. Area II
6. c. Area IV	39. b. Area II	72. a. Area II	105. a. Area V	138. c. Area VI
7. a. Area VII	40. d. Area III	73. c. Area IV	106. c. Area I	139. d. Area II
8. d. Area I	41. a. Area IV	74. d. Area VI	107. b. Area V	140. d. Area V
9. b. Area IV	42. c. Area VI	75. d. Area III	108. a. Area V	141. b. Area VI
10. c. Area III	43. d. Area III	76. a. Area III	109. d. Area V	142. a. Area V
11. a. Area III	44. b. Area V	77. b. Area IV	110. c. Area V	143. d. Area I
12. a. Area I	45. a. Area II	78. b. Area I	111. c. Area V	144. a. Area II
13. c. Area III	46. d. Area II	79. a. Area II	112. a. Area III	145. c. Area VII
14. b. Area VI	47. c. Area VII	80. c. Area II	113. c. Area V	146. b. Area IV
15. c. Area IV	48. b. Area III	81. d. Area IV	114. b. Area VII	147. d. Area VI
16. d. Area V	49. a. Area VII	82. b. Area I	115. c. Area V	148. d. Area II
17. b. Area VI	50. b. Area II	83. a. Area V	116. a. Area II	149. b. Area IV
18. a. Area V	51. d. Area IV	84. b. Area IV	117. d. Area V	150. a. Area VII
19. b. Area V	52. c. Area III	85. d. Area IV	118. d. Area V	151. a. Area V
20. b. Area V	53. d. Area V	86. c. Area I	119. b. Area III	152. c. Area VI
21. d. Area II	54. a. Area IV	87. a. Area II	120. c. Area I	153. b. Area VII
22. c. Area V	55. c. Area VII	88. b. Area IV	121. b. Area III	154. b. Area III
23. c. Area VII	56. b. Area III	89. b. Area III	122. a. Area VI	155. c. Area IV
24. b. Area I	57. b. Area II	90. a. Area II	123. c. Area II	156. c. Area III
25. d. Area I	58. d. Area III	91. c. Area V	124. a. Area VI	157. a. Area VII
26. a. Area IV	59. a. Area I	92. d. Area IV	125. c. Area III	158. d. Area VI
27. c. Area II	60. b. Area VII	93. a. Area IV	126. a. Area IV	159. c. Area III
28. b. Area VI	61. c. Area III	94. a. Area I	127. d. Area V	160. b. Area VI
29. a. Area III	62. b. Area IV	95. b. Area II	128. b. Area VI	161. b. Area VII
30. d. Area IV	63. a. Area II	96. d. Area IV	129. c. Area I	162. c. Area I
31. c. Area II	64. c. Area VII	97. d. Area II	130. c. Area IV	163. b. Area IV
32. a. Area VII	65. d. Area III	98. b. Area IV	131. b. Area VI	164. a. Area IV
33. c. Area IV	66. a. Area II	99. c. Area IV	132. a. Area V	165. a. Area VII

Author Background Information

Melissa Grim, PhD, MCHES
Associate Professor
Department of Health Education and Health Promotion
Radford University
Radford, Virginia

Cam Escoffery, PhD, MPH, CHES
Associate Professor
Rollins School of Public Health, Behavioral Sciences
and Health Education
Atlanta, Georgia

C. Suzette McClellan, MPH, MCHES
Community Systems Director
SCDHEC-Pee Dee Region
Florence Regional Office
Florence, South Carolina

Linda E. Forys, EdM, MCHES
Director, Office of Health Education and Promotion
Harris County Public Health and Environmental Services
Houston, Texas

Martha Alexander, MPH, MCHES*
Workforce & Career Development Specialist
Centers for Disease Control and Prevention
Atlanta, Georgia

Adam P. Knowlden, MBA, Ph.D. CHES
Assistant Professor
College of Human Environmental Sciences
Department of Health Science
University of Alabama
Tuscaloosa, Alabama

Leah Horn Roman, MPH, MCHES
Public Health Consultant
Roman Public Health Consulting, LLC
Havertown, Pennsylvania

Michelle Carvalho, MPH, CHES
Program Manager/Coordinator
Region IV Public Health Training Center
Emory University
Atlanta, Georgia

Stacy Robison, MPH, MCHES
President, Co-Founder
Communicate Health Inc.
Northampton, Massachusetts

Amy Thompson, PhD, CHES
Professor
University of Toledo
College of Health Sciences
Toledo, Ohio

Chris Anne Rodgers Arthur, PhD, MPH, MCHES
Professor, Department of Behavioral and
Environmental Health
Jackson State University
Associate Professor, Department of Family Medicine
The University of Mississippi Medical Center
Jackson, Mississippi

Patricia A. Frye, DrPH, MPA, MCHES
Director, Prevention Training Center
Mississippi STD/HIV Prevention Training Center
Jackson, Mississippi

Author Background Information

Maurice "Bud" Martin, PhD, MCHES
Assistant Professor of Community Health Education
Department of Community Health Education and
Recreation
University of Maine at Farmington
Farmington, Maine

Angela D. Mickalide, PhD, MCHES
Principal Investigator
EMSC National Resource Center
Silver Spring, Maryland

Christopher N. Thomas, MS, MCHES*
Public Health Advisor
Division for Heart Disease and Stroke Prevention
National Center for Chronic Disease Prevention and
Health Promotion
Centers for Disease Control and Prevention
Atlanta, Georgia

Carol Cox, PhD, MCHES
Professor, Health Science
Truman State University
Kirksville, Missouri

Kelly Wilson, PhD, MCHES
Assistant Professor of Health Education
Texas A & M University
Health & Kinesiology
College Station, Texas

* The findings and conclusions presented by these authors do not necessarily represent the official position of the Centers for Disease Control and Prevention.